UROSCOPY IN EARLY MODERN EUROPE

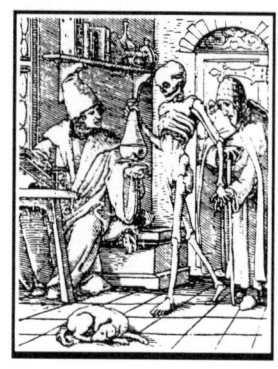

The History of Medicine in Context

Series Editors: Andrew Cunningham and Ole Peter Grell

Department of History and Philosophy of Science
University of Cambridge

Department of History
Open University

Titles in the series include

Anatomy and Anatomists in Early Modern Spain
Bjørn Okholm Skaarup

The Fate of Anatomical Collections
Edited by Rina Knoeff and Robert Zwijnenberg

Sudden Death: Medicine and Religion in Eighteenth-Century Rome
Maria Pia Donato

*Suzanne Noël: Cosmetic Surgery, Feminism and Beauty in
Early Twentieth-Century France*
Paula J. Martin

The British Pharmacopoeia, 1864 to 2014
Medicines, International Standards and the State
Anthony C. Cartwright

Uroscopy in Early Modern Europe

MICHAEL STOLBERG
University of Würzburg, Germany

Translated by
LOGAN KENNEDY and LEONHARD UNGLAUB

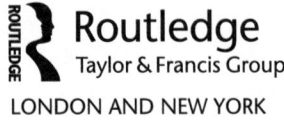

Routledge
Taylor & Francis Group

LONDON AND NEW YORK

First published 2015 by Ashgate Publishing

Published 2016 by Routledge
2 Park Square, Milton Park, Abingdon, Oxon OX14 4RN
605 Third Avenue, New York, NY 10017

First issued in paperback 2021

Routledge is an imprint of the Taylor & Francis Group, an informa business

Publisher's Note
The publisher has gone to great lengths to ensure the quality of this reprint but points out that some imperfections in the original copies may be apparent.

British Library Cataloguing in Publication Data
A catalogue record for this book is available from the British Library

The Library of Congress has cataloged the printed edition as follows:
Stolberg, Michael, 1957- , author.
  Uroscopy in Early Modern Europe / by Michael Stolberg.
    p.; cm. – (The History of Medicine in Context)
  Includes bibliographical references and index.
  I. Title. II. Series: History of medicine in context.
  [DNLM: 1. Diagnostic Techniques, Urological – history – Europe. 2. History of Medicine – Europe. 3. Urine – Europe. WJ 11 GA1]
  RC78.7.U4
  616.07'543–dc23   2015002610

ISBN 13: 978-1-03-209834-0 (pbk)
ISBN 13: 978-1-4094-5015-3 (hbk)

Contents

List of Figures   *ix*
List of Plates   *xi*

Introduction   1

1   Uroscopy in Everyday Life   **9**
    Lay Experience   9
    Consultation by Letter   11
    Uroscopy and Lay Medical Culture in the Eighteenth and
    Nineteenth Centuries   18
    Uroscopy in Learned Medical Practice   25
    Non-Academic Uroscopists   29

2   The Foundations of Uroscopy   **31**
    Consistency   32
    Colors   33
    Contents   39
    Practical Guidelines   43
    Diagnosis and Prognosis   48
    Learning Uroscopy   52
    Case Histories   58
    Uroscopy and Pulse Diagnosis   63
    Paracelsian Uroscopy   66

3   Uroscopy and Popular Culture   **71**
    Practical Advantages   76
    Diagnosing Pregnancy   82
    Making Sense of the Body   91
    Uroscopy as Ritual   97
    Uroscopy and Witchcraft   102

**4   Revealing Images: Uroscopy in Early Modern
    Genre Painting**   **105**
    The Doctor's Visit   106
    The Image of the Uroscopist in Genre Painting   110

The Uroscopist as a Truth-Seeker   114
The Secrets of Women   117

5   **The Gradual Decline of Uroscopy**   **123**
       Theoretical Contradictions   124
       Medical Authority in Jeopardy   128
       Attempting Modernization   134
       Enlightenment and Propaganda   141
       Uroscopy and the Anatomical Revolution   147
       Physicians on the Health Market   153

Epilogue: Uroscopy and the Disappearance of the Sick Man   **161**

Sources   *167*
Index   *193*

List of Figures

1.1 Bartholomäus Hübner, Michel Schüppach in his
consultation room, 1773 (Wellcome Library, London)   19

2.1 Printed black and white uroscopy wheel, in: Pinder,
Epiphanie medicorum (1506)   37

2.2 Urine flask with graduation, in: Cordus, *De urinis* (1543)   40

3.1 A uroscopist and his customers, in: Martini, *Anatomia urinae*
(1658)   81

3.2 Uroscopy note of a blacksmith, 1784 (Schwäbisch Hall,
Stadtarchiv, Best. 11, 84)   96

4.1 C.J. Visscher (after H. Goltzius), *Christus medicus* (Wellcome
Library, London)   111

4.2 Unknown artist, *Le docteur nommé le devin*, printed for
Carrington Bowles, London (Wellcome Library, London)   122

5.1a Insects in urine, in: M.A.C.D., *Système* (1726), 8f
& b Frontispiece of Johan van Dueren, *De ontdekkinge
der bedriegeryen van de gemeene pizbesienders* (1688)   143

List of Plates

The colour plate sections fall between pages 54 & 55 and pages 118 & 119. Thumbnail prints of some of the plates can be found in text.

1   Unknown painter, Cosmas and Damian (London, Wellcome Library)
2   Gerard Dou (1613–1675), *La femme hydropique* (Paris, Musée du Louvre)
3   Frans van Mieris (1635–1681), *The Doctor's Visit* (Los Angeles, Getty Museum)
4   Oil painting after Hendrik F. Herschop, 1620–1672, Uroscopist (London, Wellcome Library)
5   Contemporary copy of Adriaen Ostade (1610–1685), Physician examining a urine flask (London, Wellcome Library)
6   Gerard Thomas (1663–1721), Physician examining a urine flask (London, Wellcome Library)
7   Oil painting after Caspar Netscher (1639–1684), Uroscopist (London, Wellcome Library)
8   Late medieval uroscopy wheel (Philadelphia, Rosenbach Museum & Library, Ms. 1004)
9   Uroscopy wheel (Leipzig, Universitätsbibliothek, Ms. 1177, fol 28r)
10   Hand-colored uroscopy wheel, in: Pinder, *Epiphanie medicorum* (1506), 1v (Munich, Universitätsbibliothek, W 4 Med. 134)
11   Hand-colored uroscopy wheel, in: Ketham, *Fasciculus medicinae* (1493)
12   Uroscopy wheel, around 1420–1430 (London, Wellcome Library, Ms. 49, fol 42r)
13   Hand-colored uroscopy table, in: Pinder, *Epiphanie medicorum* (1506), 2r (Munich, Universitätsbibliothek, W 4 Med. 134)
14   Teaching uroscopy, in: Jacob Meydenbach, *Hortus sanitatis* (1491)
15   Franz Christoph Janneck (1703–1761), *The Medical Alchemist* (Philadelphia, Museum of the Chemical Heritage Foundation, Fisher Collection)
16   Oil painting after Richard Brakenburg (1650–1702), Medical practitioner feeling the pulse and holding a urine flask (London, Wellcome Library)
17   Color photolithograph after F. van Mieris (1635–1681), Physician feeling the pulse (London, Wellcome Library)

18   Jan Steen (ca 1626–1679), *The Doctor's Visit*
      (Amsterdam, Rijksmuseum)
19   Jan Steen (ca 1626–1679), *The Doctor's Visit* (Philadelphia,
      Philadelphia Museum of Art)
20   Enamel after Caspar Netscher (1639–1684), *The Doctor's Visit*
      (London, Wellcome Library)
21   Elisabet Geertruida Wassenbergh (1729–1781), Physician
      feeling the pulse of a lovesick girl (Amsterdam, Rijksmuseum)
22   Egbert van Heemskerk (ca 1700–1744), Physician at a patient's
      death-bed (London, Tate Gallery)
23   Balthasar van den Bossche (1681–1715), *The Iatrochemist*
      (Philadelphia, Museum of the Chemical Heritage Foundation,
      Eddleman Collection)
24   Gerard Thomas (1663–1721), Physician examining a urine flask
      (London, Wellcome Library)
25   Gerard Thomas (1663–1721), Physician examining a urine flask
      (variation on Plate 24) (London, Wellcome Library)
26   Godfried Schalcken (1643–1706), Uroscopic pregnancy
      diagnosis (formerly Cologne, Wallraf-Richartz Museum, Dep.
      530, current owner unknown)
27   Justus Juncker (1703–1763), Physician examining a urine flask
      (London, Wellcome Library)
28   Godfried Schalcken (1643–1706), *Het onderzoek van de dokter*
      (The Hague, Mauritshuis)
29   Oil painting by an unknown artist (around 1700?), Physician
      examining a urine flask in the presence of a young couple
      (London, Wellcome Library)
30   Gerard Dou (1613–1675), Uroscopist (Vienna,
      Kunsthistorisches Museum)
31   Oil painting by C. de Bie (?) after David Teniers (1610–1690),
      Village uroscopist (London, Wellcome Library)
32   I.T., Pregnancy diagnosis (1826), (London, Wellcome Library)

Introduction

This book is about one of the most important practices in the history of Western medicine: the visual examination of the patient's urine with the naked eye. Today we may literally turn up our noses at uroscopy, yet it played an eminent role in both medical practice and ordinary people's lives for many centuries. To highly educated professors and simple farmers alike, it was the best and most reliable means of recognizing a disease, of predicting its future course, and of devising, on this basis, a successful treatment. The belief in the revelatory power of uroscopy was so deeply rooted in contemporary culture that the procedure came to epitomize for poets and dramatists a truthful insight that penetrates the deceptive surface of things. In *Reinaert II*, for instance, Reinaert de Vos (Reynard the Fox) has his father, a physician from the Montpellier School, say that he is going to recognize the king's disease from his urine as if he saw it with his own eyes.[1] In Shakespeare's *Macbeth*, uroscopy is evoked as a metaphor: "If thou could'st Doctor, cast/ The water of my land, finde her disease/ And purge it to a sound and pristine health."[2] Innumerable medical writings dealt with uroscopy. Artists portrayed it in hundreds of miniatures, book illustrations, paintings, and prints.[3] Uroscopy had such a central place in medical practice that the urine flask, the so-called matula, became the characteristic professional attribute of the physician for centuries. It even found its way into the churches, in representations of the medical patron saints SS. Cosmas and Damian (see Plate 1).

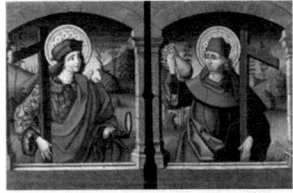 Considering the outstanding place of uroscopy in premodern medicine, medical historians have taken remarkably little interest in it. To this day, the best historical account of uroscopy is still the one by Camille Vieillard published in 1903.[4] The few more recent general surveys of

---

[1] Cit. Homblé, *Uromantie* (1974), 42f: "maect u urine, ic sal u dan segghen u pine, also saen als icse aensie mit oghen"; cf. Gils, *De dokter* (1917), 78f. The language of early modern vernacular sources is often highly revealing and illustrative of its cultural context. Since it would have been misleading to try to imitate this language in English translation, however, quotes from German, Dutch, and French sources are rendered in plain, modern English where no contemporary translation could be found.

[2] Shakespeare, *Macbeth,* act 5, scene 3.

[3] Zglinicki, *Uroskopie* (1982); Murray Jones, *Medieval medicine* (1998).

[4] Vieillard, *L'urologie* (1903); some useful earlier overviews are Osborne, *Sketch* (1820) 1–20, and Neumann, *Geschichte* (1894); see also Frisch, *Historischer Rückblick* (1907).

the history of uroscopy have added little to his work. Even worse, they have tended to describe uroscopy in anachronistic terms merely as the predecessor of modern urinalysis—a perspective that does justice neither to the very different theoretical foundations of traditional uroscopy nor to its much more wide-ranging diagnostic significance, which covered almost the entire spectrum of diseases.[5] Only the study of medieval uroscopy has developed substantially, most recently with the work of Laurence Moulinier-Brogi.[6]

One reason why uroscopy has attracted so little interest even among professional historians of medicine undoubtedly has to do with the somewhat unappetizing nature of the fluid in question. Although modern medicine found urine to be largely free of germs, it is commonly considered unsavory, disgusting even, as well as unhygienic. This aesthetic aspect seems to have combined with the little diagnostic value attributed to the visual examination of urine today. Although it has recently enjoyed some renewed popularity in natural healing circles, the claim that the whole range of human illnesses can be identified simply by inspecting the patient's urine seems rather absurd to the modern eye. It is at most in the case of inflammations, ulcers, and tumors of the efferent urinary tract, or kidney or bladder stones, and in a few very rare metabolic diseases that a simple visual examination of urine is believed to offer sufficient clues for a preliminary diagnosis. In its sweeping diagnostic and prognostic claims as well as its recognition and interpretation of what we would today consider nonexistent findings, such as blue or grey urine or purple "circles" swimming on its surface, premodern uroscopy seems little else but charlatanism and quackery.[7]

Over the past decades, the dominant approaches in the history of medicine have undergone some fundamental changes, however. Medical historians today no longer see their principal task in tracing the story of medical progress, of

---

Historians of popular culture similarly have devoted little attention to the topic (Homblé, *Uromantie* (1974), 64).

   [5]   Anonymous, *The evolution* (1911); Wershub, *Urology* (1970); for other, minor overviews which focus largely on uroscopic treatises and judge their contents based on the criteria of modern medicine: Christoffel, *Grundzüge* (1953); Berger, *Entwicklung* (1966); Bleker, *Kunst des Harnsehens* (1970); Schadewaldt, *Geschichte* (1999); Konert/Dietrich, *Illustrierte Geschichte der Urologie* (2004); more general studies on the history of medical diagnosis tend to pay little attention to uroscopy (see e.g. Nicholson, *Art of diagnosis* (1993)).

   [6]   Moulinier-Brogi, *Un flacon* (2010); eadem, *L'uroscopie au Moyen Âge* (2012). For some time already, vernacular urine treatises, in particular, have been studied. For overviews see Vieillard, *L'urologie* (1903); Keil, *Harnschriften* (2005); Moulinier-Brogi, *L'uroscopie en vulgaire* (2008); on uroscopic treatises from Byzantium see Dimitriadis, *Byzantinische Uroskopie* (1971); on the Salernitan and medieval tradition see Keil, *Urognostische Praxis* (1970); Guerrino/Kohn Loncarica, *Uroscopia* (1973).

   [7]   A typical example is Kaplan, *Robert Recorde* (1963).

the great medical discoveries and their protagonists.[8] Rather they have come to understand medical ideas and practices of the past, as cultural anthropologists would, in their own terms and in their own social, cultural, and at times political contexts.[9] Following this approach, this book will seek to reconstruct the meanings and functions of uroscopic practice in everyday life, to explore the reasons for the deep and enduring trust in it, and to point out the driving forces behind the growing criticism of uroscopy.[10]

In this respect, this book reflects a more general turn toward "practices" which has taken place in a broad range of disciplines, from sociology to the history of science.[11] These new "praxeological" approaches share the conviction that societal structures and institutions, just like scientific knowledge and procedures, are generated and perpetuated above all by concrete, individual actors, through the interaction of people with one another and with the things around them. The methodological consequences for historical analysis are far-reaching. Ordinary practice, the routine processes which have come to assume a seemingly self-evident, self-confirming authority, acquires a crucial role. Merely looking at "dominant" discourse (in our case, in particular, medical discourse) will yield an incomplete picture at best, if not a seriously distorted and biased one. It becomes as crucial and indeed indispensable to investigate also to what degree and in which manner discourse actually influences ordinary practices and how ordinary practices of people from different ranks of society influence "dominant" discourse in turn.[12] Approaching the history of uroscopy from this perspective leads us not only to analyze learned uroscopic treatises, but also to

---

[8] Rosenberg/Golden (eds): *Framing disease* (1992); Paul/Schlich (eds): *Medizingeschichte* (1998); Huisman/Warner (eds): *Locating medical history* (2004).

[9] Dinges, *Social history* (2004); Fissell, *Making meaning* (2004).

[10] From this viewpoint, premodern uroscopy proves to be a particularly rewarding object of historical inquiry. A comparison of uroscopy with early modern anatomy, to which dozens of publications have been dedicated in recent years, shows why. Looking at the numerous anatomical discoveries of the day, we must always take into account that they may have been based to some degree on "objective," factual evidence. When anatomists began to dissect human bodies in a thorough and systematic manner, one might argue, the numerous errors of traditional Galenic anatomy would have to be exposed. With uroscopy, on the other hand, it is certainly not its "objective" diagnostic superiority (according to modern standards) that explains the great, unshakable trust it enjoyed over centuries. There must have been other—social and cultural—reasons.

[11] Latour, *Science in action* (1987); Schatzki/Knorr Cetina/Savigny (eds), *Practice turn* (2001); Reichardt, *Praxeologische Geschichtswissenschaft* (2007).

[12] Vital impulses for this research agenda have come from medical ethnology and cultural anthropology (see Kleinman, *Patients and healers* (1980); Csordas, *Embodiment* (1994); Good, *Medicine* (1994); Lupton, *Medicine as culture* (1994)) and, especially in Germany, from *Alltagsgeschichte* (history of everyday life) and historical anthropology.

explore above all its role in everyday medical life and the medical culture that supported and upheld this practice.

Insofar as this book focuses on the patients and their relatives and seeks to reconstruct their interpretations and experiences, it partakes, at the same time, in endeavors to establish a history of medicine "from below," from the patient's perspective.[13] In contrast to the long-dominant history of "great doctors" and their discoveries and works, this new "history of patients" examines how sick people and their relatives experienced illness and the sick body in the past, and the ways in which they tried to make sense of their suffering. It explores the influence of dominant medical theories and how these were often selectively or creatively appropriated by ordinary people, the different strategies patients adopted to cope with their diseases, their relationship with their physicians and other healers, and related questions.[14]

Because uroscopy formed a central element in the interaction between healers on the one hand and sick people and their families on the other, uroscopic practice inevitably also reflected predominant types of the therapeutic relationship and the situation on the health market. Malcolm Nicolson's conclusion about the history of diagnosis is particularly apt when it comes to uroscopy: "What the doctor does at the bedside of the patient," writes Nicolson, "tells us a great deal about the status and power of the practitioner and about the social context within which medical knowledge is produced."[15]

A historical analysis of uroscopic practice thus also must take into account the effects of power structures, both subtle and forthright, on hegemonic discourse—in our case, above all that of the physicians—as well as on ordinary people's mental world, which frequently, especially in the realm of medical ideas and practices, proves quite resilient. It is here that social constructivist approaches prove helpful. They serve to highlight the role of power structures, market dynamics, and dominant discourses in the development, establishment, and assertion of scientific "truths." As we will see, the role of uroscopy remained relatively stable in popular medical culture but some change did take place within the learned medical world.[16] From 1600 onward, physicians slowly began to turn

---

[13] Cf. the seminal paper by Roy Porter, *The patient's view* (1985); important impulses for this approach, notwithstanding the serious limitations of her principal source, a physician's case histories, also came from Barbara Duden, *Woman* (1991), originally published in German in 1987.

[14] The relevant literature has grown substantially over the last 30 years; see in particular Porter (ed.), *Patients and practitioners* (1985); Porter/Porter, *Patient's progress* (1989); Pomata, *Promessa* (1994); Stolberg, *Experiencing illness* (2011); overviews in Wolff, *Perspektiven* (1998); Ernst, *Patientengeschichte* (1999); Condrau, *Patient's view* (2007).

[15] Nicholson, *Art of diagnosis* (1993), 801.

[16] Rosenberg/Golden (eds), *Framing disease* (1992); Lachmund/Stollberg (eds), *Social construction* (1992); Jordanova, *Social construction* (1995); Schlich, *Wissenschaft* (1998);

away from uroscopy. This gradual change of attitude cannot simply be attributed to increased critical and empirical awareness in the medical community. Rather, it must be seen in light of the highly competitive health market of the early modern era. Due to patients' high expectations, which constantly risked being disappointed, uroscopy came to be perceived as a serious threat to physicians' professional authority. Yet, at the same time, physicians found it difficult to give up uroscopy altogether. The case of uroscopy therefore offers a vivid example of how the conceptions of lay people, due to the strong position of patients in the medical market-place, were able to influence medical discourse decisively.

My analysis will be limited to the prognostic and diagnostic uses of urine. I will not discuss the prophylactic and therapeutic application of urine as a medicine.[17] In the sixteenth century, drinking one's own urine, for example, was described as a popular means to ward off the plague.[18] In the eighteenth century, Johann Friedrich Rübel, to cite another example, advised that in the case of long, drawn-out illnesses like jaundice, or at the first signs of dropsy, or when the humors were "corrupted," patients should be asked to drink, over the course of several weeks and in increasing quantities, cow's urine collected in the spring. This would often yield "very good results."[19] Compared to the overarching diagnostic significance of uroscopy in almost all cases of illness, however, the therapeutic uses of urine played a very modest role only.

This book will cover a relatively long time-span, from the late Middle Ages to the nineteenth century. Since many aspects of uroscopy remained remarkably stable over this period it is only by looking at the *longue durée* that we can trace the changing perception and place of uroscopy, first among learned physicians, and eventually also in the population at large. A fairly wide range of sources will be used. Scholarly treatises give detailed insights into the theoretical foundations and the techniques involved in its examination and interpretation. Narrative passages and case histories found in these treatises, as well as in numerous critical publications about its "abuses," offer a host of insights into the role of uroscopy in everyday life and into the activities of the barber surgeons and of the many irregular healers in towns and rural areas. Obviously, great caution must be taken when we rely on learned physicians' accounts of "popular" medical culture. These accounts were frequently self-serving, setting the physician's expertise against the alleged ignorance of non-academic uroscopists and their numerous customers.

Sarasin/Tanner (eds), *Physiologie und industrielle Gesellschaft* (1998); a decisive impetus for social constructivist approaches in the historiography of medicine and the sciences derived from the sociology of knowledge; see the seminal work by Berger/Luckmann, *Social construction* (1966); Wright/Treacher (eds), *Problem of medical knowledge* (1982).

17 Cf. Thomas (ed.), *Ein ganz besonderer Saft* (1999).

18 ÖNB Vienna, Cod. 11205, 80v; for a rich collection of recipes that used urine to treat different diseases see Willich, *Urinarum probationes* (1582), 301–34.

19 Rübel, *Von dem rechten Gebrauch* (1762), 92.

They are thus suited as sources, above all, for the perception and the professional interests of academic physicians. Yet they also offer, often incidentally, in casual remarks, valuable hints about the usual practices and conventions in uroscopy, for example the role of urine messengers or the use of mirrors in uroscopic diagnosis. Additional, particularly detailed, and presumably less selective and biased information about physicians' uroscopic practice can be gleaned from their personal unpublished journals and notebooks, such as the extensive handwritten notes of the young Bohemian physician Georg Handsch.[20]

Wherever possible, the numerous texts written by physicians will be complemented with sources that reflect the perspective of laypeople and patients. For the upper classes, we can draw on a remarkable spectrum of autobiographies, letters, and other personal testimonies. Sources that offer clues about the medical conceptions and practices of the wider, less educated population are unfortunately much rarer. For the sixteenth and seventeenth centuries we often have to rely on the writings of physicians and other educated contemporaries, reading their usually quite critical accounts against the grain, as it were. For the eighteenth century, we can also have recourse to interrogation records drawn up in the context of legal proceedings against unlicenced uroscopists. For the nineteenth century, medical topographies and ethnographies written by physicians further add to the picture, along with numerous other ethnographic accounts and, for some German areas, starting in 1870, official statistics of irregular healers.

Another important source for a cultural history of uroscopy is that of visual representations. For the early modern period, we find them first and foremost in Dutch genre painting and in prints and etchings derived from them. Many representatives of genre painting, with its frequent focus on worldly, everyday subjects, explored uroscopy, sometimes even in several variations. Among them we find some of the most famous painters of the time, such as Adriaen van Ostade (1610–1685), Jan Steen (ca 1626–1670), and Frans van Mieris (1635–1681). A fair number of these works are reproduced in this book, some of them, to the best of my knowledge, for the very first time. Some of these paintings were considered as masterpieces at the time and are still commonly perceived to possess great aesthetic quality today. The 1663 painting which became known by the title *La femme hydropique* (The Dropsical Woman) by Gerard Dou (1613–1675) is a well-known example (see Plate 2).

These paintings can contribute greatly to our historical understanding of uroscopy. Despite their realistic, sometimes even illusionist technique, these paintings, as recent art historical research has made clear, should be taken to mirror concrete,

---

20   In particular, ÖNB Vienna, Codd. 11205, 11206, 11210, 11238, 11240; Handsch's notebooks are the focus of my current work on sixteenth-century medical epistemology and practice.

everyday reality only to a limited degree. The scenes they represent are often staged and contain more or less explicit and sometimes ambiguous moral messages.[21] Yet the paintings offer important insights into the contemporary lay perception of uroscopy. The artist himself usually was a more or less educated representative of the lay medical culture of the day. In addition, Dutch genre painters frequently worked for the free market, without having been commissioned by a patron. Trade was lively and the walls of wealthier citizens were hung with dozens of paintings.[22] Obviously, an artist who wanted to survive in this market was well-advised to create paintings whose style and content met with the expectations of potential buyers; paintings, in other words, that reflected the citizens' worldview and, for our purposes, their perception of uroscopy.

Drawing mainly on personal testimonies, interrogation records, physicians' accounts, and ethnographic data, my investigation will begin with a general overview of the role of uroscopy in the daily lives of ordinary people and medical practitioners in premodern times. The second chapter will be devoted to the technique of uroscopy and the interpretation of changes in the urine, as explained and discussed in scholarly treatises, and as popularized in vernacular works written for a wider lay audience. The third chapter will pursue the reasons why uroscopy enjoyed such high esteem among the populace and for a long time also among physicians. The great popularity of uroscopy will be attributed above all to the belief in its capacity to fathom, almost like an oracle, the mysterious depths of the human body. Uroscopy will be described as a ritualized procedure whose validity seemed to be constantly confirmed in everyday life. In the fourth chapter I will turn to visual representations of uroscopy in Dutch genre painting. Among other things, I will take a critical look at the rather sweeping assessment made by some art historians that genre painters ridiculed uroscopy as an outdated procedure, and I will point out the parallels between representations of uroscopy and contemporaneous portrayals of truth-seeking alchemists. The fifth chapter will explore the reasons for the gradual decline of uroscopy in learned medicine. As I will argue, doctors did not simply recognize, finally, how unreliable uroscopy was. Many of them continued to rely on uroscopy. They only rejected the common practice of diagnosing diseases from the urine alone. Faced with tough competition from many non-academic uroscopists, who routinely diagnosed diseases from the urine alone, physicians came to perceive uroscopy as a major threat to their individual and collective standing rather than a boon. At the same time, public dissections opened up a new, more promising opportunity to successfully stage the physicians' privileged access to the secrets of the human body. The book will conclude with a comparison of early modern uroscopy to the new diagnostic techniques of the nineteenth and early twentieth centuries.

---

[21]   On the example of G. Metsu: Stone-Ferrier, *From shrew to poetess* (2003).

[22]   Zimmermann, *Arzt in der niederländischen Malerei* (1970), 28f.

The introduction of the stethoscope, of the thermometer, and of x-rays count as milestones of modern medicine. On the down-side, it has been widely lamented that these "objective" diagnostic methods devalued the patients' personal narratives of their subjective sensations. The sick person, it is claimed, became a mere medical case. As we will see, there is considerable evidence in support of this thesis but it needs some qualification in the light of the outstanding significance of uroscopy in the early modern period. After all, many patients and their families expected or explicitly demanded that the uroscopist arrive at a diagnosis without any further information about the patient and his or her complaints.

The original German edition of this book appeared in Böhlau-Verlag, Cologne/Weimar/Vienna, in 2009. For this edition, the text has been revised only slightly. Changes are largely limited to the inclusion of references to some more recent historical contributions to the topic and to the addition of material from sources which I have discovered and analyzed since then.

Chapter 1

Uroscopy in Everyday Life

Lay Experience

In his autobiography, the German pastor Wirsing (1526/27–1601) from Sinbronn recounts his wife's serious illness. The family ultimately felt compelled to seek medical advice and had their son-in-law take the wife's urine to a physician who came to the following conclusion: "This person already is bedridden or will soon be unless something is done quickly. The jaundice has laid itself tightly around the heart, making the vapors rise and weaken all the limbs. The person is to infuse St. Benedict's thistle in wine and drink from this. The person is to avoid bathing in water, as this would lead to great swelling. Also, if the person drinks from St. Benedict's thistle for a while and does not improve, consult me again." Wirsing's account is instructive and remarkable in several respects. Apparently, the physician had been told neither the patient's gender nor how sick she was. He was expected to make the diagnosis and prognosis on the basis of the urine alone—and he arrived at a surprisingly nuanced assessment: The patient suffered from jaundice and ascending "vapors." On this basis, the physician recommended specific dietetic and therapeutic measures.[1]

When Wirsing's daughter Babel had a rash, the family again relied on uroscopy: "I took Babel's urine to the physician at 9 a.m.," Wirsing noted, "who put it in his flask and told me to be back after 10 a.m." When Wirsing later returned with his daughter, "the physician said that she drinks a lot and asked if she didn't feel a stabbing pain in her left side. Babel said yes. Finally, she had to take off her bonnet. He inspected her head twice and then some of the other rashes. He looked under her tongue and pulled at her eyebrows, then finally said it was certainly not leprosy. He was hopeful that he would be able to cure [her] with God's help and wrote for me to the apothecary. For a little electuary. I gave 48 Pfennig for it."[2] In this case, the physician did follow up with a personal examination of the patient, but based on his examination of the urine he had identified complaints like a stabbing pain which had not been mentioned by the patient or her father.

Wirsing himself sought uroscopic advice shortly before his death: "In the morning, Kathrin took my urine into town to the physician Daniel Winkler,

---

[1]   Wirsing, *Altfränkisches Dorf- und Pfarrhausleben* (1952), 38.
[2]   Ibid., 21; the brackets seem to have been added by the modern editor.

told him that it was mine and that I was going to come see him shortly. [...] He told me what my urine indicated (among other things, he told me that a paralysis had affected my private parts and gave me 2 slips of paper to take to the apothecary in Nördlingen)."[3]

The case of the Wirsing family was far from unique. The memoirs of Alderman Hermann von Weinsberg of Cologne[4] also contain numerous references to uroscopy. For example, he tells of how his sister-in-law, Tringin Wolf, fell into terminal sickness in July 1553. At first, the family believed she might be pregnant but eventually Weinsberg's wife took the woman to the physician Fabri and had her urine examined. Uroscopy thus served as an essential diagnostic step when the family worried that Tringin might have fallen seriously ill. Later, in the physician's practice, the patient lost consciousness but recovered with the help of lavender water. The physician then said he did not understand what ailed her but that "[her] water was full of heat."[5]

With other cases of illness in the Weinsberg family it went without saying that before anything else, the urine—or the "water," as it was often referred to at the time—would be examined. When, in 1557, Weinsberg's wife lay dying, she seems to have called physicians to her bedside only after a uroscopy had indicated an affliction of the uterus and inner heat.[6] The alderman himself had his urine examined whenever he was unsure what might be the matter with him. According to his own account, he did not actually feel ill in May 1552 but was "unwell in the chest" ("vur de Borst ubel"). His wife took his urine to the physician and apparently did not tell him any details about the state of the patient because the physician comforted her, saying: "If he is sick, he is not so very sick after all."[7] When, in 1575, several people died of the plague and he felt unwell himself, Weinsberg sent his urine to the physician Hermann Collenberg. Collenberg advised him to have a vein on his left arm opened, and Weinsberg followed this advice.[8] And when, in 1576, he suddenly began to shake and shiver, had no appetite, and feared that he was ill with the plague, he did not call his physician right away. He first took medicine that promoted sweating and sent his urine to Dr Collenberg, who found reddish changes on the surface of the urine which he attributed to an "Überfluss" (i.e. an overflow or abundance [of humors]) of the liver. He gave Weinsberg dietetic instructions and a laxative, which produced four or five bowel movements. The ordeal cost Weinsberg one *taler*, but the shivering stopped and he remained healthy.[9]

---

3   Ibid., 39.
4   On Weinsberg see Jütte, Ärzte (1991).
5   Weinsberg, *Buch Weinsberg* (2000), vol. 2, 35.
6   Ibid., 92f.
7   Ibid., vol. 5, 9.
8   Ibid., vol. 2, 298f.
9   Ibid., 317.

In Switzerland, Johann Heinrich Hummel, a shoemaker's son (1611–1674) with a considerably more humble background, also spoke of his trust in uroscopy. After he had become pastor in Brugg, he fell ill with a serious disease which he thought he had contracted from often staying awake late to study. "My housekeeper, who loved me dearly, often travelled twice a day on foot to Baden to see Doctor Ziegler—who himself was on a sojourn at the spa there—to get help and medicine, but in vain." Eventually, he asked for help from an acquaintance who was about to travel to Berne and who promised "to show it to the physician König personally and tell him about my illness. This is what came to pass and I heard back in writing that I would not recover from this illness."[10]

His cold and his breathing difficulties had improved, the English clergyman Ralph Josselin noted in his diary in December 1648. His urine, however, was still full of "white raw phlegm," from which he concluded that he had not yet overcome the illness and was still "full of cold, watery humors."[11]

Such stories, anecdotes, and laypersons' accounts of diagnostic findings from urine turn up time and again in early modern memoirs, letters, and other personal testimonies. They show that uroscopy was ubiquitous in early modern medical culture. It was *the* central diagnostic method, and it was perfectly self-evident for patients and their relatives that they could rely on it. Even a highly educated and famous physician and botanist such as Leonhard Fuchs found himself swamped with the requests of his peasant patients for uroscopy.[12]

Consultation by Letter

Uroscopy also played an important role in epistolary consultations, a practice which was fairly widespread at the time, mainly among the upper classes.[13] The patients of Leonhard Thurneysser, a well-known Paracelsian and personal physician of the Elector of Brandenburg in late sixteenth-century Berlin, almost routinely sent their urine, as can be seen from his extensive patient correspondence. Thurneysser had acquired a certain fame for his new method of diagnosing diseases by distilling the patient's urine. But even the letters of patients and their families to orthodox physicians such as Felix Platter often make mention of the urine that was sent along with the letter and whose examination was being requested. Gregorius Krafft von Talmessingen, for example, told of the tightness around the heart and chest experienced by the sick bailiff of

---

[10] Hummel, *Historie* (1950), 40.

[11] Josselin, *Diary* (1976), 149.

[12] UB Erlangen, Trewsche Briefsammlung, undated letter to Joachim Camerarius, apparently written after 1542, according to Fichtner, *Leonhart Fuchs* (1968).

[13] Stolberg, *Patientenbriefe* (1996); idem, *Experiencing illness* (2011).

Wittnau, and as the patient wished to hear the precise cause for his physical weakness, he again sent his urine.[14] Graf von Löwenstein, too, repeatedly sent his wife's "urine so you may arrive at a better knowledge of the weakness."[15] Furthermore, uroscopy was considered an aid in choosing the right medication. Hans Georg von Reinach, for example, sent his urine to Platter with a messenger, "requesting you to prescribe me a purging agent after examining the urine."[16] In case he was unable to accompany the messenger, the sick Metternich told his personal physician Horst in Darmstadt, he would send horses and a servant and his "highly esteemed Sir could look at the water and come to a conclusion."[17] In a response that bespeaks how common and expected such requests were, Dr Georg Molther in 1648 confirmed the receipt of a letter, "including the urine,"[18] about the "weakened state" of the ill chancellor Fabritius.

Diagnosing diseases from urine that was sent from far away was somewhat problematic. The medical literature recommended that the urine be examined without much delay, that is, after six or seven hours at the latest. With a delay greater than this, the urine possibly changed and became corrupted. However, if the journey was too long and it was feared that the urine would change, there was still the option that the patient, a relative, or a local physician or healer described in their own words what they observed in the fresh urine. His urine was very cloudy, Gideon van Boetzelaar was able to tell his physician Jan van Heurne, and sometimes it also showed a certain putridity, rarely, however, any febrile boiling-up.[19] "A small pebble" was discharged with his urine, wrote Bernhardt von Wehren with similar detail to Thurneysser, and, at times, he had "made water that was fairly black."[20] Many patients spoke of color changes and clouding. His urine was "ugly," "brown and thick" as never before in his life, complained Baltzer Barfuss; he suffered from intense bodily pain, a bloated belly, and shortness of breath.[21] On one of his trips he had twice discharged urine colored

---

[14]   UB Basel, Ms. Fr. Gr. I 6 32, undated, probably around 1570.

[15]   UB Basel, Ms. Fr. Gr. I 6 123, May 13, 1570.

[16]   UB Basel, Ms. Fr. Gr. I 6 137, May 1570.

[17]   Senckenberg Archiv Frankfurt, Ms. 334, letter from Niederselters, August 12, 1657; besides "water" or, in German, "Wasser," terms like "Bronnen" or "Brunnen" ("fountain" or "well"), were widely used as synonyms for "urine."

[18]   Senckenberg Archiv Frankfurt, Ms. 334, letter from Molther, October 24, 1648; the author is probably identical with the Georg Molther who is documented as a town physician in Wetzlar during that period.

[19]   UB Leiden, Ms. Marchand 3, letter, October 13, 1591.

[20]   StB Berlin, Ms. germ. fol. 420b, 263r–v, letter from the patient, September 14, 1574.

[21]   StB Berlin, Ms. germ. fol. 420a, 81r–v, letter from the patient, Tuesday before St James [July 1571].

like chickpea broth, a patient of Alessandro Tadini reported.[22] Discussing the qualities of a patient's urine could even involve relatives and acquaintances. One patient recounted that he had made water two days earlier and that the urine had adhered to the glass in such a way that he needed a stick and cloth to clean the glass. On the cloth, he found a yellow substance that felt strange between his fingers. The people around him had never seen such a thing in their lives either.[23]

Sometimes rapid changes in the course of the disease left the patient or family hardly any choice but to describe what they saw in the urine in their own words rather than send it to the uroscopist. Another patient of Thurneysser, Georg Traupitz, looked at his urine every day. At first, it was clear, but the day after, it was all cloudy, "with a lot of stringy mucus mixed in."[24] In the case of Anna von Bassenitz, the urine even "often changed once or twice during the day"; it was red, then again clear as water, and at times resembled the urine of a healthy person.[25]

People appreciated uroscopy not just as one diagnostic method among many. They attached an importance to it that made early modern physicians increasingly uneasy. From the early sixteenth century, medical authors in a growing number of publications questioned the reliability of a diagnosis that relied solely on uroscopy.[26] They did not reject uroscopy outright as such but they declared further information about the patients indispensable: about their current complaints, lifestyle, temperament, previous diseases and therapies, and so on. Ideally, the physician saw the patient for a personal consultation. As Euricius Cordus put it: "If you are in the presence of the patient, you can tell the condition of his brain from his eyes and face, from his speech, and his movements; the condition of his lungs from his coughing and hacking up, the condition of the heart from the pulse, the condition of the stomach and intestines from the vomit and stool, the condition of the liver, the blood and other humors from the urine. Summa summarum, a physician must himself see the patient, touch him and ask questions if he is to help him. But if he treats him unseen, he does like someone who wants to shoot birds in mid-air and this is an uncertain, even dangerous thing."[27]

---

[22]   Biblioteca Trivulziana, Milan, Ms. 1709, 357, letter from a patient suffering from dysuria, 1651.

[23]   StB Berlin, Ms. germ. fol. 420b, 54r–55v, letter from sick Godhart von Kamp(e), Wednesday before St Lawrence, 1574.

[24]   Ibid., 87r–v, letter from the patient, October 7, 1571. Something was "running" in his body, he complained, and his stomach was full of winds. He also suffered from coughing in the mornings, which hardly allowed him to breathe.

[25]   StB Berlin, Ms. germ. fol. 422a, 50r–51r, letter from the patient, June 23, 1578.

[26]   One of the earliest critics was Fries, *Spiegel* (1518), LXIIIr–LXIXr.

[27]   Cordus, *De urinis* (1543), no pagination.

Indignant, at times disgusted, physicians decried the widespread and persistent conviction of people that an artful physician must be able to tell and treat everything simply by looking at the urine.[28] The "common people" had more trust in uroscopy "than in anything else," observed Lorenz Fries, for instance. They believed that urine was enough "to tell all illnesses, causes, symptoms and pains."[29] "Today, the majority of people, be they rich or poor, from higher or lower estates, educated or uneducated, women or men, have become blind in such a way that they cannot but believe that all diseases, and all dispositions of the human body as well, can be seen in the water," reported Sigmundt Kolreutter from Coburg.[30]

This firm belief in the outstanding possibilities of uroscopy, the physicians found, was not limited to the "ignorant" lower classes. That sick people sent their urine was a most common habit, according to Andreas Starck, and "not only of the common man but also of many learned and wise people," who were "all of the opinion that the physician is and must be able to tell what is wrong with the ill person by examining the patient's water."[31] Indeed, many among the often high-ranking or noble patients, for example, who wrote to Felix Platter and Leonhard Thurneysser to ask for advice, sent their urine but made hardly any mention of their medical history or their complaints.[32]

Little seems to have changed in this respect in the course of the early modern period. In the seventeenth century, Ananius Horer complained that the opinion had been "implanted not only in the common folk but also in many great people that it is well possible to know and see a patient's illness with all its circumstances simply by examining his urine, no matter whether the patient lives ten or more miles from the doctor, and now they decry anyone who refuses to work like this as a poorly trained and inexperienced doctor—try as one might to contradict."[33] And a good century later, Rübel similarly indicated at most a subtle change in the upper classes when he explained that it had "got into the minds of not only the common man but also some rather learned people that a mere examination of the urine is the best and most certain way to discover the whole constitution and the entirety of the body and its parts or the defects of the same."[34]

To the physicians' great dismay, patients often even explicitly denied them any further information in order to make sure that the physician was basing his findings exclusively on uroscopy. The doctor who wanted to learn details about

---

[28] Kolreutter, *Von rechten Gebreuchen* (1574), chapter 3.

[29] Fries, *Spiegel* (1518), LXIIIr.

[30] Kolreutter, *Von rechten Gebreuchen* (1574).

[31] Starck, *Harmspiegel* (1597), dedication.

[32] UB Basel, Ms. Fr. Gr. I 6; some letters, especially those brought by a relative, indicate, however, that the messengers also provided Platter with some oral information.

[33] Horer, *Artzney-Teuffel* (1634), 61.

[34] Rübel, *Gebrauch* (1762), 82.

the patient and his complaints, wrote Lorenz Fries in the sixteenth century, heard replies such as, "I think you should see for yourself," or even got to hear lies.[35] When asked about the patient, stormed Foreest, the peasants who brought the urine would just stand there "like sticks, as if mute, or, if their jaws do loosen a little, the first thing they say is, 'We wanted to hear (i.e. what you are desiring to know from us) from you, hoping you would see it in the water, and this is why we came to see you.'"[36] Scribonius, too, complained that only very few would say whose urine they were bringing, name the patient's sex and age, and so on. They believed it was the physician's task to "divine" everything from the urine and foresee like a soothsayer.[37]

The critics apparently spoke from experience. Writing about the time when he returned home from his studies in Montpellier, Felix Platter recounted, "I found that people had the bad custom of taking their water to the homes of the physicians; from many uncouth people who came to my home with their stinking piss and whom I asked a thing or two, I got nothing but the sullen answer: This is what we'd like to hear from you, otherwise we would not have brought you the water. If we are to tell you everything about the patient, why would you still need the water?"[38]

Physicians voiced such complaints throughout the early modern period. According to Antonius Eijgel, living in the Netherlands of the late seventeenth century, messengers "commonly" offered no further information about the illness.[39] In Germany, K.B. Behrens (1660–1736) condemned "the great naiveté of people who think they have done enough by sending the physician their water, but communicate nothing else because the messenger often does not know the patient nor has he seen him, nor is he able to pass on any message, except that he is his neighbor and happened to be going into town this morning."[40] Many of those bringing urine were so bullheaded that they simply did not answer when asked about the state of the sick person, Friedrich Hoffmann (1660–1742), professor at the University of Halle, complained.[41] His colleague and competitor in Halle, Georg Ernst Stahl (1659–1734) had the same experience: common people brought the urine, from which "the physician is to tell not only the illness but especially the present magnitude of their symptoms." They were stubborn to the extent that "they will not say a word but simply expect to see that the

[35] Fries, *Spiegel* (1518), LXIIIIr.
[36] Foreest, *Uromanteia* (1620), 228f; cf. Liphimeus, *Warnung* (1626), 40.
[37] Scribonius, *De inspectione urinarum* (1585), 36f.
[38] Foreest, *Uromanteia* (1620), 231.
[39] Eijgel, *Apologema* (1672), 39.
[40] Behrens, *Wasserbeschawen* (1688), 23f.
[41] Hoffmann, *Medicus politicus* (1708), 132; cf. Kongelige Bibliotek Copenhagen, Ms. Thottske S 4 689 (Piper, Collegium), 243r.

physician has mastered his art."[42] Certainly the country physician, according to Johann Georg Zimmermann (1728–1795), "in most cases" simply did not get to see the patient face to face. Another person would be sent who would put the matula down on the table and, "to all questions imaginable," would give "consistently the same answer: 'Well, you will be able to tell from the urine.'"[43]

In the mid-eighteenth century, Johann August Unzer gave a particularly vivid description of his encounter with a peasant who came to him and pulled out a filled matula. Unzer explained to the peasant that it would be better if he told him whose urine this was and what ailed the person and so on. But the peasant simply replied: "Can't you tell from looking at the water?" And when Unzer answered in the negative, the peasant replied "And you are supposed to be a doctor?" When Unzer insisted that he would be better able to cure the patient if he had some information about him, the peasant answered, "Oh, hogwash! I might as well guess myself what ails the patient." He then picked the flask up and left.[44]

Physicians likely exaggerated somewhat. In his extensive personal notes on his medical practice and that of his teachers and colleagues, the young Bohemian physician Georg Handsch, who was dealing with high-ranking aristocrats as well as with ordinary town folk, repeatedly complained about people's expectation that he diagnose diseases and pregnancies just from their urine. He also mentioned cases, however, in which the messengers volunteered some information. For example, the brother of a sick farmer told him that the patient had been sick for a year but was now confined to his bed and had no appetite. Having examined the urine, Handsch concluded that it was indeed an "old disease" against which various medicines had been applied which had made things rather worse. The stomach was full of mucus, obstructed, and corrupted and thus could no longer digest the food and produce the good blood needed to nourish the body, making the patient become weaker and thinner. Therefore the patient was to take medicines which would clean out and strengthen the stomach.[45] Handsch's notebooks also contain brief accounts of conversations, in which the physician examined the urine, offered a preliminary diagnosis, and then asked the patient questions in order to confirm it.[46] Patient letters and autobiographies similarly show that, at least among higher circles of society, information about the patient's medical history and present complaints—or indeed his or her identity—was not consistently denied.

---

[42]   Stahl, *Gründliche Abhandlung* (1739), 25f; original Latin edition: Stahl, *De uromantiae abusu* (1711), 18.

[43]   Zimmermann, *Von der Ruhr* (1767), 207.

[44]   Unzer, *Von der Kunst* (1760), 130.

[45]   ÖNB Vienna, Cod. 11206, 16v–17r (Innsbruck, around 1570).

[46]   ÖNB Vienna, Codd. 11205, 11206, 11210, 11238 and 11240.

Yet even Felix Platter's well-educated upper-class patients at times offered only very brief and general descriptions. It could happen that Platter was just told that the patient in question suffered from tightness of the chest and heart—and that they sent the urine so the physician could come "to a better and more thorough [understanding of the] cause" of the ailment.[47] Pastor Wirsing's above-quoted account of the examination of his wife's urine by a physician who was apparently not even told whether the urine came from a man or a woman suggests that this procedure was indeed fairly common practice. This would have been especially true when a paid messenger was used to deliver the urine, not a member of the family. In this case, complained Scribonius, patients sometimes even made sure that the messenger himself did not know the identity of the patient and was thus unable to give the physician any information.[48] In order to evade the physician's questions, Georg Ernst Stahl claimed, townspeople who had their own urine examined or that of a family member, often simply pretended the urine had been sent from the country and "nothing more had been said about it."[49]

Since a skillful uroscopist could be expected to make his diagnoses from an examination of urine alone, uroscopy, to the ordinary mind, offered a welcome opportunity to gain a reliable impression of individual healers and to identify the truly able ones among the many who were available. In some respects, finding the most competent medical practitioner was even more important to patients and their relatives in that time than it is today. In private correspondence, experiences with different doctors and the outcome of their treatments were an important topic, and understandably so. The diagnosis and treatment of diseases was standardized only to a limited degree. Contemporary textbooks recommended a plethora of different drugs for the same disease and, on top of that, educated patients expected the doctors to adapt their treatment to the patient's personal condition, to his or her temperament, diet, life-style, and so on. If one size did not fit all patients who appeared to share similar complaints, then the diagnostic and therapeutic abilities of the individual healer were all the more significant. In fact, they had to be seen as the decisive factor in determining the patient's fate.

Uroscopy therefore offered a welcome tool to test the abilities of a healer, a "vain and foolish but common way to judge a doctor," as H. Brooke put it.[50] Laypeople felt that a uroscopist and his diagnostic and therapeutic judgment could be trusted more readily if he was capable of describing the patient's complaints accurately just by examining the urine. If he was off the mark, they had better consult somebody else. As Detharding found, people sometimes

---

[47]   UB Basel, Ms. Fr. Gr. I 6 32, letter from Gregorius Krafft von Talmessingen, probably around 1570.

[48]   Scribonius, *De inspectione urinarum* (1585), 36f.

[49]   Stahl, *Gründliche Abhandlung* (1739), 26.

[50]   Brooke, *Hygieine* (1650), 196.

took this even a step further. They would "send old women to take [urine] to several physicians, and the physician who got closest would be called to attend the patient."[51]

Uroscopy and Lay Medical Culture in the Eighteenth and Nineteenth Centuries

The great trust uroscopy enjoyed among large parts of society hardly wavered during the late eighteenth and nineteenth centuries. It is "known that it has become the custom almost everywhere that the doctor [is asked] to determine the age, sex, disease, the most likely and the most unlikely cause, and the favorable or unfavorable outcome of the affliction," explained the itinerant healer Franz Anton Vogel, who traveled the Ansbach area in the 1790s, lauding his own abilities in the field.[52] In his flyer he pointed out that asking a doctor to detect age and sex, the most likely and the most unlikely cause, and the outcome of the illness from the sick person's urine was "asking too much," since "soothsaying and prophesying" was not commensurate with an "honorable physician." However, he also emphasized the manifold insights that urine revealed to the "doctor experienced in this," and invited sick people to send him their urine: "I will discover, to the extent possible, the circumstances and perhaps more than you think and might expect from me by examining [the urine], and will shed light on your illness."[53]

Uroscopy continued to be valued as a powerful diagnostic tool even in the highest circles. The Swiss uroscopist Michel Schüppach (1707–1781) acquired great fame throughout late eighteenth-century Europe for his sagacious uroscopic diagnoses and successful therapies. Patients from all over Europe, including members of the high aristocracy, came to seek his advice (see Figure 1.1).[54]

---

[51]   Detharding, *Kranken-Wärter* (1679), 69f; similarly already Foreest, *Uromanteia* (1620), 219.

[52]   Flyer, announcing the arrival of F.A. Vogel, reproduced in *Journal von und für Franken* 2:5 (1791), 590–94.

[53]   Ibid.

[54]   Cf. Archiv des Medizinhistorischen Instituts der Universität Zürich, Ms. H 11 (case book of Michel Schüppach); cf. Wehren, *Schüppach* (1985).

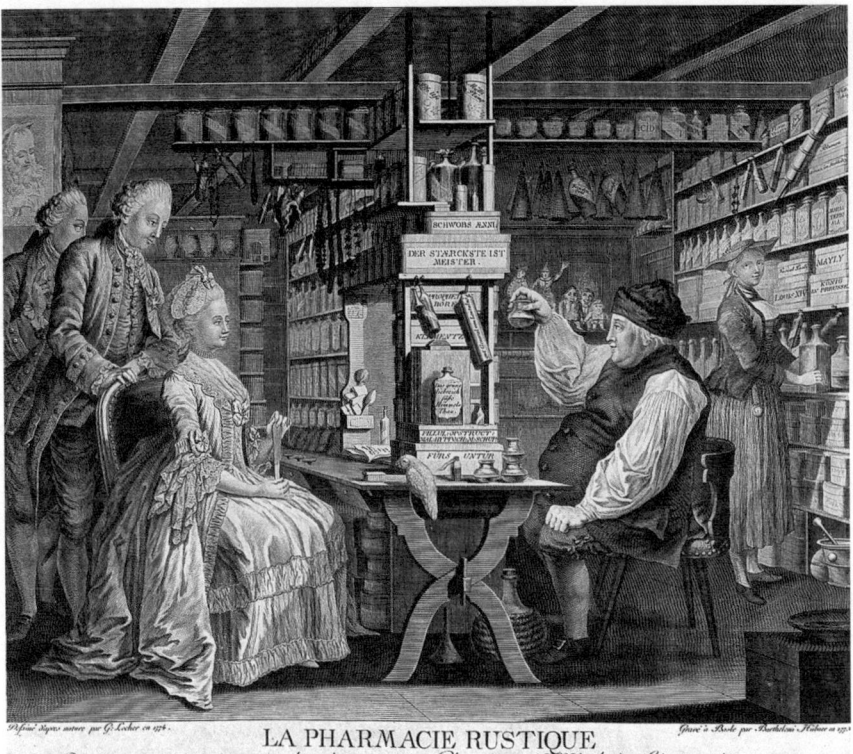

LA PHARMACIE RUSTIQUE
ou Representation exacte de l'interieur de la Chambre, où Michel Schüppach connu sous le nom du Medecin de la Montagne, tient ses Consultations.

Figure 1.1   Bartholomäus Hübner, Michel Schüppach in his ordination
room, 1773 (Wellcome Library, London)

Yet there are also signs of a gradual change. More and more, an anonymous medical author noted in 1786, people ceased to offer the urine glass or even the contents of a chamber pot to the physician, without being asked, and to imagine that all kinds of diseases could be recognized in it "just as one recognizes one's own face looking into a mirror."[55] Certainly by the late eighteenth century, letters of consultation by upper-class patients indicate a marked change. While they often provided very detailed accounts of their medical history and current

---

[55]   Anonymous, *Onomatologia* (1786), vol. 4, coll. 1533–4.

complaints, uroscopy moved into the background.[56] Wealthy and educated patients now usually expected the doctor to spend a considerable amount of time on their case. He was to inquire about their unique bodily constitution and biography and on this basis prescribe them a personalized therapy. Changes in the urine were mentioned only occasionally, and sending a flask of urine along with the initial letter was pretty much out of the question—in stark contrast to Platter's and Thurneysser's time. Presumably patients were well aware that the medical luminaries of the time would hardly have appreciated this.

However, marked changes in the urine continued to be recognized and appreciated for their diagnostic value among educated circles during the eighteenth century. And patients and their relatives were still confident that if necessary they could put these visible changes in words well enough for the distant doctor to form a diagnosis. Some were content with simply writing that their urine was "beautiful" or "healthy."[57] Others described changes in the quantity and regularity of their urination, or concomitant complaints such as pains, burning, or sensations of heat.[58] Highly educated patients also continued to write about visible contents and the coloring of their urine as well as about its consistency, and they did so not only when they or their relatives suspected a disease of the kidneys, bladder, or urinary tract, which are still associated with marked visible changes in the urine today.

In the early eighteenth century, a 52-year-old female patient of Etienne-François Geoffrey, for example, complained about bouts of intense heart palpitations. She felt very weak in these moments and on the brink of death but had also noticed an evacuation of large amounts of watery urine.[59] J.F. Stubenrauch, in a letter to the famous doctor Senckenberg in Frankfurt, mentioned a markedly darker coloration. His urine was "altered," he said and looked "like a thin beer" not "like lemon, the way it is supposed to be";[60] initially,

---

[56] This may in part be due to the fact that larger collections of pre-1800 patient letters are known to us mostly from French speaking areas, where, according to doctors' accounts, uroscopy enjoyed less popularity. However, in the patient correspondence of Senckenberg, too, urine is mentioned only occasionally.

[57] BCU Lausanne, Fonds Tissot.

[58] BIM Paris 5242, 82r–v (case 29), undated letter, delivered by philosophy professor Poitevin in Beauvais, concerning a patient in her late twenties. Her urine caused a burning sensation and she also suffered from intense itching and her period felt unusually hot—all symptoms that fit with an accumulation and evacuation of hot, acrid morbid matter; cf. ibid. 5241, 119r–125v, letters from a 24-year-old nun, 1729–1730, who suffered from nausea, exhaustion, and stomach pain.

[59] BIM Paris 5241, 139r–140r, undated letter of an unnamed female patient (reply dated July 1730).

[60] Senckenberg Archiv Frankfurt, Senckenberg correspondence, letter from Mainz, December 4, 1726.

he had described his urine as "quite cloudy" with "quite a lot of matter" in it.[61] Hellenist and Bishop Mordecai Cary (1687–1751), who sought the advice of the famous English physician James Jurin concerning the chest ailment of his sick wife, repeatedly described the properties of her urine in detail. Initially, when her left breast had become painfully swollen after a cold, he found her urine to be "thick and cloudy until, after standing for a while, a coarse sediment settles, which looks like the lime on the bottom of tea crockery."[62] A few days later, he supplied additional information which shows that he also examined the urine with his fingers: "her urine, which looks like the sediment of a small wheat beer, leaves on the entire walls of a large glass a white deposit that appears fatty to the eye but is coarse to the touch, and indeed, when you rub along the side of the glass you hear the sound of sand."[63] Her menstruation—which Cary, like most laypeople at the time, seems to have understood as a vitally important, health-preserving excretion of impure, morbid substances[64]—had become disturbed as well, and Cary worried that his wife might suffer from breast cancer.[65] Breast cancer was a widely feared consequence of an insufficient expulsion of menstrual blood, which was, in that case, believed to accumulate in the body, spoil and become "acrimonious." However, after she took the various drugs that Jurin had recommended, Cary was happy to be able to write: "The period came in an appropriate amount and the urine was right again too."[66] In another "gynecological" case, Gräfin von Wedel, an elderly lady at the Danish court who was quite knowledgeable in medical matters, wrote to the famous Swiss doctor Tissot. She described in much detail her sometimes intensely bloody and sometimes sanious and stinking vaginal discharge of the past 18 months, while also referring to the properties of her urine as "not cooked" and bad smelling.[67]

Some laypeople even followed the physicians' example and observed how their urine changed when they left it standing. His urine, wrote stonemason Johann Michel Schmidt from Mainz, was "at first, when still warm, a nice urine, that is of bright lemon color; but when it is cold, it is white as milk and has a thick white deposit on the bottom."[68] Others ventured into an interpretation of their own. Adam Bernd wrote in his biography about his famulus, who

---

[61] Ibid., letter dated November 26, 1726.

[62] Rusnock, *Jurin* (1996), 396f, letter from Cary, early June 1733.

[63] Ibid., 398, letter from Cary, June 6, 1733.

[64] Stolberg, *Erfahrungen* (2004).

[65] Rusnock, *Jurin* (1996), 399, letter from Cary, June 12, 1733.

[66] Ibid., 402–5, letter from Cary, March 28, 1733.

[67] BCU Lausanne, Fonds Tissot, letter from the Countess of Wedel, November 12, 1784.

[68] Senckenberg Archiv Frankfurt, Senckenberg correspondence, letter to Senckenberg, December 22, 1726.

began acting "very strange and gloomy" in the summer of 1714, said "fantastical things," and whose sleep was agitated. Although the servant drank nothing but water, Bernd noticed to his astonishment that "his urine nevertheless looked like blood." Bernd therefore suspected "an excessive heat in the head and great mental alienation."[69] A 31-year-old patient from the French town of Aix-en-Provence who was plagued by seizures wrote in 1772 that his urine was sometimes of a natural, lemon-yellow color but sometimes mixed with a very thick, mealy substance that could be cut with a knife after it had settled. He also believed he knew the cause of this. By his own admission, he had given himself to masturbation early on in his life, and now he suffered from a feeble constitution and in particular from a weakness of the nerves and the stomach.[70]

Uroscopy was thus far from being considered obsolete among the educated upper classes of the eighteenth century. Basic knowledge about the diagnostic conclusions that could be drawn from certain changes in urine remained current. As late as 1831, Ernst Joseph Gustav de Valenti, in his *Medicina clerica*, praised specialists in uroscopy: "Someone who concerns himself with the exclusive study of one single symptom all his life ultimately has the advantage that one-sidedness offers, i.e. he sees in this one vessel, the matula, more than even Boerhaave and Sydenham."[71] Nevertheless, the significance of uroscopy ostensibly waned among the upper classes during the eighteenth and nineteenth centuries—certainly when it came to using the method as the sole basis of diagnosis. Presumably this loss of significance was also a reflection of the growing skepticism toward uroscopy among the learned doctors whose services these social classes preferred and with whom they were in close exchange. Long-term changes in the dominant concepts of the body and its diseases may also have played an important role, however. Among physicians, the focus shifted from notions of humors and mobile morbid matter—on which uroscopy was based—toward an understanding of diseases as resulting from pathological changes in the various solid parts of the body. The rapid spread of the new doctrine of the irritability of the nerves and "nervous complaints" among the upper classes of the eighteenth century—which largely supplanted older notions of mobile vapors and fumes—illustrates how readily such changes in medical theories could be accepted by educated laypeople.

The vast majority of the population, however, continued to adhere to uroscopy as a key to all knowledge about illness, just as they did with the traditional concepts of humoralism. They could not imagine a medicine without uroscopy.

---

[69]   Bernd, *Lebens-Beschreibung* (1738), 315; Bernd used the term "Gemüts-Krankheit."

[70]   BCU Lausanne, Fonds Tissot, letter from sick M. Dauphin, June 1772. His complaints matched well those which the enlightened anti-masturbation campaign, of which Tissot was one of the most influential protagonists, ascribed to "onanism"; on the driving forces behind this campaign and on its effects see cf. Stolberg, *Unmanly vice* (2000).

[71]   Valenti, *Medicina clerica* (1831), 113f.

A good illustration of what uroscopy continued to mean in the everyday life of the population at large can be gained from interrogations of patients and their relatives who sought the advice of irregular practitioners. In the 1770s there was, for example, an official inquest into the so-called "doctress" of Schozach, who was a non-licensed, irregular healer from the Heilbronn area.[72] It had come to the attention of the authorities that many people from the area consulted the woman and praised her skills even though there was a physician with a doctoral degree in the nearby town who received a salary from the government and was thus allowed to ask only moderate fees. After several patients had died in the care of the "doctress,"[73] people who went to see her were intercepted and questioned to find out the names of more of her clients. Of course, those interrogated would have been eager to present themselves in a good light. Still their stories yield illuminating insights into the practice of the "doctress," and into the reasons why her advice was sought.

Many of those questioned were relatives who had served as messengers to deliver urine and pick up a prescription or a medicine. They came from Ottmarsheim, Gemmrigheim, and other places within a radius of around 10 kilometers. To justify their having taking recourse to an irregular healer, they commonly emphasized that they had acted out of Christian charity. They had no longer been able to deny the wishes of the sick, once all efforts undertaken by legitimate, officially approved healers had failed. His wife had "not given him peace until he went to the doctress from Schozach, because reports had it that the doctress had helped many local people," recounted Johannes Schunz. So he had not been able to deny her wish "without a bad conscience." He took his wife's urine to the doctress "in a small flask," where he found six or eight people present. He was "unable to tell [the doctress] about the illness of his wife," but she "examined the water and said his wife had consumptive fever" and gave him a flask with medicine.[74] Another witness, the vintner Johannes Finkk, even found around 30 people at the house of the "doctress" when he brought her the urine of his 30-year-old brother. According to the interrogation protocol, Finkk excused his own action by saying that his "brother had forced him, and anyway, everybody went to Schozach."[75] Others likewise justified carrying the urine of a sick person to the doctress by saying that everybody was seeking advice from the "doctress." The baker Konrad Nägeli, whose wealth would have easily permitted him to consult a doctor, explained that "because the entire neighborhood and

---

[72] HStA Stuttgart A 213 Bü. 6734.

[73] Ultimately, the authorities were unable to prove that the "doctress" was directly responsible for the deaths.

[74] HStA Stuttgart A 213 Bü. 6734, interrogation of Johannes Schunz, March 3, 1780.

[75] Ibid., interrogation of Johannes Finkk, March 3, 1780

simply everyone was going to Schozach without any qualms, he believed the woman was licensed as a healer."[76]

The numerous ethnographic accounts penned by mid-nineteenth-century physicians in southern Germany still described uroscopy as very popular.[77] According to Dr Lingl from Oberdorf, everyone, in fact, "who went to the doctor on behalf of a sick person" brought urine in a flask and "it would be the end of the doctor's reputation if he did not pay attention to it or rejected it as unimportant."[78] People in the countryside were even found to travel long distances to consult a particularly famous uroscopist.[79] The popular appeal of uroscopy waned, at most, only gradually. Some irregular healers were still explicitly characterized as uroscopists in the so-called "quack statistics" ("Kurpfuscherstatistik"), which were compiled regularly in the Kingdom of Bavaria, starting in 1874, after legal restrictions on the practice of medicine had been lifted in the German Reich. According to the new regulation, anyone was allowed to treat patients, with no need for medical training or a license.[80] Some of the uroscopists listed in the statistics came from an agricultural background and the preponderance of women is striking. For instance, it was said about the widow of vintner Lochmayer from the Palatinate that she gave advice "based on urine examination." She enjoyed "great trust" and was visited frequently at her home "especially by those with chronic internal diseases." Anna Maria Hofstetter, a field laborer in the Palatinate village of Speyerdorf, who also relied on uroscopy to give "advice concerning all kinds of illness," sometimes traveled to see patients who lived farther away. Another occupational group which ranked prominently among the listed "quack" uroscopists was the knackers. About Georg Kaiser, a knacker in the Upper Franconian town of Kulmbach, it was said that he cured "everything with or without sympathy, is a uroscopist and also hands out drugs." Sick people even came from the neighboring county to ask his advice. Similarly, it was said about a knacker's wife from Bachhofen, Barbara Pechtner, that she made her diagnosis "by examining urine" and administered

---

[76]   Ibid., interrogation of Konrad Nägeli, March 4, 1780.

[77]   Valenti, *Medicina clerica* (1831), 113f; Buck, *Medicinischer Volksglauben* (1865), 29.

[78]   BSB Munich, Cgm 6874/129, medical topography and ethnography of Oberdorf; similarly BSB Munich, Cgm 6874/111, Mindelheim; BSB Munich, Cgm 6874/155, Rothenburg ob der Tauber. "Brunnen" – a term frequently used for "urine" literally means "well" but it also sounds similar to the colloquial "brunzen" for urinating.

[79]   StA Bamberg KIII 1481, medical topography of Höchstadt (Dr G.H. Bruder).

[80]   HStA Munich, MInn 61355, Kurpfuscherstatistik. Also, many a "quack," whose practice was described only in general terms, as in "oversteps his authority" or "heals internal and external diseases," is likely to have used uroscopy. As the data collection served mainly to assess the negative impact on the practice of doctors caused by the abolition of licensing requirements in the German Reich, the focus was on the therapeutic, not on the diagnostic preferences of healers.

medication. And there were others: a constable's wife from Deggendorf, who was an "uroscopist for women's and children's diseases"; a "mason's wife"; a landlady, who "gave medical advice based on the examination of urine"; and the wife of a brickyard owner, who practiced "uroscopy" and treated illnesses with herbs she gathered. But it seems likely that those captured in the statistics were only the tip of the iceberg. Only the healers whose practice became known to the county doctors were recorded, and since such healing activities had been prohibited and punishable until very recently, many healers probably continued to work in secret. They were all the more difficult to uncover, explained Dr Bruder in Höchstadt, as the "quacks" did not themselves administer medicines to the same extent as before but limited themselves "to uroscopy and oral advice" and made the necessary drugs available to their customers through out-of-town sellers.[81]

In France during the same period the situation appears to have been quite similar. In 1821, Mérat agreed that uromancy, that is divination from urine, could be found predominantly among the lower classes, but even the more educated patients with incurable diseases and melancholics—he was probably referring to patients with psychiatric disorders in general—resorted to it. Indeed, according to Mérat, the belief in uromancy was still so widespread in France that there was hardly a village where not at least one person practiced it. Every county had at least one "urine doctor" to whom people flocked from the whole area, matula in hand. Even in Paris, the palladium of good taste, sophistication, and modern knowledge, uroscopists advertised their services in broad daylight.[82]

Uroscopy in Learned Medical Practice

Learned medical writing, since the sixteenth century, expressed considerable doubts about the diagnostic power of uroscopy and warned of the widespread custom of diagnosing illness by examining nothing but the urine. Hardly any medical writer until far into the eighteenth century challenged the usefulness of uroscopy as such, however, as long as the physician also took the patients' complaints and their history and present circumstances into account. Some authors even warned critics not to throw the baby out with the bathwater and condemn uroscopy simply because it was "misused" by "quacks" and "old crones."[83]

Uroscopy's central place in ordinary medical practice was also acknowledged in official regulations. In sixteenth-century Wurttemberg, for example, an ordinance on medical taxes distinguished only three kinds of medical fees: one

---

[81]   StA Bamberg KIII 1481, medical topography of Höchstadt.

[82]   Mérat, *Uromancie* (1821), 344f.

[83]   Cf. e.g. the detailed criticism in Pleier, *Examen tractatus Guil. Adolphi Scribonii* (1617); similarly Horst, *Manuductio* (1648), 103.

for uroscopy and the advice based upon it, one for a house call, and one, finally, for a house call when the physician also examined the urine.[84] In employment contracts of city and hospital doctors as well, it was commonplace that performing uroscopy was listed among their duties.[85] Not least of all, we find that urine examination frequently figures in medical case histories of the time. Thus Dr Frank from Ulm wrote in the seventeenth century about "raw urine" as the central symptom of a 24-year-old maidservant,[86] or about the "thick, cloudy urine" of a woman who at the age of 22 had never had her period.[87] He concluded from the cloudy urine of a wealthy Blaubeuren man that his blood was raw and undigested.[88] In the "white" urine of a weaver woman from the country, whose husband had the urine taken to him "according to Swabian custom," he found "chyle" and red sediment that "suggested rawness due to spoiled acid." He therefore surmised that the patient had a lot of air in her belly (it seems he presumed a process of fermentation), "which the messenger confirmed."[89]

Only very gradually did uroscopy lose some of its overarching significance in learned medicine. In the eighteenth century this loss in significance was still only relative. Thus, around 1700, the famous German professor of medicine Friedrich Hoffmann from Halle vociferously condemned the "empirical and divining art" of uneducated uroscopists. But at the same time he pointed out how valuable uroscopy was in the hands of an experienced physician to help diagnose acute as well as chronic diseases.[90] In this spirit, a group of doctors from Breslau around this time described their practical experience of the typical changes in urine, for example in cases of dropsy or hysteria, and more generally with patients suffering from spasmodic, convulsive complaints such as asthma and epilepsy.[91] Many held that "no sure judgment could be gained from urine," noted Hygiander in a text which was first published in 1720. But, he continued, if they arrived at unreliable judgments, this was above all because they did not respect the rules and drew incorrect conclusions.[92] Practicing in Leuven, H.J. Rega likewise attacked the widespread custom of taking the urine to the doctor's home, expressing at the

---

[84]   HStA Stuttgart A 282 Bü. 1299, *Ordnung der* Ärzte *und Apotheker im Fürstentum* Württemberg, December 7, 1566.

[85]   Cf. e.g. Jankrift, *Krankheit* (2003), 65.

[86]   Stadtarchiv Ulm, Ms. Franc 8b, 247v.

[87]   Ibid., 231r, on the daughter of Joh. Hirns.

[88]   Stadtarchiv Ulm, Ms. Franc 8a, 26r

[89]   Ibid., 29r–v.

[90]   Hoffmann, *Medicina rationalis* (1729), 218.

[91]   Academia Leopoldina, *Historia morborum* (1746), 195 and 437.

[92]   Hygiander, *Regeln* (1744), preface.

same time his great appreciation of artfully executed uroscopy that shed light on the causes, symptoms, and consequences of illnesses.[93]

For all his skepticism, even Herman Boerhaave—one of the most noted and influential representatives of a new, empirically oriented clinical medicine in the eighteenth century—praised the virtues of uroscopy in certain cases. He confided to his students that when faced with a patient with many different complaints and unsure which symptoms were predominant, "I casually look at and examine the urine, and immediately find what I am looking for."[94] He explained in another context that urine did not only offer valuable clues about diseases of the kidneys, the efferent urinary tract, and the seminal vessels, as well as about various illnesses that had their origin in the bile; he claimed that the nature, the impetus, and the *symptomata* of the blood, the state of the disease, its crisis, concoction, and secretions, could also be indicated by the urine—all things that were central to the conception of illness at the time.[95] In 1797, Karl Arnold Kortum spoke out against the "doctors and instructors of the people," who "out of an exaggerated fervor, want to abolish uroscopy as a whole, although it has its place in the teaching of medical symptomatology."[96]

Only in the course of the nineteenth century did the traditional visual examination of urine with the naked eye lose much of its former importance in the physicians' practice. They continued to seek diagnostic information from examining the urine[97] but increasingly they relied on chemical analysis.[98] For Germany, this development is strikingly illustrated, from the 1860s, in the different editions of Carl Neubauer's *Anleitung zur qualitativen und quantitativen Analyse des Harns* (Instruction on the Qualitative and Quantitative Analysis of Urine), on which he later collaborated with Julius Vogel. While the book grew substantially in size—the tenth edition, which came out in 1898, stretched over 900 pages—the color of urine took up less and less space. The first editions of the work still featured a small color chart of nine basic colors, ranging from pale yellow to a brownish black. However, these colors were interpreted merely to express different concentrations of urine.[99] Later editions no longer contained this chart and instead the reader was given only black and white illustrations of spectrophotometric analysis in which individual lines indicated the various

---

[93]   Rega, *Tractatus* (1733), preface to the first treatise and ibid. second treatise, *De urina ut signo* (separate pagination).

[94]   Boerhaave, *Introductio* (1740), 16; cf. Probst, *Weg* (1972), 41f.

[95]   Boerhaave, *Institutiones medicae* (1747), 464.

[96]   Kortum, *Vom Urin* (1793), preface.

[97]   See e.g. Ziegler, *Uroscopie am Krankenbette* (1865).

[98]   Becquerel, *Séméiotique* (1841); Neubauer, *Anleitung* (1854).

[99]   Neubauer/Vogel, *Anleitung*, 7th edn (1876), 174–6 and table IV.

chemical components.[100] Because of the very specific proportions of different substances and their permeability in regard to particular light frequencies, this process provided a superior means of "determining and proving with certainty the presence of such substances for which a given proportion is known and to distinguish them from other, seemingly similar ones, while also determining the coincidental presence or absence of other colored substances."[101] The skilled gaze of the uroscopist had been replaced by modern technology.

In the large majority of cases, however, chemical and photometric analysis contributed only little to diagnosis. Its value remained largely restricted to diagnosing and charting the progression of particular metabolic dysfunctions and of diseases of the kidneys and the efferent urinary tract. Modern chemical urinalysis could not come near the paramount position uroscopy had held in premodern medicine. Far from offering a key to virtually all known illnesses of the human body, as traditional uroscopy had done, it has remained a diagnostic procedure that provides valuable insights for only a very limited number of specific diseases.

Even in the light of modern laboratory analysis, some authors incidentally saw no reason to ban outright the tried and tested practice of examination with the naked eye from their medical practice. They attempted to uphold uroscopy's place in medical diagnostics, or even sought to provide it with a new theoretical foundation, drawing on contemporary science. In the early nineteenth century, the path to choose for such an endeavor was that of high philosophical standards. Only on a solid theoretical footing, writes Joseph Loew in his 250-page dissertation of 1808, could "urinary semiotics practiced as uromancy flourish again in its old, admired dignity, which it affirmed time and again in past epochs of pathological medicine." The main question guiding his interest was "how the quiddity and form-giving principle, the soul of any disease, must reveal itself within the urinary organs and become visible in the urine."[102] In the 650 or so pages of his 1829 work on Hippocratic uroscopy, J.C.F. Baehrens presented uroscopy on the basis of contemporary natural philosophy.[103] Drawing on his professional experience of 16 years, Johann Grosshauser published his *Practical Hints for an Easy Identification of Illnesses in the Urine* in 1901. A second edition came out only two years after the first.[104] As late as 1937, Dr Pfleiderer of Ulm issued a reprint of Hygiander's *Rules to Be Unmistakably Established from Urine*,

---

[100] Neubauer/Vogel, *Anleitung*, 7th edn (1876), 141f; iidem, *Anleitung*, 10th edn (1898), 680–98 and ibid., appendix with tables.

[101] Neubauer/Vogel, *Anleitung*, 10th edn (1898), 681.

[102] Loew, *Ueber den Harn* ([1808]), 7f.

[103] Baehrens, *Harnlehre* (1829).

[104] Grosshauser, *Praktische Winke* (1901).

specifically advising his colleagues to continue practicing traditional uroscopy alongside chemical analysis.[105]

Non-Academic Uroscopists

Uroscopists did not constitute a separate medical profession in the early modern period. Uroscopy was so ubiquitous that virtually every medical practitioner performed it. At best, individual healers were known and particularly sought after for their uroscopic abilities. If we want to get a better idea of the professional figure of the early modern uroscopist, we therefore need to look at the different groups of medical practitioners in general that were active in premodern societies.[106]

Though their number grew substantially from the sixteenth century, learned physicians played only a minor role in the medical care of most people. Much more numerous, at least on the European continent, were the barber-surgeons who acquired their medical knowledge and skills in the course of an apprenticeship. They cared for the vast majority of the rural and urban population into the nineteenth century. In many places, regulations stipulated that they only treat injuries and external diseases such as ulcers and abscesses. In practice, however, barber-surgeons frequently also diagnosed and treated internal diseases. Among the licensed medical practitioners they were thus the largest group that practiced uroscopy. Some of them earned such an outstanding reputation that patients would send their urine from faraway places.[107]

Though they were, in principle, barred from any therapeutic activity, some apothecaries also ran a flourishing medical practice.[108] In the early seventeenth century, for example, an inquest was held into the medical activities of the apothecary Lietscher from the German town of Memmingen. The apothecary assured the court that he had sent anyone asking him for an examination of urine back to the doctors, as the court scribe of Kellmünz could confirm, "who himself came to me with the urine of his wife." When, however, the treatment by the academic physicians had not helped, he conceded, and the patients or their

---

[105] Hygiander, *Regeln* (1744), preface to the reprint of 1937.

[106] Overviews in Jütte, Ärzte (1991); Kinzelbach, *Gesundbleiben* (1995).

[107] Cf. e.g. Staatsarchiv Ludwigsburg B 412 37, on a highly popular barber-surgeon in Essingen, 1765.

[108] Landesarchiv Schwerin, Altes Archiv 2.12–2/3, 178, report to the Duke, November 15, 1702, concerning an apothecary who, according to the husband's statement, had examined his wife's urine and had incorrectly told the patient—who then died shortly after delivering prematurely—that she was definitely not pregnant; we will come back to this case.

relatives had urged him, he did give his advice out of Christian charity, free of charge and with good results.[109]

Midwives traditionally not only delivered babies but also played an important role in the medical care of newborns and women in childbed. It is unclear, however, to what extent they practiced uroscopy. They may have been asked for a uroscopic judgment particularly when a pregnancy was suspected.[110]

Especially in the countryside, unlicensed, irregular healers are known to have played a major role in the health care of ordinary people. Sources which reflect their actual practice and the place of uroscopy in it are scant. They tended to hide their activities from the authorities. Most of our knowledge comes from the descriptions of educated contemporaries and, occasionally, from interrogation protocols. They could be ordinary members of the community, farmers, artisans, or clergymen. Yet, there were some professions that lent themselves particularly well to medical activites. First and foremost of these were the executioners, knackers, and shepherds, who, as we have seen, were still playing a prominent role in the "quack" statistics of the late nineteenth century.

Much more visible were the itinerant healers who traveled the land and advertised their services and medicines at fairs.[111] In 1733, the medical professor H.J. Rega from Leuven, for example, wrote indignantly about an itinerant female uroscopist who knew how to impress people to such a degree that not only common folk flocked to her but also clergy and nobility, who praised her art, put their own lives, and the lives of their relatives, into her hands, and conferred "authority" on her.[112]

---

[109] Stadtarchiv Memmingen, Bestand A Reichsstadt, Schubl. 408 Nr. 9.
[110] Cf. Stukenbrock, *Abtreibung* (1993), 98f.
[111] Cf. Probst, *Fahrende Heiler* (1992).
[112] Rega, *Tractatus*, I (1733), preface.

Chapter 2
The Foundations of Uroscopy

The examination of urine with the naked eye remained a central diagnostic procedure even in learned medicine until far into the eighteenth century. Indeed, it continued to be appreciated by most doctors as a highly valuable way of gaining essential insights into the nature and causes of illness. Among the general public and among parts of the medical profession it did not lose significance until well into the nineteenth century. Such a tenacious belief may seem puzzling. Why would highly educated physicians with years of scientific and philosophical training have believed that a visual examination of urine held the key to insights into the mysterious processes of disease inside the body, and that it pointed the way to an effective treatment? And what fed the unwaning belief of patients and families in this method at a time when doctors began to grow more skeptical? In order to answer these puzzling questions, we first need to take a closer look at what uroscopists actually did, what they looked out for, and how they underpinned their diagnostic reasoning. In a second step, we will examine how uroscopy worked in ordinary medical practice and how it seemed to prove its worth over and again in various ways.

Uroscopy has a long history.[1] It is already mentioned in the Hippocratic writings, where changes in the urine are described for different diseases. According to the Hippocratic *Epidemic diseases*, Pythius, who lived near the shrine of the earth goddess and had come down with intense fever, tremors, and vomiting, emitted urine that was, from the onset of his illness, thin, colorless, and with "cloudy patches beneath the surface."[2] The text gives a similar description of the urine of acutely feverish Hermocrates, which, however, was sometimes also thick and reddish in color and had no sediment when it sat for some time.[3] In addition, a number of more general diagnostic and prognostic propositions about diagnosing from urine have survived in the Hippocratic *Aphorisms*. For example: "With all who pass translucent white urine, the course of illness will be wearisome; this is most obvious with those who are ill in the brain."[4] In Galen—antiquity's other eminent medical authority—numerous references to

---

[1]   Uroscopy was already being used as a means to diagnose diseases in ancient Mesopotamia and Egypt.

[2]   Hippocrates, *Epidemics* 3.1 (Littré, vol. 3, 24–9).

[3]   Hippocrates, *Epidemics* 3.2 (Littré, vol. 3, 32–9)

[4]   Hippocrates, *Aphorisms* 4.72 (Littré, vol. 4, 528f).

the diagnostic significance of different urinary changes are found.[5] While Galen still deemed pulse diagnosis more significant than uroscopy, this relationship became inverted in the Middle Ages, mostly due to the influence of Arab medical writers. Uroscopy became the central diagnostic means. In particular, Constantinus Africanus's (ca. 1020–1087) Latin translation of a work by Isaac Judaeus (ca. 900) and the *Canon medicinae* by Avicenna (Ibn Sina) had an outstanding and lasting impact on Western uroscopy.[6]

Thanks to these works, Latin translations of other ancient writings, and a range of contributions by Arab, Byzantine, and Latin authors during the Middle Ages, numerous Latin and vernacular writings on urine were available to early modern doctors and literate laypeople. They offered their readers more or less detailed instructions on how to interpret the manifold changes in the urine, often complemented with theoretical elaborations from natural philosophy, explaining the formation and emission of urine and the reasons for its change with different illnesses.

How did the uroscopist proceed according to these writings? While the different authors sometimes arrived at conflicting conclusions when it came to the details, they largely agreed on the fundamentals. The characteristic changes concerned consistency or "substance," color, and contents. In addition, some authors mention further criteria such as the amount of urine, its taste and smell, and sometimes even the haptic sensation when urine came into contact with one's skin,[7] and the sound when passing water—presumably into a chamber pot.[8]

Consistency

The consistency or "substance" of urine was described as thick or coarse (*crassa*), thin (*tenuis*), or in between (*mediocris*), which was typical of healthy urine but could also occur in certain illnesses.[9] Only rarely do we find mention of "oily" urine, comparable to the color and consistency of olive oil, which Galen had described as a symptom of liquefaction of body substance.[10] What exactly was meant by "thick" and "thin" urine and how this was judged often remains somewhat obscure. It seems that, for one thing, what mattered was the degree of viscosity. Healthy urine resembled regular water in this respect, and was only

---

[5]   Galen, *De crisibus* (1825), 594–607 (book 1, ch. 12).

[6]   Isaac Judaeus, *De urinis* ([1515]); Avicenna, *Canon* (1595).

[7]   Avicenna, *Canon* (1595), 47v.

[8]   Da Monte, *De excrementis* (1554), 6r; British Library, Ms. Sloane 94 (uroscopic manuscript written around 1500); Bonacursius, *De humano sero* (1650), 37f.

[9]   Avicenna, *Canon* (1595), 49r; Anonymous, *Seinge of urynes* (around 1550), no pagination; Argenterio, *De urinis* (1591), 13.

[10]   Bonacursius, *De humano sero* (1650), 64; Galen, *De crisibus* (1825), 604.

slightly more viscous owing to its somewhat coarser constituents. According to Bellini, also the sound of making water had to be like that of water being poured from a comparable height into a container filled with water.[11] In a similar sense, Bonacursius compared the sound of healthy urine with that of good wine. A muted or noiseless urine indicated insufficient concoction or else sticky or fatty humors.[12]

Another factor in determining the consistency of urine was what today we would call color density. Thick urine was characterized by strong colors, thin urine by pale, watery colors. Thick urine, explained Da Monte—using a comparison that likely resonated with his Italian readers—was like wine from Padua; thin urine on the other hand was fine like wine that was watery in substance.[13] Thick urine could have the same color as thin urine but transmitted less light; it looked less transparent. A rule of thumb was that the uroscopist holding a flask of "thin" urine in his hand could make out his finger joints through the liquid.[14] This might indicate a cold, weak stomach.[15] Later, when distillation was increasingly used to examine the different elements of urine, a thick or thin consistency was also ascribed to the urine's concentration of salts and other solid substances.

Colors

The most important and most obvious characteristic to which the uroscopist had to pay attention was color. Following medieval tradition, most authors distinguished 19 or 20 different shades.[16] The color spectrum ranged from light/ watery to yellow, red, green, blue, grey, and all the way to black. Some of the colors were subdivided into two versions, one of a stronger (*non remissus*) and one of a lesser (*remissus*) color intensity. Usually, the colors were identified by names taken from a well-established century-old canon and illustrated by comparing them with everyday liquids or objects, comparisons which themselves were passed down as part of a century-old tradition and showed very little variance. In addition, the different colors were sometimes illustrated in uroscopy charts and

---

[11] Bellini, *De urina* (1718), 3f; according to Walaeus, *Medica* (1660), 76, healthy urine made no sound.

[12] Bonacursius, *De humano sero* (1650), 37f.

[13] Da Monte distinguished not only the *substantia* but also the *liquor* and the *corpulentia*, referring primarily to the degree of opacity, it seems. Urine could be glistening (*splendida*), luminous and bright (*candida, lucida*), or else dark (*obscura, opaca*).

[14] ÖNB Vienna, Cod. 11205, 68v and 79v–80r.

[15] Anonymous, *Seinge of urynes* (around 1550), no pagination.

[16] The number of colors was usually 20 because two different kinds of "black" were listed.

wheels (see Plates 8–13).[17] Such visual representations of the different colors of urine were quite frequent and can be found in portable medical vademecums, which suggests that they were indeed used at the sickbed.[18] Foreest explicitly mentions uroscopists who relied on charts "on which all waters are shown in life-like colors, holding their matulae with the water up to them."[19]

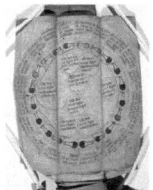

Descriptions and images of urine color were usually organized from light to dark, from pale and translucent colors to the darker and more intense shades, and concluded with black. Showing only very little variation, this arrangement was also based on a tradition that remained consistent for centuries.[20]

The following list gives an overview of the different color terms and the comparisons commonly used to illustrate them. They are taken from Latin inscriptions which accompanied the uroscopy wheel in *Manuscript no. 1177* in the Library of the University of Leipzig (see Plate 9), from Apollinaris's German *Tractätlein*,[21] and from the anonymous *Seinge of urynes*.[22] I have added the English translations for German terms where they differ considerably from those in the *Seinge of urynes*.

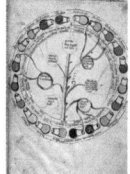

1. *albus*, "ut aqua putrida," "weiß als Wasser," "whyte as claye water of a well"
2. *lacteus*, "ut serum,"[23] "weiß als Milch, da das Schmaltz von gemacht ist" ("white as milk from which concentrated butter is made"), "whyte as whay"

---

   [17]   Cf. Sudhoff, *Harnglasscheibe* (1907); Pergens-Maeseyck, *Urinschautafel* (1908); Murray Jones, *Medieval medicine* (1998); sometimes uroscopic texts were also illustrated with single urine flasks in different colors; see e.g. Wellcome Library, London, Western manuscripts 7117/36 fol. 119r–122v, *Practical uroscopy*.

   [18]   Cf. Talbot, *Vade mecum* (1961); cf. e.g. the folded uroscopic color tables in British Library, Ms. Harley 5311 and Rosenbach Museum & Library, Philadelphia, Ms. 1004.

   [19]   Foreest, *Uromanteia* (1620), 203.

   [20]   Bonacursius, *De humano sero* (1650) even refers to Plato and Aristotle in his use of color terms like *cruentus, puniceus, passeus, purpureus, ferrugineus*, or *oleagineus*.

   [21]   Apollinaris, *Tractätlein* (1663), 79f.

   [22]   Anonymous, *Seinge of urynes* (around 1550), no pagination. An English translation of Vassaeus's treatise arrived at somewhat different comparisons, namely: whyte as cristall, clere as water, meane white, white as mylke, gray as the heres of a camell, clere lyke horne, pale, flaren, yelow as golde, lyght yelow, light saffron, full saffron, redde, clarett, crymsyn, purple, blew, grene, pale, blake (Vassaeus, *Litel treatise* (1553)). On Spanish and Italian terms see Zaun/Geisler, *Harnfarbenbezeichnungen* (2011).

   [23]   Some authors, such as Apollinaris, listed *lacteus* or the corresponding vernacular term after *glaucus*.

3. *glaucus*, "ut cornu lucidum," "weiß als ein durchsichtig Horn," "a whytysshe yeallowe, almoste as bryghte as the horne of a lanterne"

4. *karopos*,[24] "ut vellus cameli," "bleich als eines Kamels Farb" ("pale as the color of a camel), "as a whyte ruffet"

5. *subpallidus*, "ut brodium carnis semicrude," "bleich als Brüh, so Fleisch halb gekocht ist," "as it were the brothe of flesshe, that is halfe sodden"

6. *pallidus*, "ut item remissior," "bleich als Fleischwasser," "as brothe of flesshe that is well sodden"

7. *subcitrinus*, "ut color pomi citrini remissus," "gelb als ein bleicher Apfel," "nat [sic] fullye so yelowe as the yelowe apple"

8. *citrinus*, "ut color pomi citrini non remissus," "gelb als schöne Quitten" ("yellow like beautiful quints"), "as a yelowe apple"

9. *subrufus*, "ut aurum remissum," "roth als bleich Gold," "as whyte golde"

10. *rufus*, "ut aurum non remissum," "roth als schön Gold," "as reed golde"

11. *subrubeus*,[25] "ut crocus occidentalis," "roth als liechter Saffran," "nygh as yelowe as saffron of the garden"

12. *rubeus*,[26] "ut crocus orientalis," "roth als satter Saffran," "red as anye safron"

13. *subrubicundus*, "ut flamma ignis remissa," "roth als Flamme des Feuers" ("red like the flame of a fire"),[27] "reed as a rose"

14. *rubicundus*, "ut flamma ignis non remissa," "roth als Flamme des Feuers," "reed as a brennynge cole"

15. *ynopos*,[28] "ut color epatis vel vinum nigrum," "Leberfarb," "a swartish reed as it were ye liver of a beast"

16. *kyanos*, "ut sanguis putrefactus," "eine Farb als dicker rother Wein" ("like thick red wine"), "as blacke wine or rotten bloud"

17. *viridis*, "ut caules," "grün als Krautsafft" ("green like cole juice"), "green as wortes"

18. *plumbeus* (in some treatises *lividus*), "ut plumbum," "grau als Bley," "is wanne as leade"

19. *niger adustionis*, "ut incaustum," "schwartz als ein Horn" ("black as a horn"), "black and shynynge as a Ravens fether"

20. *niger incensitationis*,[29] "ut cornu bui nigrum," "schwartzfarb als ein Dinten" ("like black ink") or "wie schwarzes Rinderhorn" ("like black beef horn"), "black as a cole."

---

24 Sometimes also spelled *karipos*, *karapos*, or *caropus*.

25 Sometimes also *subrubicundus*.

26 Sometimes also *rubicundus*.

27 Apollinaris has only one entry for "fire-red"; though he claims there are 20 different colors he only names 19.

28 Sometimes also *inopos*.

29 Frequently also *mortificationis*.

Numerous Latin texts in particular list the above color terms and illustrative comparisons nearly identically. Even Greek color terms such as *kyanos* and *ynopos* continued to be used for centuries to come, including the comparison with camel hair to illustrate *karopos*—which presumably reflects Arab origins—though few people, at the time, will ever have seen camel hair.[30] Though otherwise aspiring to originality, even Davach de la Rivière's voluminous eighteenth-century treatise on urine still employs the traditional terms, and merely illustrates and specifies them with further comparisons. Davach de la Rivière's most striking departure from the canon is his translation of *karopos* as "grey," and his comparison of this color with that of an ass or with the whitish grey hair of humans, which would have been much closer to the experience of his readership than the classic reference to camel hair.[31]

A closer look at the many different charts and treatises on urine reveals some differences and conflicting details. Only minor variation can be found in the color terms, when for instance *plumbeus* is used instead of *lividus*. The order in which the colors were presented, ranging from *albus* to *niger*, also was subject to change only to a very limited degree. A case in point is the different shades of reddish and yellow urine: *Subrubeus* and *rubeus* sometimes preceded and sometimes followed *subrubicundus* and *rubicundus*; also, *lacteus* and *glaucus* occasionally swapped places. The greatest variance is found in the comparisons used to illustrate the color terms. Especially in vernacular writings such as *Seinge of urynes,* attempts were made to make the comparisons closer to people's everyday experience. Two different shades of black, for instance, are compared in *Seinge of urynes* with raven feathers and coal, respectively, two different shades of red with roses and glowing embers.

Most striking, by far, is the variation in the coloring of contemporary uroscopic color charts and wheels. We find differences that cannot be sufficiently explained by the ageing of the paint and pigments that were used. At times, the verbal description and the coloring of the depicted matula do not seem to match at all. A matula colored in with a shade of brownish/black may be described as "reddish, like the color of the strong flame of a fire" (*rubicundus color ut flamma ignis non remissa*).[32] On closer inspection, such inconsistencies are not all that surprising, however. We only need to consider how the charts or wheels got their coloring: Those in manuscripts had to be colored in by hand. At best, the illustrator could try to copy as well as he could the colored chart he found in another manuscript. Things did not become any easier or more standardized

---

[30]   As Georg Handsch suggests in his notes on Fracanzani's lectures in Padua, however, the term may have been familiar from another context: the color of the Franciscan monks' frock was called "caropos" (ÖNB Vienna, Cod. 11210, 83r).

[31]   Rivière, *Miroir* (1722), 40.

[32]   Rosenbach Library & Museum, Ms. 1004.

with the invention of book printing, but rather, more difficult: printing at the time was usually monochrome. Someone who bought a treatise on uroscopy therefore could not expect colored charts in it. What he usually found were 20 perfectly identical black and white matulae arranged in a circle or a table (see Figure 2.1).

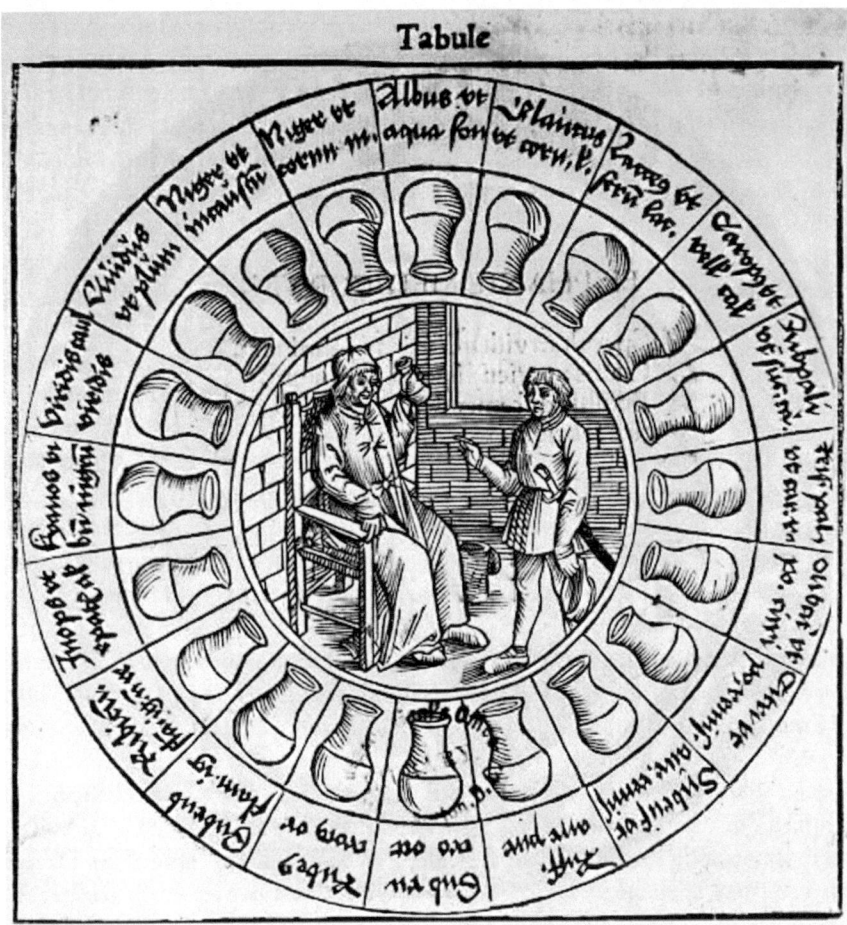

Figure 2.1   Printed black and white uroscopy wheel, in: Pinder, *Epiphanie medicorum* (1506)

Presented with these printed images of matulae, the buyer had to color them in by hand himself or assign someone else the task. Unlike for a scribe who copied colored manuscripts, there usually was not even a colored copy to work from. One could only go by the written descriptions of the different urine colors and their illustration by comparison with liquids or objects from everyday life. In other words, as aesthetically pleasing as the urine color charts may strike us today and as much as they may seem to try to be true to reality, the essential information was not conveyed by them but by the written descriptions and comparisons—which the experienced uroscopist could supplement from his own personal observations.

Under these circumstances, coloring the charts inevitably could produce very different results. For one thing, some of the comparisons referred to substances or objects such as flames or apples which came in a wide range of colors. For another, some of the comparisons were somewhat at odds with the color they were meant to exemplify. As many doctors knew from their Greek studies, the word *kyanos*, for example, denoted "blue"; yet it was commonly compared to dark wine. *Glaucus*—known today from the term "glaucoma"—means "greenish" in classical Latin and not "yellow."[33] *Rufus* was a familiar term (with a proper name derived from it) denoting red hair color, while the common comparison with the color of gold pointed, again, in a different direction. Whoever colored in the black and white charts could thus arrive at very different results depending on how he interpreted the color terms and the comparisons commonly used to illustrate them. It remains an open question whether these differences were also owed to people's empirical observation, which would have told them in the case of *kyanos,* for instance, that urine could hardly be "sky-blue" but certainly claret-red. In this sense, a hand-colored copy of an Italian edition of the late fifteenth-century *Fasciculus medicinae* exhibits above all different shades of yellow, a tint that we would expect people to have encountered most commonly.[34] The coloration of this edition is strikingly different from the much more colorful manuscript no. 1004, held at the Rosenbach Library & Museum in Philadelphia (see Plate 8), in which yellow is hardly present at all.

]Thumbnail 8 near here[

Reading late medieval and early modern uroscopic treatises from today's perspective, we are presented with still another difficulty. Color designations from those times are not as self-evident as they may seem at first glance. This is most obvious in the case of the color "white," in Latin "albus." As Davach de la Rivière explained, "white" could be understood to mean more or less the color of milk. But "white," at the time, could also denote the color of water or crystal—liquids that are today described as transparent.[35] Consequently, the famous *Fasciculus medicinae* from the late fifteenth century illustrates *color albus*

---

[33]   The term can also indicate a light grey or a watery color, however.

[34]   Ketham, *Fasciculus medicinae* (1493).

[35]   Foreest, *Uromanteia* (1620), 148 compares "white" urine with water from a fountain; according to Avicenna, *Canon* (1595), 48v, the common folks used the term "white" to describe transparent fluids.

with a reference to the color of "fine water."[36] As Konrad Horlacher explained in 1691, the commonly encountered *albedo* (whiteness) strictly speaking was nothing but the absence of the natural color of urine.[37] In the same vein, when they recommended the use of "white" glass for uroscopy, writers obviously meant clear, transparent—and not milky—glass.[38] Equating "red" with "the color of gold" is hardly less surprising to modern eyes. And similarly accounts of "black" urine probably have to be understood as referring more generally to a dark coloration of urine.[39]

Contents

A third important diagnostic criterion was the presence of visible material contents. Since Hippocratic times, uroscopy treatises had usually distinguished three different kinds, depending on their location in the matula. Some contents stayed on the surface, others sank as a sediment or "hypostasis" to the bottom of the flask, and others—the so-called *enairomena*—remained floating in the liquid. Some authors assigned the individual sections of the matula to the body area that was presumably ailing. Contents that swam on the surface were thought to indicate diseases of the head, the *enairomena* in the middle of the matula indicated chest ailments, and sediment pointed to afflictions below the ribs.[40] Sometimes matulae were given graduation marks (see Figure 2.2) to allow for an even more subtle diagnosis of the affected part.

---

[36] Ketham, *Fasciculus medicinae* (1493).

[37] Horlacher, *Methodus* (1691), 35.

[38] Fernel/Cole/Culpeper, *Two treatises* (1662), 37.

[39] Voswinckel, *Der schwarze Urin* (1993), uses uroscopy to emphasize the central significance of a finely differentiated perception of color with the senses in medicine and criticizes that this has largely been lost today. However, he takes the mention of "black urine" in premodern literature too literally when he understands it as an indication of rare diseases such as alkaptonuria. The historical idea of "black urine" was closely related to widespread notions of excessive heat and burning inside the body; and the sources show clearly that, in many cases, reference was made simply to fairly dark—not black—urine.

[40] Fries, *Spiegel* (1518), LXXr.

De vrinis/das

ist/võ rechter besichtigunge des harns/vnd jhrem miß-
brauch/etwan durch D. E. Cor-
dum Medicum gesetzet/ytzt
vbersehen/vnd in truck
verfertiget.

Durch J. Dryandern genent Eych-
man medicum Marpurgeñ.

Vrteyl Dominici Burgawer von
besichtigunge der wasser.

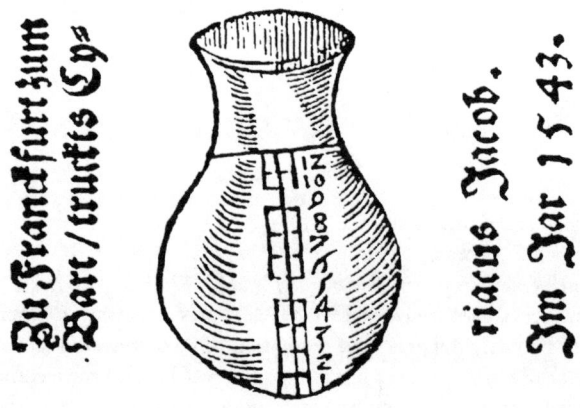

Figure 2.2   Urine flask with graduation, in: Cordus, *De urinis* (1543)

Uroscopic treatises listed a remarkable range of possible contents. Sometimes, a *circulus* or "crown" (*corona*) of a different color than the urine was found floating on the surface.[41] According to Apollinaris, different types of *circuli* indicated different diseases of the head. If the circle quivered, this signified "an apoplexy." If a green circle was visible on the urine of a patient with high fever, this pointed to a *phrenesis*.[42] Bubbles usually indicated an accumulation or expulsion of fine, volatile morbid matter. They came in different sizes and shapes. For example, if small bubbles covered the entire surface of the urine, the uroscopist could conclude that a headache was present; if they covered only half the surface, it was safe to assume a *hemicrania*, i.e. a migraine.[43] Following Galen, foamy urine could be attributed to heated humors that caused volatile matter to rise up. However, one had to make sure that the urine in the flask had not simply been shaken up in transit.[44] Also, foam could result from the winds that arose inside the body, for example due to a hot liver.[45] In this case, foam or bubbles pointed as much to the known symptoms, such as colic or the painful expansion of the stomach and intestines, as they did to the immediate cause, namely insufficiently concocted food or the ingestion of fruit, beans, and other flatulent food.[46] If the bubbles remained on the urine's surface for a long time, this indicated thick, mucous humors. If the bubbles burst easily, thin humors and light winds could be assumed.[47] Sometimes fat collected on the surface and gave rise to fears that the body's own substance was melting away, as it typically occurred in consumption or hectic fever.

The liquid itself could contain clouds, *nubes* or *nubeculae*. If they appeared in the lower part of the matula and assumed the color of lead, they signaled consumption. Yellow or green clouds formed in the case of superfluous bile.[48] Hair or hair-like shapes could also be found in urine. "The urine is still red and [...] small fibers swim in it," reads one patient letter from 1579.[49] The presence of hairs made doctors and patients fear an illness of the kidneys above all. An excessive heating of the kidneys found expression in yellow or red hairs. Hairs of a fatty appearance pointed to a "liquefaction of the kidneys." Coarse hairs that dissolved with shaking indicated a congestion of the kidneys "with a coarse and

---

[41] Horst, *De urinis* (1607), no pagination.

[42] Apollinaris, *Tractätlein* (1663), 88f.

[43] Fernel/Cole/Culpeper, *Two treatises* (1662), 60.

[44] Apollinaris, *Tractätlein* (1663), 89f.

[45] Ibid., 89; Wellcome Library, London, Western manuscripts 94, uroscopic treatise (partially in German).

[46] Beverwijk, *Schat der ongesontheyt* (1672), 10.

[47] Ibid.

[48] Apollinaris, *Tractätlein* (1663), 94.

[49] StB Berlin, Ms. germ. fol. 422b, 71r, letter from Dr Salomon Teichner (?), August 30, 1579.

stringy humor."[50] If hairs were found in urine the color of oil, consumption was diagnosed. Minute grains of sand pointed to one of the humors being viscous and overly heated.[51]

Pus was seen above all with diseases of the bladder and kidneys. If it was accompanied by pains in the right upper abdomen, this indicated a liver ulcer, while large amounts of putrescent pus in the urine were caused by a uterine ulcer.[52] This probably reflects the apparently widespread notion that the urethra and vagina shared a common exit, a view that was upheld even in the writings of the famous anatomist Vesalius. A contemporary German summary of Vesalius's anatomy explicitly spoke of a "part of the bladder neck" that was "implanted in the uterine cervix and ejected the urine into the same."[53]

Occasionally, male and/or female semen in the urine was described. Small, separated amounts of semen meant, as the anonymous *De judicio urinarum* put it, that the man and the woman had "joked" with one another. If, on the other hand, the semen appeared "coarse and lumpy," the person in question had "lived purely" and had not disposed of the semen against nature, "which may cause many a disease."[54]

Mentioned only by some authors but noteworthy for historians of science, the *atomi* or *atoma* formed a very fine and subtle variety of contents. In the medicine of the day they were understood in a general sense as very small particles[55] which, due to their extremely small size, could travel from all body parts to the liver or to the kidneys. They showed up in urine as a fine, dust-like turbidity. They were sometimes likened to the appearance of very fine dust when suspended in the air and illuminated by oblique rays of sunlight.[56] Such "small matter like dust in the sun"[57] lying on the bottom of the matula suggested joint pains or podagra.[58] Dust like this, found in the middle region of the flask indicated—in analogy to the regions of the body—a disease of the lungs and shortness of breath.[59]

---

[50]   Apollinaris, *Tractätlein* (1663), 94f.

[51]   Horst, *De urinis* (1607), no pagination.

[52]   Apollinaris, *Tractätlein* (1663), 97.

[53]   Vesal, *Anatomia Deudsch* (1551), Lr; cf. ibid., LXVIr.

[54]   Apollinaris, *Tractätlein* (1663), 97 and 92f.

[55]   Cf. e.g. the definition in the chapter *De atomis urinae* in Savonarola, *De urinis* (1561), 102v: "Atoma sunt corpuscula parva humoralia nondum terrestrificata."

[56]   According to Giovanni Argenterio, the up and down motion of smallest particles in the matula, "more atomorum," i.e. "in the manner of atoms," was an important distinguishing feature that allowed the doctor to judge whether or not a liquid was actually urine (*De urinis* (1591), 92). Walaeus, in *Medica* (1660), 76, states that such atom-like particles distinguished the urine of healthy women from that of healthy men.

[57]   Apollinaris, *Tractätlein* (1663), 95.

[58]   Ibid.

[59]   Ibid.

Studies on the history of atomism so far seem to have completely overlooked the role of *atoma* in early modern uroscopy.[60] Since this concept of the smallest mobile particles was well known among physicians, it seems quite plausible, however, that from there the term and idea would have spread to authors such as Girolamo Fracastoro and Daniel Sennert, who are credited today with the introduction of atomist thought in early modern natural philosophy.

Lastly, there was sedimentation. It had diagnostic significance most of all when it presented itself as sand, which could indicate kidney or bladder stones.[61] However, soft red sand also occurred in conjunction with fevers or coagulated humors.[62] If the patient suffered from neither fever nor loin pains, red sand indicated an excessive heating of the liver.[63]

Practical Guidelines

Medieval and early modern authors agreed that an exact and reliable urinary diagnosis had to be made with great diligence. Carelessness in procuring, transporting, or examining the urine could lead to serious misjudgments. For this reason treatises on uroscopy frequently listed various points that the uroscopist had to observe closely.

Such advice was more than just practical instruction. It also provided an excuse when the diagnosis or prognosis proved wrong. According to medical writings of the day, the crucial mistakes were made before the doctor even had a chance to look at the urine. Consequently, patients and urine carriers were to blame for any misjudgments arising from these mistakes, not the doctor. Despite the normative and apologetic character of this advice in the many versions in which it came, a vivid image arises of the concrete, everyday practice of uroscopy, an image that we essentially find confirmed in other written and pictorial sources.

First of all, the urine had to be procured at the correct time of day. It was commonly recommended to take it first thing in the morning,[64] "toward 6 o'clock, when we usually get up," as Piper clarified.[65] The reason lay in the physiology of urine formation. During the night, the body and its innate heat could focus entirely on the concoction and assimilation of food. For this reason, the morning urine best reflected these processes. If necessary, the urine could

---

[60]   For recent overviews of early modern atomism see Pyle, *Atomism* (1997); Clericuzio, *Elements* (2000).

[61]   Apollinaris, *Tractätlein* (1663), 92.

[62]   Ibid.

[63]   Ibid.

[64]   Isaac Judaeus, *De urinis* ([1515]), 157v; Apollinaris, *Tractätlein* (1663), 76f.

[65]   Kongelige Bibliotek Copenhagen, Ms. Thottske S 4 689 (Piper, *Collegium*), 245r.

also be collected at 5 or 6 o'clock at night, just before supper.[66] Georg Handsch, in the sixteenth century, almost routinely mentioned two different glasses of urine which the physician was to examine.[67] And some authors recommended taking several samples throughout the day and keeping them in separate flasks to observe any changes.[68]

It was pointed out repeatedly that patients collecting urine should always empty their bladder completely, though cultural norms of the day sometimes stood in the way. Recent body and gender history has shed light on the widespread premodern image of the woman as a "leaky vessel."[69] In this sense, some contemporary authors were convinced that "women made more water than men," the reason being women's natural, colder, and more humid constitution.[70] But we know from doctors' accounts that women, for their part, were embarrassed about producing large amounts of urine and wanted to avoid creating the impression of having an excessive, "cow-like" excretion. Thus Da Monte warned his colleagues about women who made more water than three cows taken together but "showed the doctor only a tiny portion to appear more respectable."[71] Cordus tells us that in Germany, too, there were "many, namely women" who "are ashamed of having a lot of urine,"[72] while Johan Hayne even maintained that it "was the custom among women and girls," to pour out some of their urine.[73]

Another point was to avoid contamination. Both the chamber pot, which might be used to collect the urine, and the flask in which it was subsequently taken to the physician had to be clean. Otherwise the physician might find contents that did not originate in the patient's body. In line with the topos of the lack of cleanliness among the country folk, medical authors outperformed one another in describing insufficiently clean, even downright dirty vessels, in which urine was collected or transported.[74] In Lorenz Schönefeldt's particularly drastic words, "completely ignorant people" would often bring their urine in a flask in which the dirt was three times as thick as the glass itself.[75]

Further, the flask itself had to be suitable for uroscopy to avoid having to first pour the urine into a different vessel, which could result in further corruption of the sample. Vessels made of tin or lead were condemned as absolutely unsuitable.

---

[66] Ibid.

[67] ÖNB Vienna, Codd. 11205, 11206, 11210, 11238 and 11240.

[68] Detharding, *Kranken-Wärter* (1679), 71.

[69] Paster, *Body embarrassed* (1993), 23–63.

[70] Kongelige Bibliotek Copenhagen, Ms. Thottske S 4 689 (Piper, *Collegium*), 248r.

[71] Da Monte, *Lectiones* (1552), no pagination.

[72] Cordus, *De urinis* (1543), no pagination.

[73] Hayne, *Drey Tractätlein* (1620), 214.

[74] Clauser, *Betrachtung* ([1531]), no pagination.

[75] Schönefeldt, *Ein gantz fruchtbar underricht* (1534), [C2v].

But doctors also complained that the colored glass vessels that were sometimes used by patients to send their urine created a false picture.[76] The best material was thin, transparent glass. The reader could see the difference, Lorenz Schönefeldt explained, if he gazed first through a green glass window and then through a window made of clear Flemish glass.[77]

The shape of the flask mattered as well. Ideally, it featured a round belly and a long neck that was neither too wide nor too narrow. This specific shape, together with the name of the vessel, which contemporary sources knew as "urinal" or "matula," also suggests that it was made specifically for this purpose. It was supposed to be of about the same shape and size as the human bladder, big enough to hold the full amount of someone's morning urine.[78] In practice, contemporary illustrations suggest that urine flasks varied greatly in size, however, and in the length and width of the neck.

Families who did not own a flask may have been able to borrow one. Pictures of uroscopists sometimes show several empty flasks lined up. In the more distinguished families, matulae seem to have been among the household effects. Elisabeth Enenkel, in 1611, mentioned four matulae that she wanted to send in a chest along with a lye pitcher, a blood-letting bowl, and other objects.[79] According to Brian, urine was commonly transported in matulae in English towns, while ordinary bottles were used in the countryside.[80] In those cases, the uroscopist first had to pour the urine into a suitable urine flask.[81]

The common practice of transporting urine to the home of the uroscopist posed another source of corruption, which could result in error. Doctors told numerous stories and anecdotes to this effect. A messenger might spill some of the urine. A well-corked flask helped prevent this and furthermore ensured that the vital spirits contained in the urine did not escape.[82] However, sealing the flask incorrectly, for example with a bunch of grass, could lead to an even more serious distortion.[83] In the winter, complained the doctors, the urine could even turn to ice. It had to be thawed but then this changed its constitution.[84] Urine also had to be shielded from wind; otherwise the resulting airy contents might

76 Da Monte, *Lectiones* (1552), no pagination; Rhenanus, *Urocriterium* (1614), 6f.
77 Schönefeldt, *Ein gantz fruchtbar underricht* (1534), [C2v].
78 Isaac Judaeus, *De urinis* ([1515]), 163r.
79 Letter from Elisabeth Enenkel née Kirchberg (1554–1620), September 1611 (Haus-, Hof- und Staatsarchiv Wien, HA Rosenau, Karton 71) (www.univie.ac.at/Geschichte/Frauenbriefe/briefliste1.htm).
80 Brian, *Pisse-prophet* (1655), 14.
81 Cf. van Dueren, *Ontdekkinge* (1688), 92.
82 Rhenanus, *Urocriterium* (1614), 4.
83 Foreest, *Uromanteia* (1620), 227; Beverwijk, *Schat der ongesontheyt* (1672), 11.
84 Cordus, *De urinis* (1543), no pagination. G.E. Stahl still recommended that one return cooled-down urine to its "first state" by heating it (*Gründliche Abhandlung* (1739),

be interpreted erroneously as winds or *flatus* from inside the patient's body.[85] For this reason, and to prevent breakage, wicker baskets and casings were often used to transport urine flasks. As a number of the illustrations in this book also show (see Plates 4, 6, 11, 21, 24 and 25), they can frequently be found in medieval and early modern visual representations of uroscopy.[86]

In the worst case, the messenger fell and the flask broke. If he admitted his mishap, there was not much of a problem. The doctor simply could not examine the urine. But doctors worried that the messenger, for example the patient's maid, fearing punishment, might replace the spilled urine with her own or even worse with that of a cow. Some authors advised not to have the urine carried at all and to examine it in the patient's home, because the inevitable agitation of the urine on the road would lead to misleading changes, especially regarding the appearance of bubbles and of other signs suggesting volatile contents. Another factor was time. On the one hand, when the urine was too fresh, the heat that had gone into it during its passage through the urinary tract was still active in it and caused the material contents to remain distributed and invisible. Only after a certain time, when nothing but the urine's intrinsic warmth was still active, did they collect and form sediment.[87] For this reason the physician Senger from late sixteenth-century Ansbach, for example, had the urine brought to him and then asked the messengers or patients to come back an hour later.[88] If, on the other hand, the urine was too old, it underwent further changes which could mislead the physician. Many authors considered six to seven hours the maximum.[89] Accordingly, the sixteenth-century author of *Le traicté des urines* cautioned that when examining urine that was brought from far away, a doctor could only offer guesswork, a *jugement extimatif*.[90] He claimed that the consistency would change, that sediments could dissolve again, and that the urine could become thicker.[91]

There were still other ways in which urine could be altered, and physicians needed to be aware of them in order to avoid an embarrassing misdiagnosis: certain foods and drugs caused the urine to change. Cassia, for instance, a

---

32); Kräutermann also mentioned this option but cautioned that the urine would "lose a lot of its color and substance" (*Curieuser und vernünfftiger Urin-Artzt* (1732), 9).

[85]   Cordus, *De urinis* (1543); Da Monte, *Lectiones* (1552), no pagination.

[86]   Cf. Sudhoff, *Harnglas* (1925), 292–8, with illustrations; Sudhoff has traced the earliest illustrations of such baskets to shortly after 1300; see also the frontispiece of Starck, *Krancken Spiegel* (1598).

[87]   Da Monte, *Lectiones* (1552), no pagination.

[88]   Wirsing, *Altfränkisches Pfarrhausleben* (1952), 21.

[89]   Scribonius, *De inspectione urinarum* (1585), 33; Rhenanus, *Urocriterium* (1614), 2f.

[90]   Anonymous, *Traicté des urines* (before 1567), VIr.

[91]   Scribonius, *De inspectione urinarum* (1585), 33.

popular laxative, made the urine darker, while rhubarb—another common laxative—increased its yellow tint.[92]

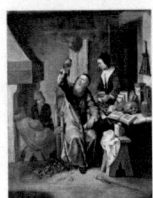

Once a patient's urine had arrived at the uroscopist's office—hopefully uncorrupted, in the full amount, and in a suitable vessel—several rules had to be observed with regard to the examination itself. A correct evaluation of the consistency, the many potential shades, and the contents required great care. The uroscopist had to allow some time for the task and remain alert to all disruptive and deceptive influences. He was advised to raise the flask in his hand and hold it against the light or a bright wall. Candle light alone was not enough. Direct sunlight, on the other hand, was too bright and weakened the urine's color.[93] As an anonymous French treatise explained, direct sunlight impeded proper sight because it scattered the *spiritus*, which were responsible for proper vision.[94] Ideally, the uroscopist held the matula into the subdued light, of a window for example, in such a way that it was illuminated from one side (cf. for example, Plate 7). Also, he was to cover the opposite side of the matula with his hand or a black cloth.[95] Using his hand, his clothing, or a piece of cloth in this way, he created a contrast. Da Monte explained that this allowed the air contained in the urine to collect rays of light much like a (parabolic) mirror, which made the subtle changes in the urine visible.[96] To be sure, the correct distance between eye and matula had to be observed as well;[97] it was roughly defined by the doctor's extended arm. Seen from up close, the urine might appear exceedingly dense. When viewed at a distance, on the other hand, it could easily seem too thin and the doctor also could not clearly see the consistency and the *contenta*.[98] Holding the matula at an angle and carefully moving its base in a circular motion while looking at it from slightly below allowed the uroscopist to judge the sediments more closely.[99] This practice is documented in many images of the period. Individual authors further suggested

---

92   Argenterio, *De urinis* (1591), 91.

93   Rhenanus, *Urocriterium* (1614), 8; Hayne, *Drey Tractätlein* (1620), 214; cf. Liessell, *Konsten* (1668), 18.

94   Anonymous, *Traicté des urines* (before 1567), IIIv; very similarly: Apollinaris, *Tractätlein* (1663), 76f.

95   Isaac Judaeus, *De urinis* ([1515]), 163r; Rhenanus, *Urocriterium* (1614), 8; Hayne, *Drey Tractätlein* (1620), 214; Fletcher, *Differences* (1641), 2.

96   Da Monte, *Lectiones* (1552), no pagination.

97   Avicenna, *Canon* (1595), 47v.

98   Anonymous, *Traicté des urines* (before 1567), IVr, however, thought the reason for this lay in the physiology of the eye and explained it as a result of a rarefying of the spirits.

99   Isaac Judaeus, *De urinis* ([1515]), 163r; Vermeer, *Iudicium urinarum* (1970) (edition of a *iudicium* by Augustin Streicher, here 64v); Anonymous, *Traicté des urines* (before 1567), IVr.

dipping a piece of linen in the urine to help determine its inherent color more accurately. They claimed that the urine of a jaundiced patient, for example, might seem dark at first glance, while the test with linen showed that it was intensely yellow or saffron-colored (*crocea*).[100]

Diagnosis and Prognosis

According to a misconception that is widespread even among medical historians today, uroscopy was an empirical procedure whose theoretical sophistication was minimal. Very much the opposite is true. Uroscopy, the way it was presented in academic uroscopic treatises and taught at universities, was guided by theory to a high degree. The meaning attributed to individual colors and contents originated not simply in tradition or empirical observation. It was founded on the basic principles of humoral pathology and physiology, which, in turn, were more complex and variable than is often assumed.

In order to understand and explain the manifold changes that could be observed in urine, one had to know how urine was produced in the human body. While there were differences in some details, it was widely acknowledged that urine—like all other substances and excretions of the body—resulted from the digestion, that is, the "concoction" of food.[101] According to the traditional Galenic teachings, ingested raw food was concocted in the body in various stages, in which it was assimilated to the body's substance, that is, literally made similar to it. The notion of concocting food, too, was understood literally. In the Galenic tradition, the intriguing processes of food assimilation—vegetables or eggs became human skin and muscles—were communicated principally with the image of a kitchen fire. While there is little evidence to show this was true for laypeople, several steps were distinguished by the doctors:[102] First, the stomach, with the help of vital heat, formed chyle, while coarse waste matter contained in the food was excreted via the intestines as feces. The chyle then moved from the stomach to the liver where it was concocted a second time. The result was good, nutritious blood. The parts which could not be assimilated collected in the gallbladder as yellow bile or flowed to the spleen as black bile, and the watery parts reached the kidneys (or were attracted by them). The kidneys strained these watery parts and passed them on as urine to the bladder, and the urethra. The third step of food concoction took place throughout the body and

---

[100] Württembergische Landesbibliothek Stuttgart, Cod. med. et phys. 4° 13, *Historiae aegrotorum XXV*.

[101] On the following see the classical account by Isaac Judaeus, *De urinis* ([1515]), 158v–162r.

[102] Stolberg, *Experiencing illness* (2011), 122–6.

did not directly involve the formation of urine. Nutritious blood reached the individual body parts and organs, which each took what they required for their nourishment and what they were able to assimilate to their own substance. The resulting waste left the body via the skin as sweat and transpiration or, if the body lacked the necessary strength to eliminate waste matter in this manner, with the urine where it might show up as sediment.[103]

The principal site of the formation of the watery excrements which eventually issued forth as urine was thus the liver.[104] Some authors described the formation of urine and other waste more precisely, locating it in different places within the liver or even postulating two different concoctions in the liver, or claiming that urine was formed in the *gibbus* of the liver, that is, in its humped, upper part,[105] while yellow and black bile were formed in the liver's lower, concave part. Still others rejected this position saying that there were no more than three steps of concoction, the second of which happened in the liver.[106]

Leaving the liver, urine moved with the blood and reached the kidneys which strained it.[107] This corresponded with the widespread definition of urine as a *colatura*, a filtration of blood.[108] Urine was "water that is strained from blood and other humors," Fries wrote,[109] or as Hornung put it, "a watery humor, which is filtered out from the blood in the kidneys, secreted from it."[110] In this, urine was similar to the watery whey, a by-product of the production of butter and cheese, a comparison that had been passed down since antiquity.[111] Etymologically, the term "urine" may even derive from the Greek word *uros* for "whey."[112] The Latin word for "whey," on the other hand, was *serum*, a term that is still used today to refer to the cell-free liquid seen when blood coagulates in a glasstube. In this sense some late medieval and early modern authors defined urine as a "serum humorum in venis contentorum"[113] and understood it as nearly identical to the light-colored excess liquid that accumulated when blood from a bloodletting

---

[103]   Pinder, *Epiphanie medicorum* (1506), 7r.

[104]   Opinions that differ from this are found only rarely. According to Salvianus (*De urinarum differentiis*, 1587), urine was already formed in the first concoction and was further changed in the liver only *per accidens*.

[105]   Avicenna, *Canon* (1595), 47v; ÖNB Vienna, Cod. 11210, notes on A. Fracanzani's lectures on uroscopy in Padua, 81r.

[106]   Da Monte, *Lectiones* (1552), no pagination.

[107]   Savonarola, *De urinis* (1561), 93v–94r.

[108]   Hornung, *Uroscopia fraudulenta* (1611), 13.

[109]   Fries, *Spiegel* (1518), LXIIIv.

[110]   Hornung, *Uroscopia fraudulenta* (1611), 12.

[111]   Anonymous, *Judycyall* (1530); Savonarola, *De urinis* (1561), 93v.

[112]   Cf. Siegel, *Galen's system* (1968), 126.

[113]   Vassaeus, *De iudiciis urinarum* (1553), 4.

was left to stand for a while.[114] Citing Bernard de Gordon, Bonacursius even gave his uroscopic treatise the title *De humano sero*.[115]

The most important diagnostic conclusions that could be drawn from the different colors and consistencies of urine had their theoretical underpinnings in the understanding that urine resulted from blood that had been concocted from food. The color of urine above all indicated the degree of "digestion," "concoction," or "heating" of the urine. It reflected the overall digestive strength and vital heat of the body and especially that of the organs involved in the concoction of food and the formation and excretion of urine: the stomach, the liver, and the kidneys. Urine the color of a ripe, yellow apple indicated a normal, natural digestion or concoction.[116] A lack of digestion or concoction was indicated by pale, thin urine. Excessive heat, on the other hand, became manifest in dark yellow, orange-colored, or red, rather condensed urine. Thus, based on her "reddish" urine, Rembertus Dodonaues, for example, diagnosed a woman who felt intense pain in her upper right abdomen with an *inflammatio iecoris*, that is, literally with an inflammation of the liver.[117] In the case of excessive, pathological heat, urine could turn the color of burnt food, that is, very dark, even black.

These notions were central to uroscopy and found expression in many urine wheels and charts (see Plates 8–13). Charts and wheels often grouped two, three, or four similar colors, with each group designating a different degree of digestion or concoction. The spectrum ranged from the watery urine resulting from a lack of concoction or digestion to the pale and lemony/bright urine of a beginning or medium concoction, and on to the gold or saffron-colored urine that indicated complete concoction. If chyle was heated even further, this resulted in an excessive concoction which produced first red urine and then liver-colored, blue, green, lead-colored, or even black urine, which indicated a complete combustion.

In the course of the early modern period the explanation for the causes of different urinary color shifted somewhat. Increasingly the notion came to the fore that the color of urine did not so much indicate the degree of concoction or heating, which changed the urine itself, but instead was caused by the addition of natural and unnatural bodily humors of different colors. This notion can be found even in older literature.[118] According to Michele Savonarola, for example, the color of urine (along with its "salty" quality), originated in bad yellow or red

---

[114] Pinder, *Epiphanie medicorum* (1506), 10r.

[115] Bonacursius, *De humano sero* (1650).

[116] Bellini, *De urina* (1718), 3.

[117] Dodonaeus, *Medicinalium observationum* (1581), 69, case 28.

[118] Tentzelius, *De urinis* (1609), paragraph 26, citing Jean Fernel, pointed out both possibilities.

bile which had been mixed in.[119] In the course of the seventeenth and eighteenth centuries, academic uroscopic literature attached increasing importance to this difference between the intrinsic color of the urine proper and the color of added particles.[120] In the first case, intensely yellow urine might indicate healthy concoction, while in the other it could result from an excess of yellow bile in the blood.[121] Black urine traditionally was thought to indicate excessive, burning heat which was likely to cause fatal consumption and ultimately the extinction of the natural heat. If the same color merely resulted from an admixture of black bile it was much less critical.[122]

A second explanatory level came to bear above all in the interpretation of cloudiness and other contents that were discernible with the naked eye. In early modern medicine—and this holds as much for doctors as for laypeople—illness was usually not explained by a disturbed equilibrium of the humors or qualities, as even recent writings in the history of medicine continue wrongly to assume. Rather, most illnesses were attributed to harmful, spoiled, pathological substances which the body disposed of with its excretions—not least of all urine.[123] From the ingested food, foreign to the body, but also from spoiled natural humors, morbid matter could accrue within the body. In addition, there were more or less specific pathological substances that were associated with particular diseases, including the *contagia* which caused plague or smallpox. They were transmitted by air but also by physical contact with sick people or with objects they had contaminated.

According to the prevailing belief, morbid matter could spread throughout the blood or settle in certain body parts. In the latter case, it gave rise to so-called fluxes, which presented themselves as localized pain and other complaints. Morbid matter was also thought to harden and form tumors and cancer or, when exposed to the body's heat, to release pathological fumes or vapors.

To ward off disease, the body had to render the morbid matter innocuous, usually by concocting and/or by eliminating it via its natural routes: through the feces, often by way of diarrhea, through sweat, and through urine, but also via bleeding from the lungs or from hemorrhoids, rashes, running sores, and similar lesions, whose secretions often looked unpleasant and were malodorous, underlining their pathological nature.

The crucial role of secretions and excrements in liberating the body of morbid matter constituted the second and vitally important theoretical basis of uroscopy, next to the theory of concoction. If the body used urine to eliminate

---

[119] Savonarola, *De urinis* (1561), 93v.

[120] E.g. Rivière, *Miroir* (1722).

[121] Beverwijk, *Schat der ongesontheyt* (1672), 9.

[122] Ibid.

[123] Stolberg, *Experiencing illness* (2011), esp. 95–142; idem, *Der gesunde Leib* (2001).

pathological substances, these could be detected directly in the urine. But even if the body chose other routes, the illness—at least according to the prevailing opinion (we will come to the critique later)—still showed in the urine. This was above all because urine, on its way from the liver to the kidneys, mixed with the blood. In addition, residues from the third step of concoction which were usually excreted as sweat could reenter the blood and ultimately leave the body with the urine. Therefore, changes in the urine reflected the constitution of the blood or indeed of all humors in the body and of the solid parts as well.[124] A melting of body substance was indicated by fat. The release of volatile morbid matter caused bubbles and foam. Heavier pathological substances settled as sediment.

Lastly, a third level of interpretation—more readily appreciated today—addressed contents that originated in the kidneys and in the urinary tract and were washed out with the urine: blood and pus from ulcers and injuries, as well as matter that had come loose in the kidneys, the ureters, the bladder, or the urethra.

Learning Uroscopy

As we have seen, uroscopy rested on a set of complex theoretical principles. Theoretical knowledge was by no means sufficient, however. A successful uroscopist also needed extensive practical experience. Just knowing what healthy urine could look like—an essential prerequisite[125]—already took considerable experience which was not easy to gain, since uroscopists commonly only got to see the urine of sick people.[126] The uroscopy treatises never tired of underlining how greatly even healthy urine could vary depending on the temperament, age, sex, and lifestyle of the person.[127] The variety of patients and uroscopic findings was virtually infinite.

We know little about the ways in which medical students and physicians—let alone their non-academic competitors—acquired uroscopic knowledge and skills. Books must have played a significant role. Even some of the learned, theoretical treatises on uroscopy focused on what was useful in ordinary practice, limiting themselves to common finds and their most likely significance. Particularly pronounced was this focus on practice in works of the *Medicus Politicus* tradition. This was a genre of writing aimed at equipping the doctor not so much with academic knowledge but with the necessary professional *savoir faire*. He was meant to learn how to stand his ground at the sick bed and

---

124 Beverwijk, *Schat der ongesontheyt* (1672), 8.
125 E.g. Liessell, *Konste* (1668), 29.
126 Scribonius, *De inspectione urinarum* (1585), 28.
127 E.g. Saxonia, *De urinis* (1639), 59.

prosper economically thanks to his medical skills and his ability to communicate well with his clients.[128] When it came to uroscopy, the reader was instructed to recognize the most common and therefore most probable symptoms or complaints in the changes of urine and to use his skills to impress his patients and their families.

A fine example is the *Medicus Politicus* by Roderigo da Castro, a Portuguese-born physician who practiced in Hamburg.[129] In his widely read work, he listed the most important urinary changes doctors commonly encountered in their practice along with the most plausible explanation for each. From this, he surmised which symptoms a patient might experience, which the doctor could then tell the messenger without having received any further information. In terms of colors, da Castro focused on the whitish (or clear), the gold-colored, and the orange or light red tints of urine, adding the parameters thin, thick, or cloudy, but omitting rarer findings like green, livid, dark red, blue, and black urine. Likewise he offered only a small selection of interpretations for each type of finding. Whitish or straw-colored urine indicated that the liver and stomach were weak and cold. It could be surmised in such cases that the patient suffered from eructation, especially if the urine was foamy. The patient probably also complained of a stomachache after eating. If this was an illness of long standing—this information might have to be requested—it could be assumed that the patient had lost his healthy color and the uroscopist could state that edema of the foot and cachexia loomed. If light-colored urine was coarse or turbid, this indicated a preponderance of coarse, stringy mucus.

Da Castro's account of the various possible contents was more comprehensive, probably because here, individual findings allowed for a fairly specific diagnosis. He mentioned a circle the color of lead, which could indicate a pathological melancholy or negative affects when occurring on thin or clear urine. Fat in urine indicated an existing or looming consumption or else greatly heated kidneys, which liquefied the fat. Foam pointed to winds, while bubbles on the surface indicated pains in, or a disease of, the head—presumably due to rising vapors which collected underneath the skull. Scales indicated a bladder ailment, and filaments pointed to trouble with the urethra and "groin."

The way Piper, an archiater in Riga, phrased his practical "rules" of uroscopy in his manuscript *Collegium Medicum* resembles that of da Castro.[130] Piper's descriptions, in turn, were almost identical to some of the advice that Friedrich Hoffmann gave his students in the early eighteenth century and later published

---

128 Cf. Elkeles, *Aussagen* (1979).

129 Castro, *Medicus politicus* (1662).

130 Kongelige Bibliotek Copenhagen, Ms. Thottske S 4 689 (Piper, *Collegium*); the text may even be based directly on notes on Hoffmann's lectures.

in his *Medicus Politicus*.[131] Different from da Castro, these two authors no longer focused so much on identifying the patient's subjective complaints from the urine, but rather strove to name the underlying disease. This may indicate that the custom of leaving the uroscopist in the dark about the identity and the state of the patient was waning among the upper classes of their day. With virgins, Piper and Hoffmann claimed, thin, watery urine indicated a so-called chlorosis or love sickness.[132] With children, a white, whey-like urine with a white sediment usually suggested worms.[133] While reddish urinary color commonly pointed to a strong innate heat,[134] reddish urine that was not accompanied by heat was a sign of scurvy, and the more intense its color, the more serious the disease.[135] Reddish and slightly cloudy urine with bubbles but no sediment usually indicated ailments of the chest, asthma, or an irregular heartbeat, with the bubbles arising merely from ordinary air mixed in with the urine.[136]

Vernacular publications also tended to focus on concrete and practical uroscopic instructions. Some simply provided a list of short maxims or "rules"[137] which linked common urinary changes with certain diseases. Clear urine with a black circle on the surface indicated that the patient suffered from consumption, as could be read in the several editions of Owen Wood's *Epitomie of most experienced, excellent and profitable secrets*, a publication aimed specifically at "ladies of understanding" and others who aspired to do good things in this field.[138] Thick, cloudy urine, resembling that of horses, by contrast, indicated headaches; urine with fat at the bottom, a white tint in the middle, and a red color on top signaled a quartan fever.[139]

As brief as these vernacular instructions were, broken down to succinct maxims, the complexity of urinary diagnostics remains tangible. Wood listed as many as 32 urinary findings and what they indicated, with nine additional findings that were particular to women.[140] If urine had the color of white lead, for example, the woman was carrying a dead child in her womb. Pregnancy excluded, lead-colored, malodorous urine was understood to indicate that the uterus was disintegrating or rotting.[141]

---

[131] Hoffmann, *Medicus politicus* (1708).

[132] Ibid., 141; Kongelige Bibliotek Copenhagen, Ms. Thottske S 4 689 (Piper, *Collegium*), 247r.

[133] Kongelige Bibliotek Copenhagen, Ms. Thottske S 4 689 (Piper, *Collegium*), 248v.

[134] Hoffmann, *Medicus politicus* (1708), 149.

[135] Kongelige Bibliotek Copenhagen, Ms. Thottske S 4 689 (Piper, *Collegium*), 249r–v.

[136] Ibid., 250r–v.

[137] Fries, *Spiegel* (1518).

[138] Wood, *Epitomie* (1653), 230.

[139] Ibid., 230.

[140] Ibid., 230–34.

[141] Ibid., 234.

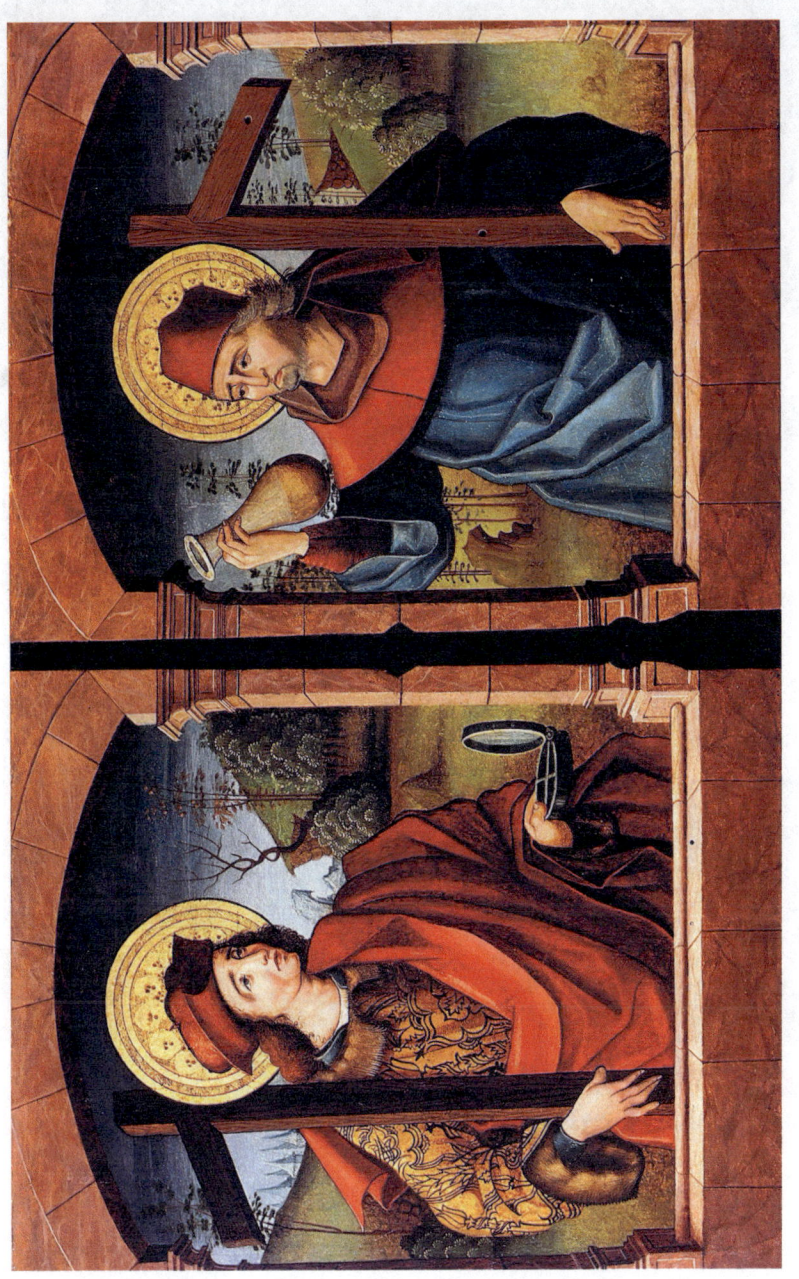

Plate 1   Unknown painter, Cosmas and Damian (London, Wellcome Library)

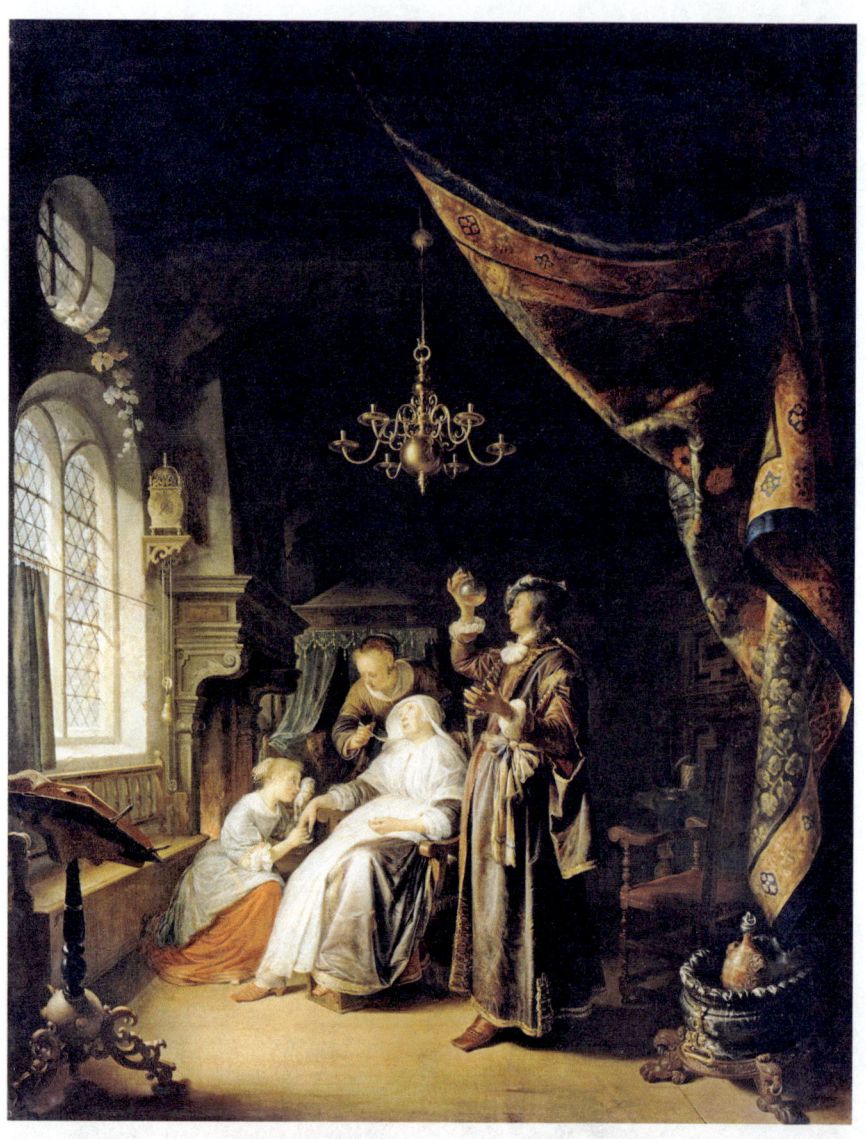

Plate 2   Gerard Dou (1613–1675), *La femme hydropique* (Paris, Musée du Louvre)

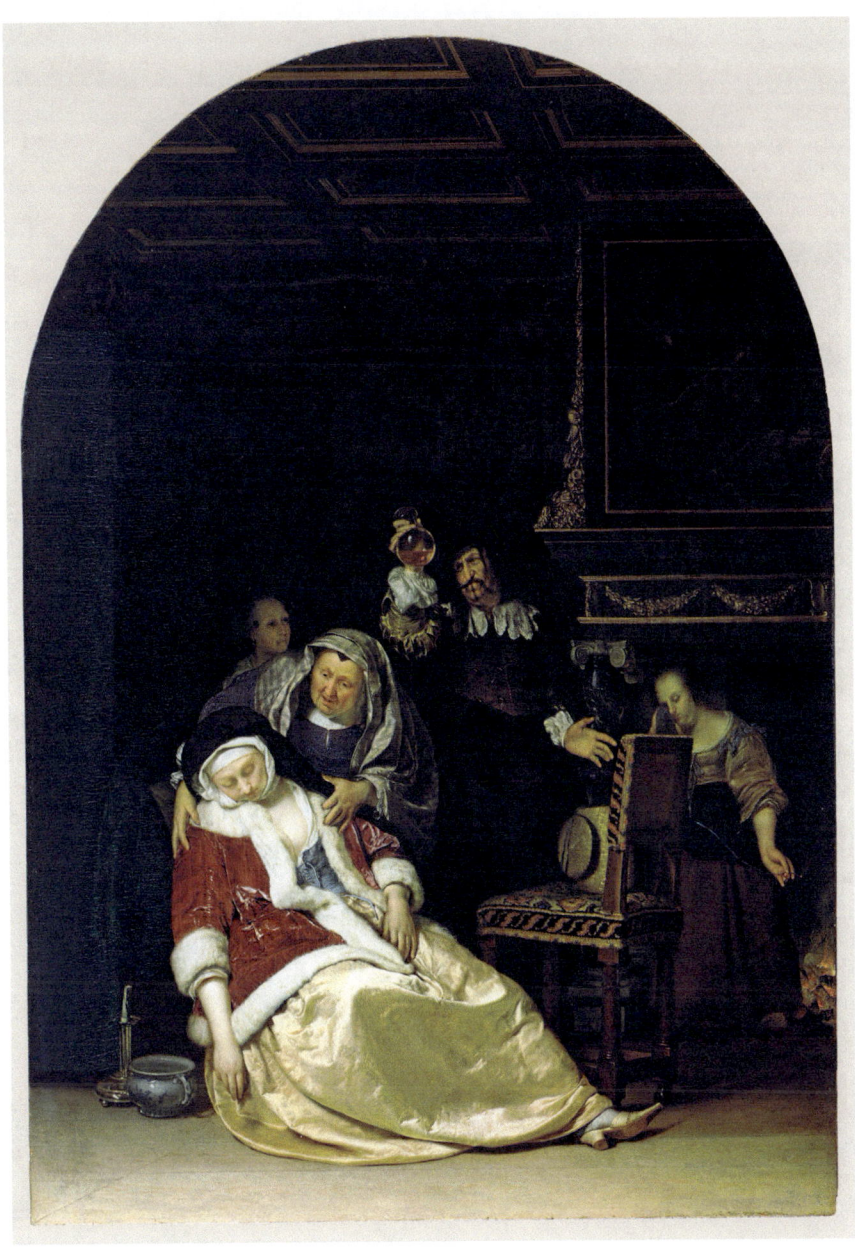

Plate 3   Frans van Mieris (1635–1681), *The Doctor's Visit* (Los Angeles, Getty Museum)

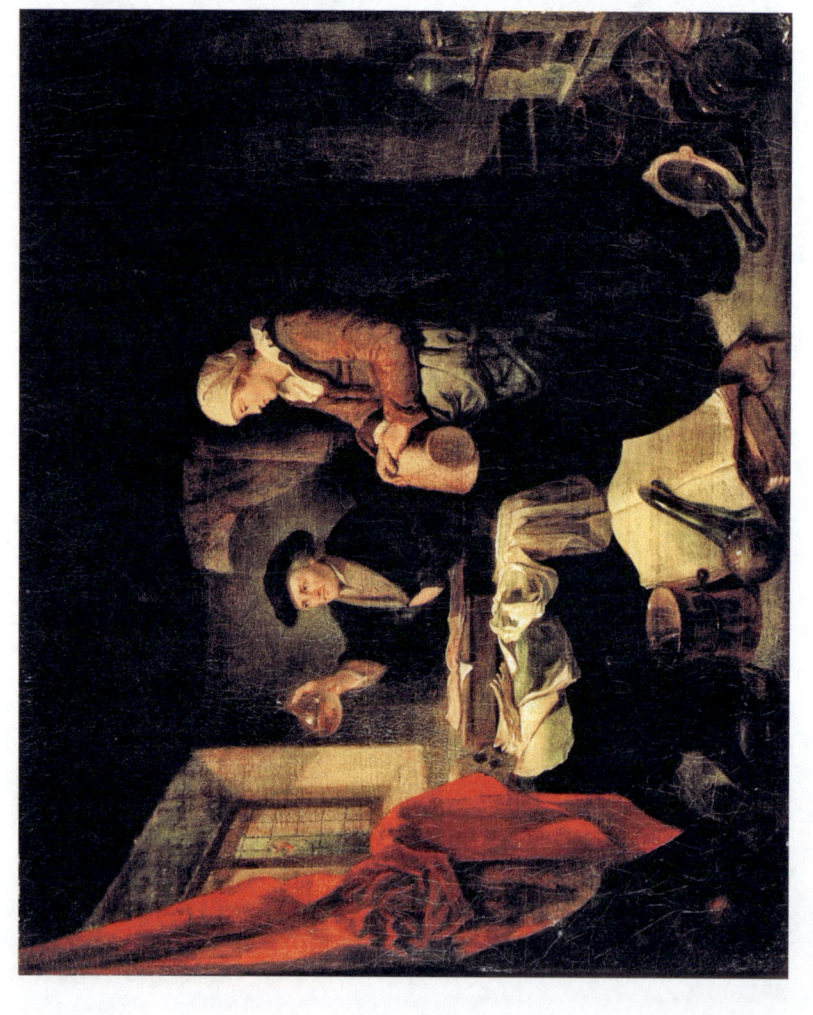

Plate 4   Oil painting after Hendrik F. Herschop, 1620–1672, Uroscopist (London, Wellcome Library)

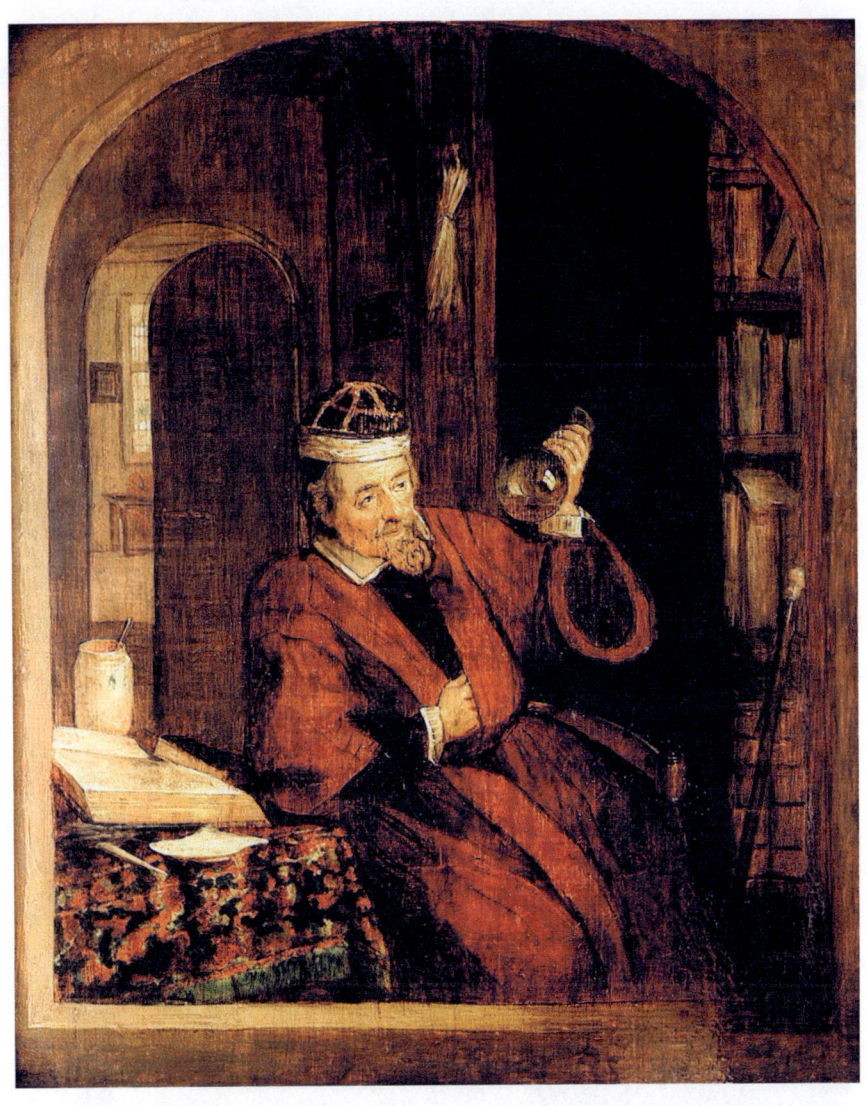

Plate 5   Contemporary copy of Adriaen Ostade (1610–1685), Physician examining a urine flask (London, Wellcome Library)

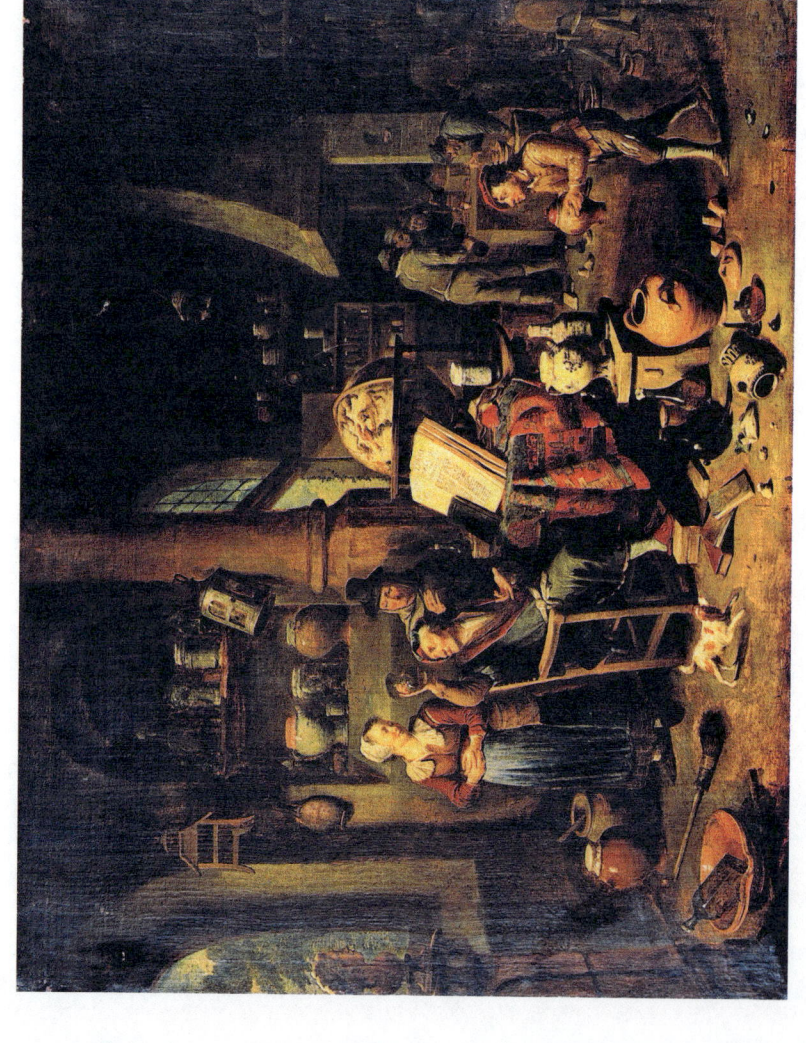

Plate 6   Gerard Thomas (1663–1721), Physician examining a urine flask (London, Wellcome Library)

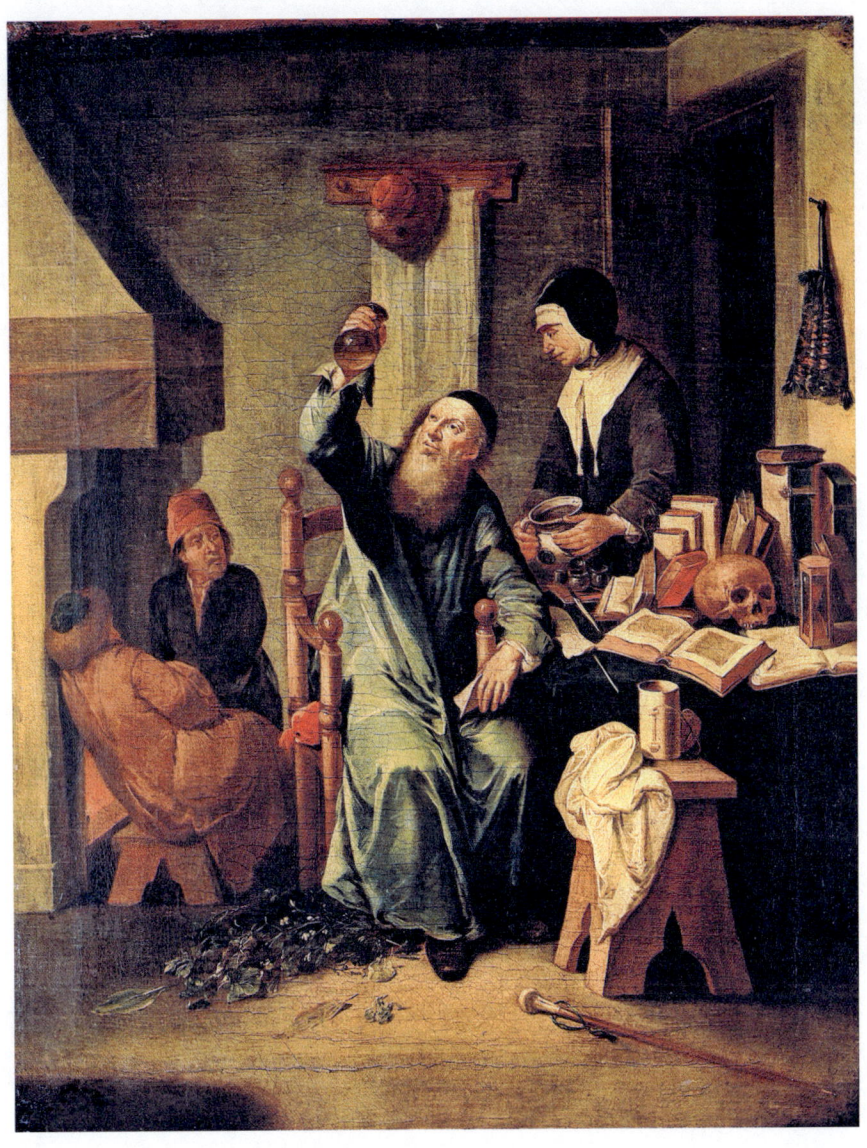

Plate 7   Oil painting after Caspar Netscher (1639–1684), Uroscopist
(London, Wellcome Library)

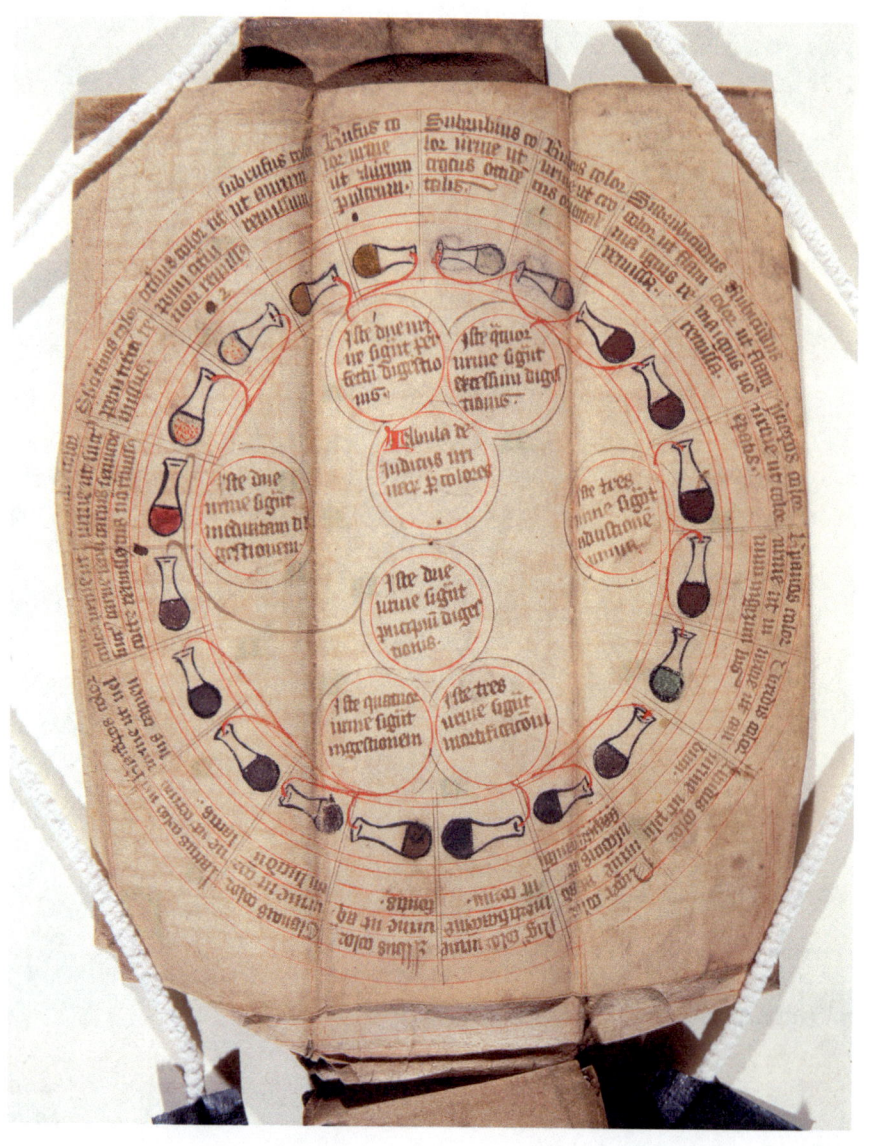

Plate 8   Late medieval uroscopy wheel (Philadelphia, Rosenbach Museum & Library, Ms. 1004)

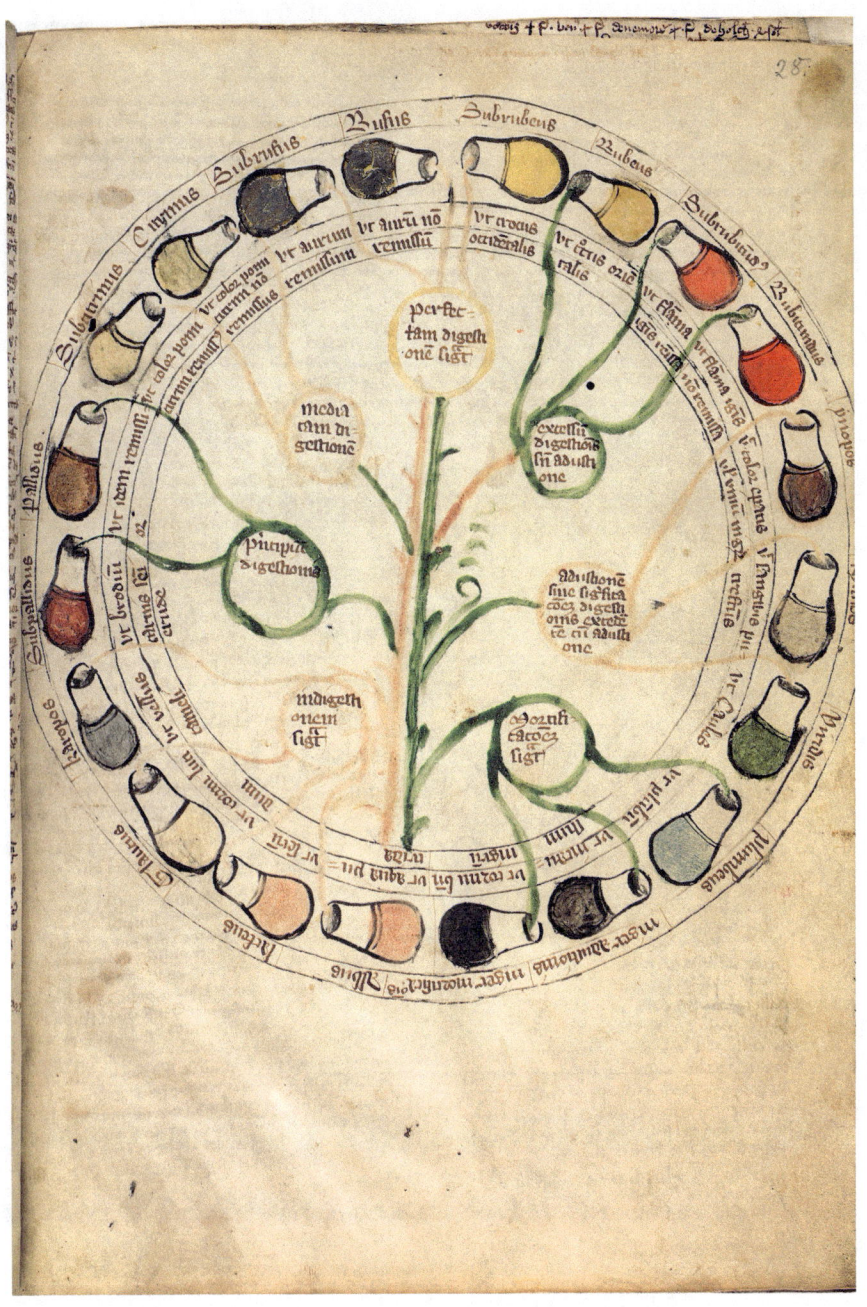

Plate 9   Uroscopy wheel (Leipzig, Universitätsbibliothek, Ms. 1177, fol 28r)

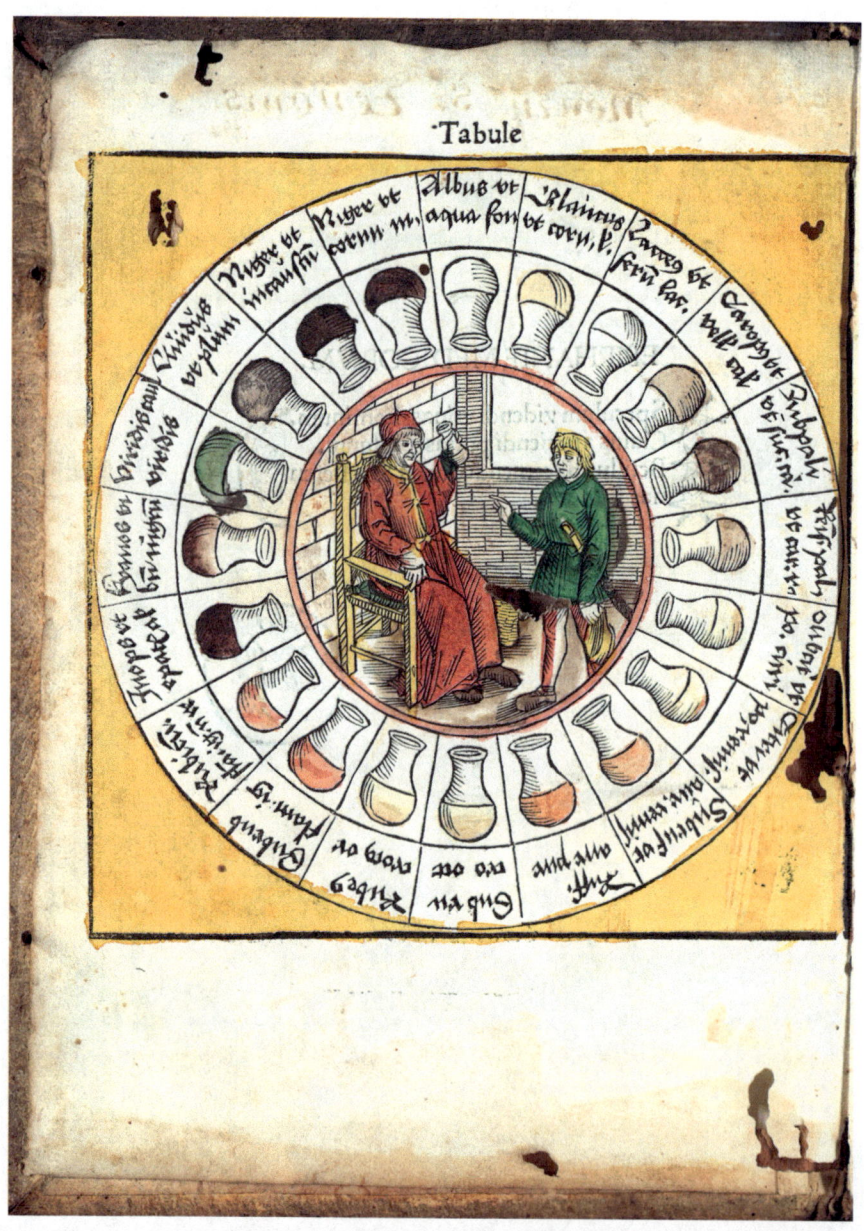

Plate 10   Hand-colored uroscopy wheel, in: Pinder, *Epiphanie medicorum* (1506), 1v (Munich, Universitätsbibliothek, W 4 Med. 134)

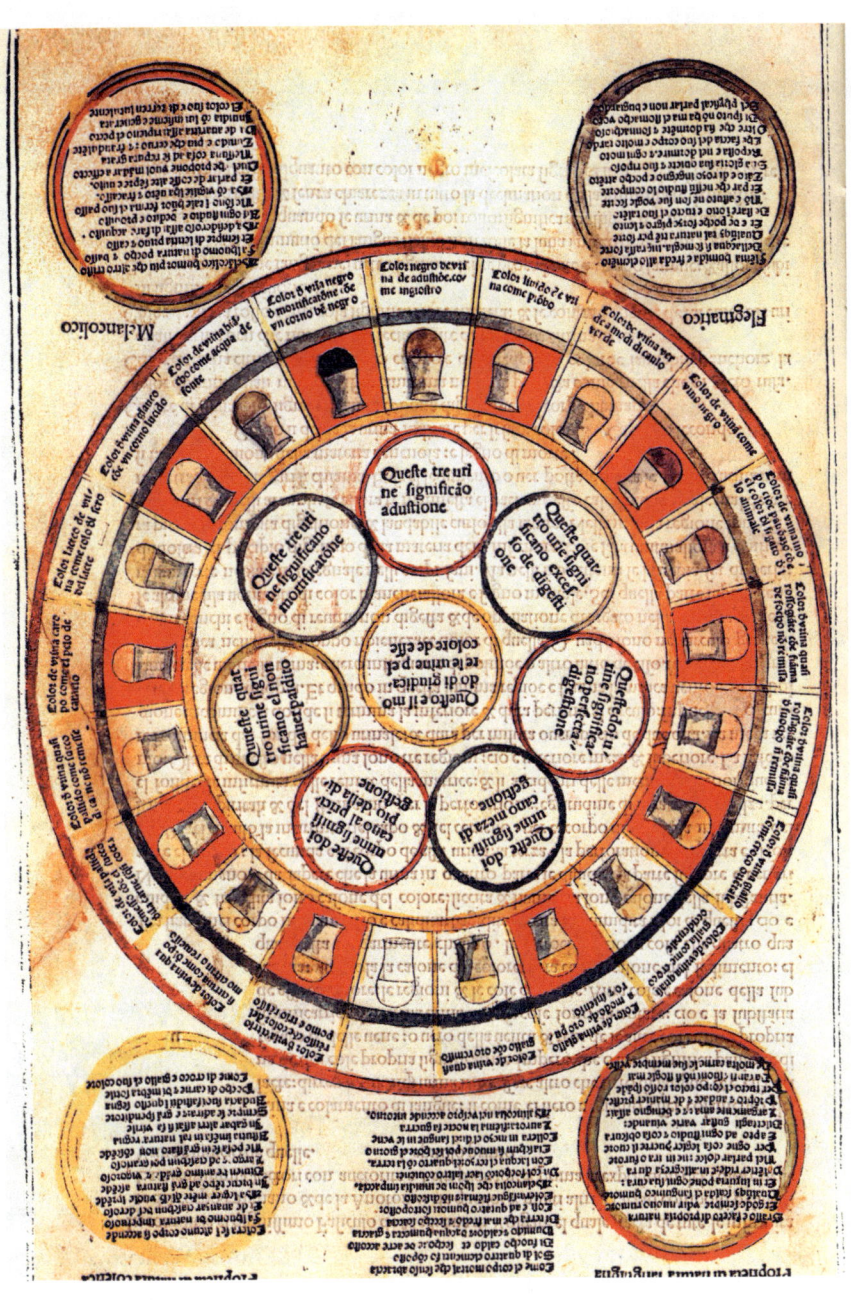

Plate 11   Hand-colored uroscopy wheel, in: Ketham, *Fasciculus medicinae* (1493)

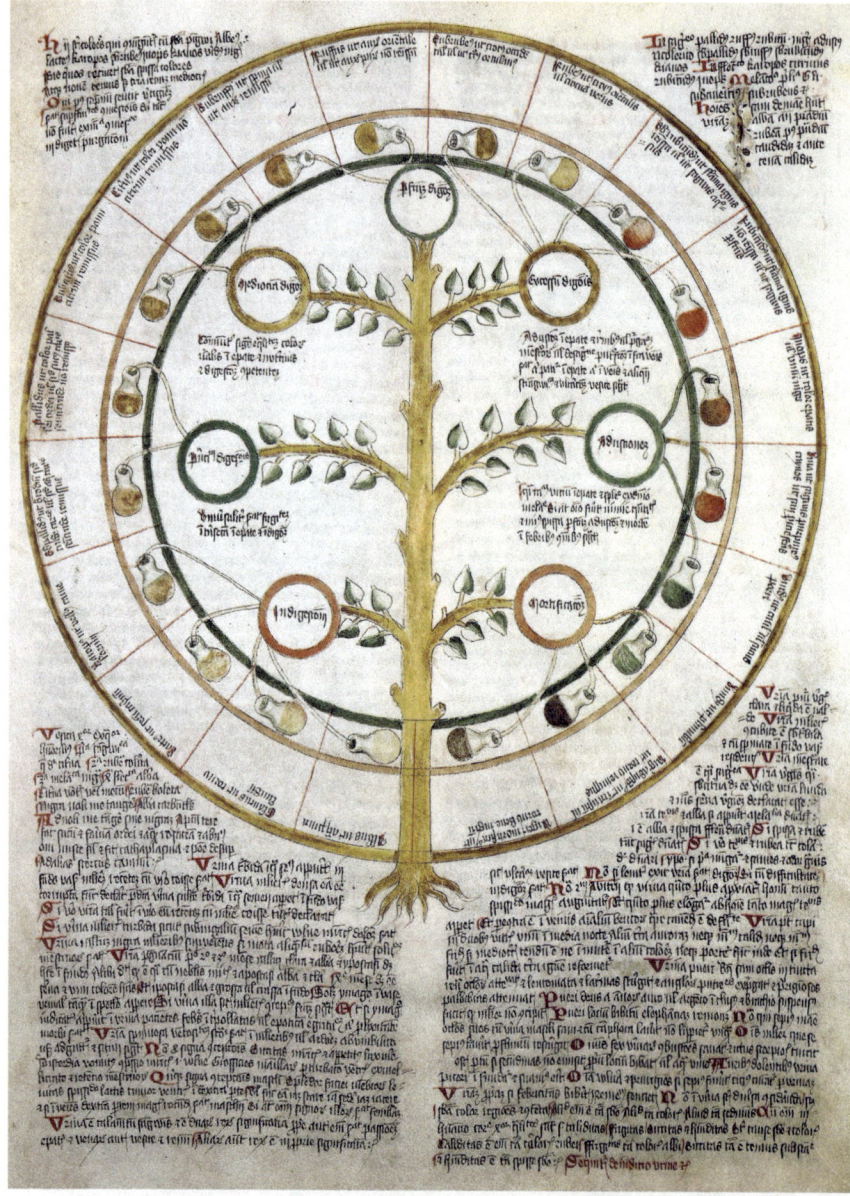

Plate 12   Uroscopy wheel, around 1420–1430 (London, Wellcome Library, Ms. 49, fol 42r)

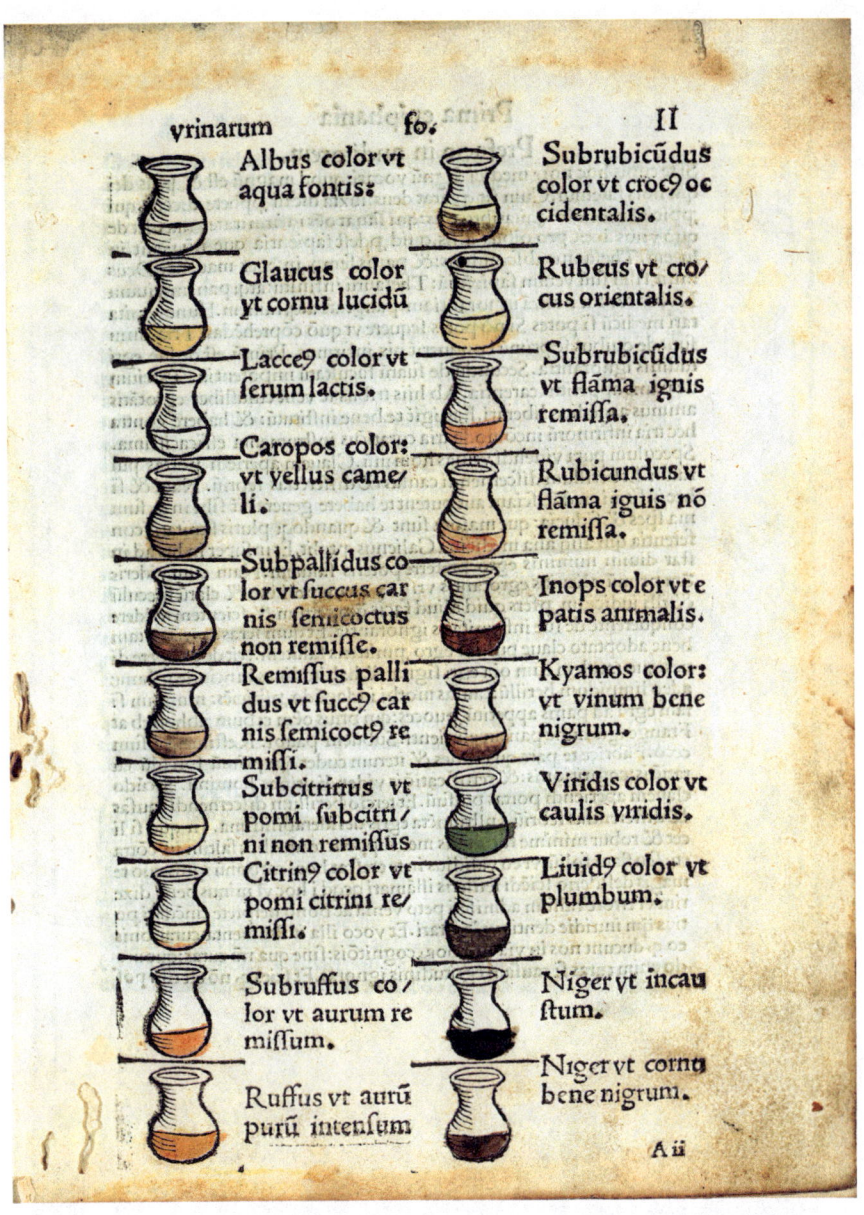

Albus color vt
aqua fontis:

Subrubicũdus
color vt croc9 oc
cidentalis.

Glaucus color
yt cornu lucidũ

Rubeus vt cro/
cus orientalis.

Lacce9 color vt
serum lactis.

Subrubicũdus
vt fláma ignis
remissa.

Caropos color:
vt vellus came/
li.

Rubicundus vt
fláma iguis nõ
remissa.

Subpallidus co
lor vt succus car
nis semicoctus
non remisse.

Inops color vt e
patis animalis.

Remissus palli
dus vt succ9 car
nis semicoct9 re
missi.

Kyamos color:
vt vinum bene
nigrum.

Subcitrinus vt
pomi subcitri/
ni non remissus

Viridis color vt
caulis viridis.

Citrin9 color vt
pomi citrini re
missi.

Liuid9 color vt
plumbum.

Subruffus co/
lor vt aurum re
missum.

Niger vt incau
stum.

Ruffus vt aurũ
purũ intensum

Niger vt cornu
bene nigrum.

A ii

Plate 13   Hand-colored uroscopy table, in: Pinder, *Epiphanie medicorum* (1506), 2r (Munich, Universitätsbibliothek, W 4 Med. 134)

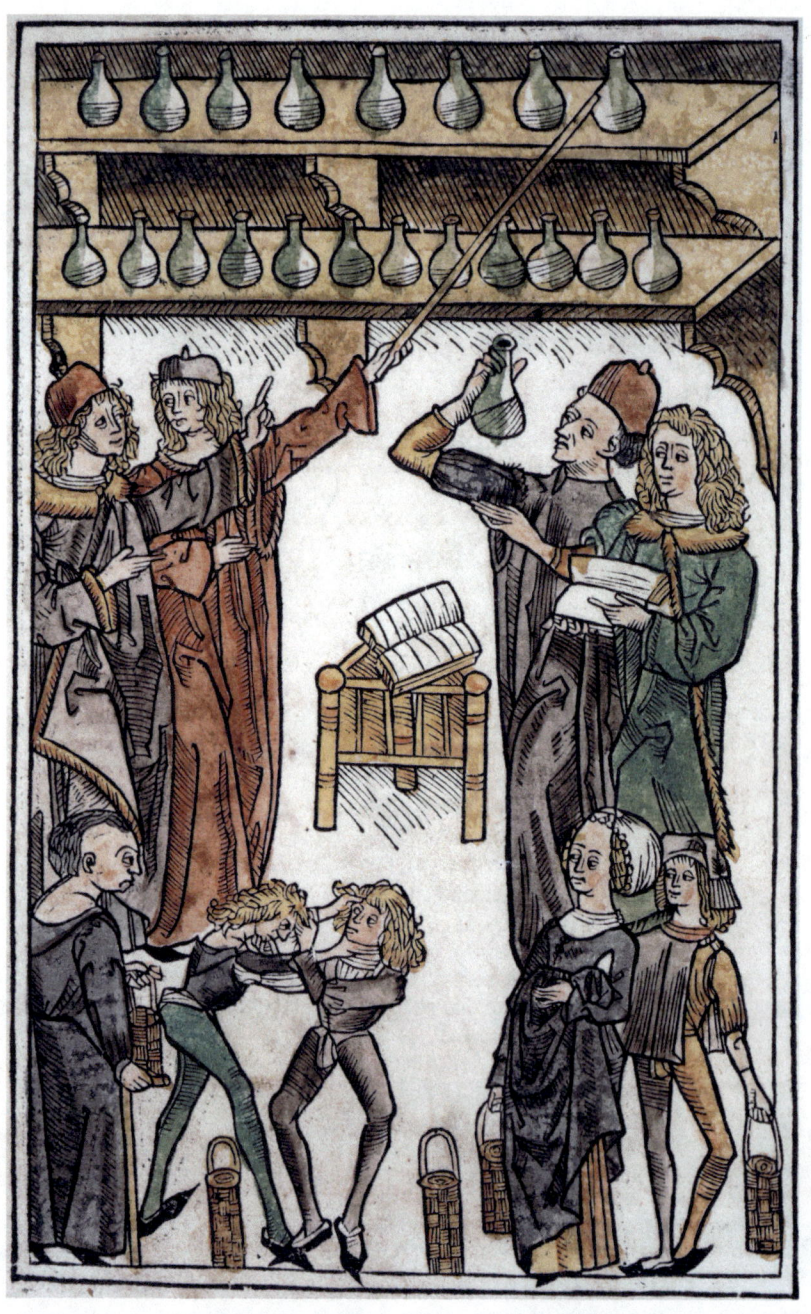

Plate 14   Teaching uroscopy, in: Jacob Meydenbach, *Hortus sanitatis* (1491)

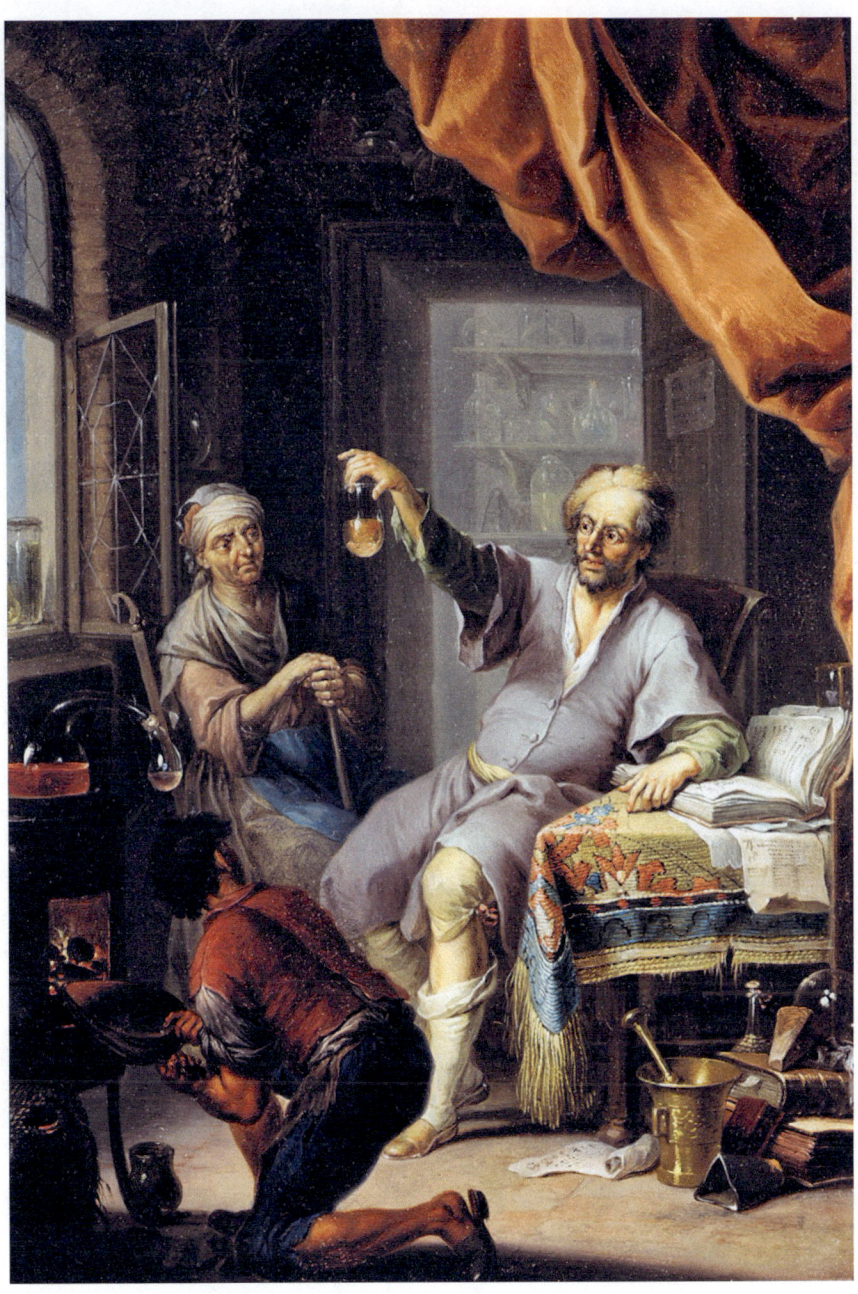

Plate 15   Franz Christoph Janneck (1703–1761), *The Medical Alchemist*
(Philadelphia, Museum of the Chemical Heritage Foundation,
Fisher Collection)

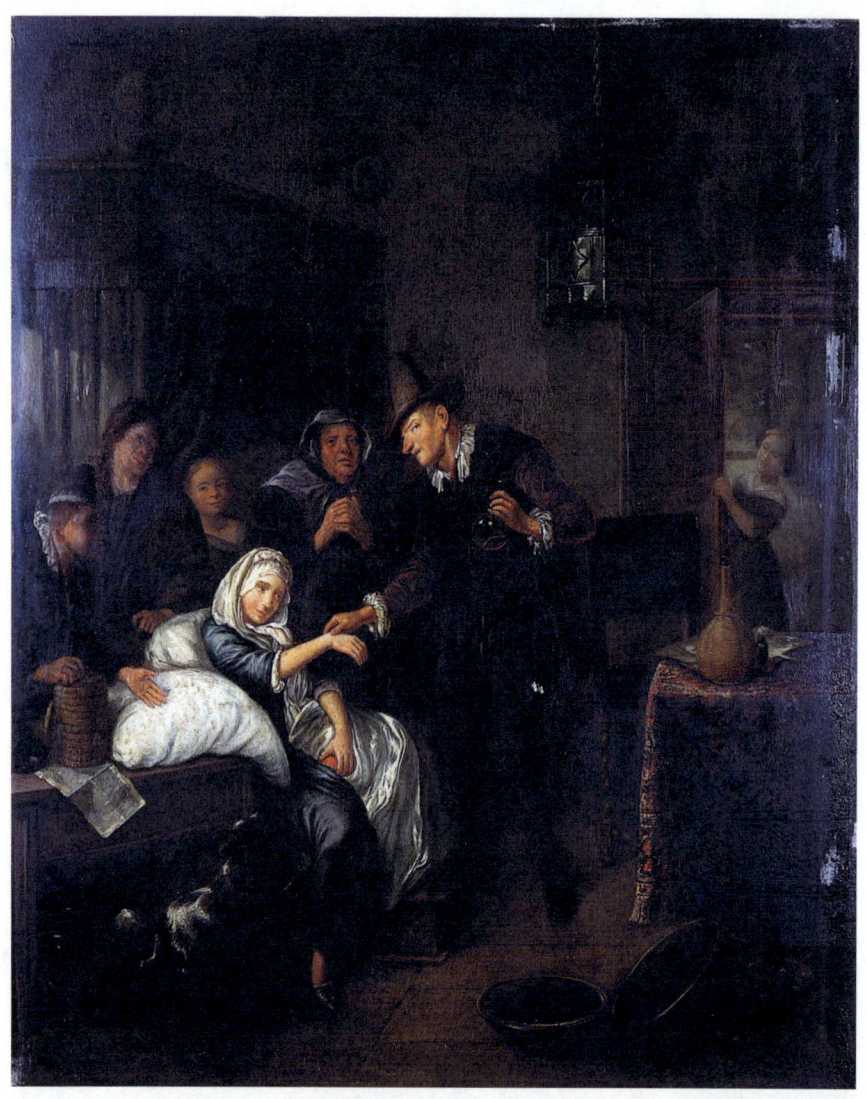

Plate 16   Oil painting after Richard Brakenburg (1650–1702), Medical
            practitioner feeling the pulse and holding a urine flask (London,
            Wellcome Library)

Advice literature sometimes even pointed out how a very probable and convincing diagnosis could be made taking clues from external circumstances without actually considering any visible urinary changes. One English instruction book published in 1662 under the names of Jean Fernel, Abdiah Cole, and Nicholas Culpeper advised the academic physician to take into account the time of year, the weather, and the illnesses that currently held sway. After all, the diseases that befell many people were to be expected most often.[142] In addition, the physician was to find out the patient's sex and constitution, if possible. With an old man living in a humid country in the winter, it was fairly safe to surmise that he had a cough and catarrh, and, especially if he was inclined to drinking and gluttony, a heavy and weak stomach as well. With a young choleric man in hot weather in a hot country who had eaten hot and spicy food and then exercised extensively, a "burning fever," dysentery, or an inflammation of the pleura seemed likely, as these were diseases to which such people were prone and which were most common among the populace.[143]

For the "vainglorious," the authors had further advice to give. When the uroscopist was presented with light-colored, thin urine—one of the most common findings—he was supposed to say that the stomach and liver were cold, that the patient hated to eat meat, had little appetite, frequent sour eructation, and a lot of winds, felt cold, had a heavy head, and felt weak in all his body. All these were indeed symptoms that the dominant school of thought claimed were to be expected with a weak stomach and accordingly weak digestion—as indicated by the urine. And as urine of this kind was also present in the case of melancholy and a swollen spleen, the uroscopist was to name the symptoms of those conditions as well when describing the presumed complaints of the patient: sadness, anxiety, somber dreams, noises on the left side, heartburn, and impaired vision.[144] In the same vein, thin but gold-colored urine, for example, allowed the uroscopist to surmise a heated liver and conclude from this the typical symptomatic consequences: thirst, thin stature, bad sleep, and hot palms and soles.[145] Thick, golden urine, by contrast, did not simply indicate heat but bile: presumably, the patient was vomiting, and had a bilious bitter taste in his mouth; his vital spirits were weak, his stomach hot from thirst, his abdomen was painful or he had diarrhea, possibly turning into dysentery, or his skin might itch.[146]

In vernacular compilations that targeted a broader readership, the prognostic side was emphasized even more than in writings by and for doctors. Nicholas

---

[142] Fernel/Cole/Culpeper, *Two treatises* (1662), 75.
[143] Ibid., 75f.
[144] Ibid., 77.
[145] Ibid., 77.
[146] Ibid., 78.

Culpeper—one of the best-known authors of "popular" medical and medico-astrological literature in seventeenth-century England—gave the central chapter of his *Semeiotica Uranica*, which addressed only the most important kind of illness, the fevers, the title *Presages by the urine in a fever*, or "Foretelling from urine in the case of a fever." Among his terse statements in the book is: "Slimy, swampy, black, tan, dirty, and stinking urine is usually fatal." Other examples are: "Urine that is white and clear points to melancholy and is very bad" and "A cloud floating in urine means health if it is white; danger looms if it is black." Only few of the total of 12 maxims that Culpeper listed pointed explicitly to a diagnosis. And even in those cases, the diagnosis clearly implied also a prognostic judgment, as in the case of "consumption," which was known to lead almost inevitably to increasing weakness and emaciation and, ultimately, to death.[147]

Diagnostic maxims of this kind were sometimes accompanied by therapeutic commentary in the style of a dispensary. For each urinary finding, the reader learned about the drugs that promised to be most successful. A section with the heading *The Acute Judgement of Urines* that appeared in the appendix of a popular medical advice book of 1656, for instance, stated that thick, rosy urine indicated a burning fever. Under the sub-heading *Medicine*, the advice read: "Let him have a bloodletting below his ankle or from his arm vein; take aloe [and] 1 dram of liverwort and boil it in a pint of white wine [for him to] drink a spoonful in the morning and at night."[148] By contrast, urinary findings that had essentially only prognostic value were not accompanied by therapeutic advice of this kind. For example, the book stated bluntly that coal-black, fatty, and stinking urine announces death.[149] Authors might even just pair up different urinary colors with different medicines without mentioning the underlying illness, for example, "the best drugs" for a "camel hair colored urine."[150]

Even if they focused on practical advice, uroscopy could hardly be learned from treatises alone. Much like pulse diagnosis, uroscopy was an eminently practical skill and the copious literature on uroscopy was only of limited value when the physician had to arrive at a judgment which—if it proved erroneous—might seriously damage his authority. Galen himself had professed that he was unable to express the changing nature of healthy urine in words; one had to be shown by someone or learn from one's own experience.[151] This aspect of hands-on practice was emphasized particularly strongly in the Paracelsian tradition. "All this is better shown and learned with [actual] urine [samples],"

---

[147]   Ibid., 78.

[148]   Turner, *Compleat bone-setter* (1656); the section on uroscopy (175) seems to have been written by Turner. In a second, and longer, part of this section (366–75), which was likely borrowed from another author, such therapeutic advice is missing.

[149]   Ibid.

[150]   Anonymous, *Judgment of all urynes* ([around 1555]).

[151]   Galen, *De crisibus* (1825), 599.

wrote Johan Hayne, for example, in his instruction book on uroscopy (which nevertheless amounted to 150 pages).[152]

The necessary skills were best acquired by accompanying and assisting his more experienced colleagues. For barber surgeons and barbers—who made up the lion's share of licensed healers up into the nineteenth century—this was part of their technical training, first as apprentices, then as journeymen. But medical students and assistant doctors, it seems, also learned the art of uroscopy, like many other aspects of medical practice, above all through personal instruction. The significant role practical instruction by experienced doctors played in the education of medical students from as early as the sixteenth century has often been underestimated. Historians have too narrowly focused on formal clinical teaching, a development that tends to be associated with Herman Boerhaave in the Dutch town of Leiden during the early eighteenth century. Yet already in the sixteenth and seventeenth centuries many German doctors who studied at Italian universities shouldered the additional costs and effort of studying abroad not only because the anatomy classes were better there but also because the practical training was superior. In Italy, students were able to go on house calls with their professors, and the large hospitals of northern Italy were particularly rich sources of illustrative examples. Georg Handsch, in mid-sixteenth-century Padua, reported listening to Antonio Fracanzani's lectures on uroscopy in the hospital and seeing up to 30 different patients' urine on his almost daily visits in the hospital.[153] However, doctors who received their education north of the Alps seem also to have acquired more than theoretical knowledge, accompanying experienced practitioners on their calls. As the number of academically trained doctors grew, practical training along these lines seems to have become virtually the norm. Without any practical experience to show, a young, budding doctor had little hope of winning the trust of patients and their relatives or of holding his own amidst competition from more experienced physicians.[154]

Already illuminations in late medieval manuscripts indicate such practical training in uroscopy, though we must take caution, of course, not to interpret them as a one-to-one reflection of common teaching practice. One of the best-known examples is found in *Hortus sanitatis* (see Plate 14) and shows a teacher or professor in front of 20 urine flasks lined up on a shelf who seems to be explaining to three students the different colors of urine. One of the students is holding an additional flask—presumably the one being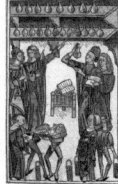

---

[152] Hayne, *Drey Tractätlein* (1620), 215.

[153] ÖNB Vienna, Cod. 11210, 80r–92v, *De uromantias sive iudicio urinarum. Lectio D. Anthonij Frankenzani Paduae in hospitali aegrorum*; ibid., Cod. 11206, 26r–v; cf. Stolberg, *Bed-side teaching* (2013).

[154] Schlegelmilch, "What a magnificent work a good physician is" (2015).

evaluated—and examining it while his companion reads in a book, which we may assume to be a learned uroscopy treatise.

Case Histories

The complex and at times highly sophisticated diagnostic pronouncements of skilled uroscopists and the pathophysiological concepts on which they relied are best illustrated with concrete examples. Considering the outstanding significance of uroscopy in late medieval and early modern medical culture, concrete uroscopic diagnoses are relatively rarely documented, however, and uroscopic diagnoses by non-academic practitioners have hardly survived at all.[155] Detailed descriptions and interpretations of the patients' urine are virtually absent in the numerous published medical *observationes* or *curationes*, a highly popular genre from the late sixteenth century onward.[156] This may reflect the focus of this genre on causal explanation and/or treatment but their authors also may not have been keen to associate themselves with what the medical profession increasingly regarded as a somewhat undignified and unreliable method. This may explain why uroscopic judgments are more commonly found in manuscript sources. They provide important insights into how early modern doctors practiced uroscopy. In what follows, we will take a closer look at some of them to learn about their typical features and about what they can tell us about the author's diagnostic reasoning.

We will start with a fairly detailed consultation by a certain Doctor Johann Lasster in the early sixteenth century. The folded sheet of paper bears neither the patient's name nor his place of residence. We may therefore assume that it was given to the patient or his relatives personally or by a messenger.[157] The German original is not easy to understand today, even for native speakers, because of its unfamiliar phrasing and diction. However, a close reading proves rewarding. Following the salutation, Lasster describes the illness along with the complaints it causes: the patient has been sick for a long time. He suffers no pain but feels tired and weak and lacks appetite. A description of symptoms like this might seem superfluous. After all, the patient is well aware of what ails him. So it must have served a different purpose. What Lasster is doing here is proving his skill at deducing from the quality of the urine the complaints and the physical constitution of the patient. Provided that his description was correct (the messenger might have had some helpful remarks too), this would have helped to

---

[155] Cf. *Making Sense of the Body* in chapter 3.

[156] Stolberg, *Formen* (2007); Pomata, *Observation rising* (2011).

[157] ÖNB Vienna, Cod. 11198, 307r; cf. the edition in Sudhoff, *Ein ärztlicher Brief* (1915).

establish the patient's trust in the uroscopist's ability also to identify the illness itself and suggest a specific treatment. Lasster's account of the patient's present state is followed by predictions for the future course of the disease: the patient would become thinner and his limbs would tire and become unfit to perform their functions. He could also expect to have pain in the back and loins, and the winter would be hard on him by making his breathing difficult.

This description of present and future complaints is followed by some brief dietetic advice on the need to avoid water, beer or new wine, as well as fruit, and the recommendation to take an electuary to warm the stomach and fight indigestion.[158] Otherwise the disease might develop into an "inner" fever, which (as opposed to common attacks of fever) would not be accompanied by a sensation of heat or chills but would instead "consume" the body and leave the patient depleted of strength. Without using that term, Lasster was clearly referring to consumptive fever or *febris hectica*, which was widely accepted in the academic medicine of the day as a disease characterized by progressive weakness and weight loss. This is quite typical of other extant medical uroscopy consultations. Determining a particular disease category or type was often not central to the uroscopic diagnosis. Attention focused on providing a causal, "pathophysiological" interpretation of the genesis and course of the disease, delivered in a way that was accessible to laypeople and which justified the prescribed treatment.

In the case at hand, Lasster thought the disease had its origin in the stomach, which was "cold" and "full of slime." This was one of the most common diagnoses in early modern medicine and a large number of symptoms could be explained in this way. As we have seen, the stomach was considered the site where the first stage of "concocting" and assimilating food took place. For this task, the stomach required sufficient heat. If the stomach or its heat were too weak, "slime" or phlegm—a moist, cold, raw, uncooked substance—began to accumulate in it. The phlegm in turn cooled or weakened the stomach further and could form deposits in the stomach and in the rest of the body. The long-term consequences could be devastating. When the stomach was blocked by "slime" in this way, this lessened its desire for food, leaving the body with insufficient nutrition. And of the little food that was still being ingested, the stomach could only produce smaller amounts of valuable chyle, resulting in smaller amounts of blood concocted in the liver and ultimately to be assimilated by the individual body parts. The patient literally wasted away. Cold, moist slime would accumulate even more during the winter, and "breathing" was likely to become more difficult when catarrh and mucus collected in the air passages.

---

[158] An electuarium or electuary is a drug preparation, usually sweetened with honey or sugar, that comes in the form of a paste or thin pulp.

Water, beer and new wine, and fruit were considered "cold" and "watery" as well as "raw" or "undigested" and were therefore bound to weaken the stomach's heat even further. The electuary, on the other hand, was to foster the stomach's "heat" and thus counteract the poor concoction of food and the accumulation of phlegm. For the time being, Lasster advised against strong "expelling" agents—presumably he meant laxatives and emetics—likely fearing that the body would be further weakened. However, he conceded that it might be advisable to take such drugs in the cold and humid autumn, when phlegm threatened to accumulate in the stomach and body.

Karl Sudhoff rightly referred to this consultation as a "contemporary document of medical thinking and acting."[159] It aptly demonstrates to what degree consultations were framed and pervaded by theoretical assumptions about the nature of physiological and pathological processes in the human body. Understanding these assumptions, in turn, is necessary if we are to make sense of the consultations. Lasster's uroscopic judgment, for example, is anything but random or arbitrary. On the contrary, on closer analysis it is very coherent and stringently argued, even if he did not make all his deductions and logical connections explicit to the patient. At the same time, his consultation shows clearly how well theories of humoral pathology could be applied in practice to explain and make pathological processes plausible to laypeople.

However, one important element is missing in this account, and this is typical of many premodern uroscopic consultations. Like most of his colleagues, Lasster foregoes giving any details about the urine itself and the changes he noticed, as if he wanted to keep his cards close to his chest, to avoid giving the patient instructions on how to do a uroscopic self-diagnosis.

We will now examine one of the rare published uroscopic judgments that included a description of the urine itself. In 1560, doctor Johannes Pontanus from Saxony gave his medical advice to an unidentified theologian who had asked for help because his vision was deteriorating.[160] For a clergyman who had to read every day, this was a tragedy. But Pontanus was able to dispel the patient's worry, without seeing him personally. The urine he had been sent, claimed Pontanus, clearly showed that the problem was not in the eyes, as the patient feared. The urine was "thick, raw, cloudy and turbid" and interspersed with contents. This indicated "without a doubt" a considerable accumulation and turmoil of "viscous and slow humors" in the "natural body parts," namely in the stomach, the liver, and the blood vessels. Due to the connection to the brain and the "consensus" of the natural parts with it, the brain could easily fill with coarse and vaporous smoke. He was confident that the images that danced

---

[159] Sudhoff, *Ein ärztlicher Brief* (1915), 451.

[160] Epistolary council by Johannes Pontanus, June 20, 1560, in: Wittich, *Consilia* (1604), 196–9.

before the eyes of the patient like small insects and his weakened vision did not originate in the eyes themselves, *per essentiam*, but in those trails of smoke and vapors sent up to the brain from the humors in the stomach, the liver, and their surrounding veins.

Like Lasster, Pontanus did not identify the disease with a specific name. Instead he focused on the presumable causes of the complaints, which, in turn, would point the way to an effective treatment. His interpretation, too, addressed those organs that were responsible for the concoction of food and its transformation into blood. Yet, the assumed disorder was a different one. Pontanus concluded that mucous, yet mobile, turbid humors were present in the stomach and the liver, and in the surrounding veins into which the liver—it was commonly assumed—released the nutritious blood that resulted from the second concoction. The patient was not informed about the presumed origin of the mucous humors. Perhaps Pontanus felt that the explanation, which he only hinted at between the lines, would have appeared too complicated to the patient. Though "raw" urine usually indicated an insufficient concoction of food due to a lack of heat, the thickening and turbidity of the urine in this specific case suggested an excessive heat.[161] This excessive heat condensed the humors, slowed their flow, and made them emit vapors and trails of smoke which, due to their higher temperature and volatility, rose all the way up to the cranium, from where they could not escape.[162]

This imagery of rising vapors and trails of smoke may seem very foreign to us today. During the early modern period, however, the role of the so-called *vapores* was widely acknowledged. An educated theologian who had possibly studied Melanchthon's *De anima*[163]—in which *spirits* and *vapors* played a paramount role—was very likely familiar with the concept. Vapors could quite literally "cloud" one's thinking. In the cerebral ventricles they became mixed with the clear lucid spirits of the soul, the *spiritus animales*, which, contaminated and darkened in this manner, could no longer adequately fulfill their tasks as the immediate tools of the immaterial soul. Obviously turbid vapors and trails of smoke interspersed with particles of soot could have a similar effect on the eyes.

Detailed uroscopic *judicia* such as these, by learned physicians, have rarely survived. Much more common are shorter urine diagnoses or brief hints at urinary changes as one among many pathological findings which, taken together, led to diagnosis. Yet, when considered collectively they too give rise to a differentiated image. Several urine findings are included, for example, in a collection of 25

---

[161] Anonymous, *Traicté des urines* (before 1567), VIr.

[162] On the concept of "vapors" see Stolberg, *Experiencing illness* (2011), 164–70; idem, *Lukas Cranachs "Melancholia"-Darstellungen* (2007).

[163] The animal spirits and their purity played a central role in Melanchthon's profoundly Galenist commentary on *De anima*; cf. Melanchthon, *Commentarius* (1540); idem, *Liber* (1552); Helm, *Galenrezeption* (1996).

case histories compiled by the Dutch physician Johannes Antonides van der Linden (1609–1664) mainly for the purpose of training students.[164] Urine is described and discussed in 12 of the cases. These were notably cases of fever, hypochondria—then understood as a physical disease located in the right upper abdomen—jaundice, and a suspected kidney stone. In the other cases the findings in the urine seem to have been unremarkable.

To van der Linden, the first distinctive feature of importance was the urine's consistency (*substantia*). Thick, coarse urine (*urinae crassae*) pointed to larger amounts of pathological humors or substances being present, while fine, thin urine (*urinae tenues*) indicated, if at all, only minor admixtures. They primarily showed that a person's innate heat (*calor nativus*) was overtaxed or, in the case of bubbles or foam, that it had set free volatile pathological vapors.

The spectrum of different hues of urinary color described by van der Linden is considerable, given the small number of only 12 cases in total, which may reflect the didactic impetus behind his selection of cases. It ranged from white (*alba*), to different shades of yellow and orange (*coloratior, crocea, flammea*), to black (*nigra*). As we have seen, this spectrum corresponded roughly with the way dominant doctrine portrayed different degrees of food concoction and the impact of heat on urine. "Whitish" urine—which would have referred to near-transparent, watery urine—indicated raw, undigested humors and thus signaled a weak innate heat. Sylvius found such "whitish" and thin urine, for example, with a young woman who, during her period, had left her house barefoot and saw her period suppressed as a result.[165] In van der Linden's view, the cold had hindered the physiological fermentation in the blood that, according to Sylvius's doctrine of menstruation, produced the period.[166] The woman experienced intense headaches and suffered from nausea and sour eructation—a sign that food was not concocted sufficiently in the stomach. Her weak innate heat, indicated by her whitish, thin urine, was not the primary cause of her complaint but was an expression of her body being burdened with raw, cold humors. He seems to have interpreted the fact that she had eaten ginger everyday throughout the winter as a sign that she desired heat. Ginger with its spicy taste was traditionally considered heat inducing and digestive. Van der Linden diagnosed an intermittent tertian fever, basing his judgment, it seems, on the overall disease pattern.

When larger amounts of undigested, raw humors had amassed in the body and blood, van der Linden's cases describe that this resulted in coarser, thicker urine.[167] In the case of a weak stomach (*debilitas ventriculi*), the whitish color

---

[164] I am quoting from a manuscript in Württembergische Landesbibliothek Stuttgart, Cod. med. et phys. 4° 13, *Historiae aegrotorum XXV*; the same case histories appeared in print, in a different version, under the title *Historiae aegrotorum vigintiquinque* (1651).

[165] *Historiae aegrotorum*, case 2.

[166] Cf. Stolberg, *Monthly malady* (2000).

[167] *Historiae aegrotorum*, case 3.

of urine could thus be explained with a diminished innate heat, while its thick consistency followed from an accumulation of raw matter (*cumulatio cruditatum*).[168] Similarly, the whitish, thick, and also turbid urine of a young girl with *febris alba*, that is, chlorosis, indicated "raw" matter and a lack of innate heat.[169] Van der Linden interpreted thick, black urine in post-menopausal women as a sign of burnt blood.[170]

The transition from very thick urine laden with pathological substances to urine with visible contents was fluid. Van der Linden described the urine of a merchant of around 40 years of age; it appeared stirred-up and cloudy and he compared it to that of cattle, explaining that urine like this indicated a great accumulation of humors which the body or Nature was trying in vain to concoct. Undissolved contents identifiable with the naked eye were found especially with kidney and bladder stones, which we can easily understand from today's perspective. Not only doctors but also patients reported sand-like contents in such cases. Van der Linden, for example, said about the "thick" (*crassa*) urine of a patient with suspected kidney stones that it seemed "earthy" (*terreus*), as if finely ground earth had been mixed into the urine.[171] Of the many other kinds of visible contents—presented and explained in detail in the contemporary uroscopy treatises—van der Linden only mentioned one more: the "cloudlets" (*nubecula*) in the flame-colored (*flammea*) urine of a lunatic. He did not give any details as to their origin, likely presuming the same cause as for the red color, that is, an excessive heating of the blood.[172]

Uroscopy and Pulse Diagnosis

In summary, we can say that especially from the perspective of academically trained doctors and other educated contemporaries, uroscopy was in no way a primitive, inferior empirical procedure. On the contrary, its validity was warranted by the leading medical authorities, from Hippocrates and Galen to Avicenna and Constantinus Africanus,[173] and it was firmly rooted in rational, natural philosophical principles. It was based on a complex theory about the multi-stage concoction of food, the formation of the different excretions, and their changes caused by pathological processes in the body. The doctrine of uroscopy stood out in that it followed a "method"; it followed the path of reason and thus possessed the key feature of true science. In this sense, Giovanni

---

[168] Ibid., case 6.
[169] Ibid., case 13.
[170] Ibid., case 11.
[171] Ibid., case 19.
[172] Ibid., case 7.
[173] Fuchs, *Institutionum* (1555), 483–506.

Battista da Monte (1498–1551), one of the leading clinicians of his day, claimed that uroscopy yielded rational, certain, and well-founded insight. And he went on to say that there was no indication that was more reliable than that from urine, since urine came directly from the blood. Any intelligent and wise doctor would be able to deduce any disease from it.[174] In the same vein, Hieronymus Cappivaccius explained to his listeners that nothing in medicine was as useful as uroscopy or contributed more to arriving at a prognosis.[175] Uroscopy led to the highest degree of knowledge about any illness, emphasized the Swiss physician Conrad Gessner as well.[176] The Welsh doctor Robert Record (1510?–1558) said that without uroscopy (and pulse diagnosis) all medical knowledge was "doubtful, murky, and uncertain."[177] Alessandro Massaria (1510–1598) added that among all medical treatises those about urine were the "most noble and excellent."[178] It comes as no surprise then if physicians in their own illnesses heavily relied on uroscopic diagnosis.[179]

Uroscopy's privileged position emerges all the more clearly when we look at the alternatives. It seemed far superior to all other diagnostic options. Compared to other excretions, urine exhibited the greatest number of perceptible changes (*differentias*) and yielded the most information (*indicationes*).[180] Coproscopy, that is, the visual examination of the stool, was in no position to compete with uroscopy—and was even more unpleasant and offensive. According to da Monte, servants and maids refused to bring a stick that the doctor could use to stir the feces.[181] Hematoscopy, that is, the inspection of the patient's blood, also was of more limited value,[182] and could only be done when a bloodletting was performed. In this case, the blood-letter could make patients and families see first-hand how "burnt" or "slimy" the blood was.[183] Academic doctors, however, had long ceded the manual labor of bloodletting to surgeons and had

---

[174] Da Monte, *De excrementis* (1554), 5v: "quoniam nulla ars est, nullaque scientia tradita sine methodo"; idem, *Lectiones* (1552), no pagination.

[175] Capivaccius, *De urinis* (1595); this is a printed publication of lecture notes, edited by Laurentius Scholz, a student of Capivaccius. The many underlined passages and contemporary notes in the margins that are found in the copy I used at the library in Wolfenbüttel indicate that someone studied the text in depth.

[176] Gesnerus, *Compendium* ([around 1541]), 1r.

[177] Record, *Urinal* (1651), To the reader.

[178] Massaria, *Tractatus* (1608), 152.

[179] ÖNB Vienna, Cod. 11205, 63v–69r, Georg Handsch on his own disease around 1554.

[180] Da Monte, *Lectiones* (1552), no pagination.

[181] Ibid.

[182] Cf. Lenhardt, *Blutschau* (1986); Riha, *Blutschau* (2005).

[183] Ackermann, *Glaubens-Bekenntniß* (1783), 72.

thus largely robbed themselves even of the modest possibility of using it to such effect, except if they took care to be present that moment.

Only feeling the pulse could claim a similar diagnostic significance. In the works of Galen and in the medicine of the High Middle Ages it had still held the first position. However, from the sixteenth century onward most authors put it second to uroscopy.[184] Before William Harvey's new theory of blood circulation was accepted, pulse diagnosis was perceived as much more limited in scope. The pulse, it was generally agreed, reflected the movements of the warm, mobile vital spirits, which flowed from the heart through the arteries and from there into the rest of the body. Consequently, by feeling the pulse, only changes or illnesses that had an impact on the movement of the spirits in the arteries could be identified. Such changes were, first of all, the affects of the soul, the emotions, which were, at the time, understood literally as "movements of the heart" causing (or caused by) movements of the vital spirits. When someone had a fright, for instance, the spirits fled toward the inside, to the heart, filling it to the point of bursting. A feeling of physical oppression spread, while the limbs hardly answered to the person's will because the soul could no longer communicate with them sufficiently via the spirits, the immediate tools of the immaterial soul and the agents of its commands.[185] In terms of diagnosing emotions, pulse diagnosis was therefore superior to uroscopy. If, for example, a doctor noticed a sudden change in a young woman's pulse at the mention of a certain young man, this provided the crucial diagnostic clue that the patient was "lovesick."[186] As we will see, this scenario became a popular subject of seventeenth- and eighteenth-century genre painting.

In most diseases, however, unveiling the patient's current emotions was of little use for diagnostic or therapeutic purposes, and there were few other physical changes that had a similar immediate impact on the movement of the spirits and therefore on the pulse. Fever ranked highest among them. Fever, following the classical definition by Avicenna, was a "foreign" heat that ignited in the heart and then spread with the vital spirits through the arteries to the entire body.[187] Fevers thus influenced the movement of the vital spirits which could be identified primarily by a change of pulse. Indeed, an accelerated pulse and not body temperature, which only started to be routinely measured in the nineteenth century, was considered the crucial diagnostic sign of a fever. The patient might feel hot or cold, he might suffer from chills, yet his accelerated pulse indicated a fever.

---

[184] For a brief assessment of contemporary views see Ulianus, *Difficiliora problemata* (1602), ch. III.

[185] On the decidedly "somatic" interpretation of emotions in early modern medicine see Stolberg, *Zorn* (2005).

[186] Da Monte, *De excrementis* (1554), 2v.

[187] Bynum/Nutton (eds), *Fever theories* (1981).

Even to diagnose a fever, however, an examination of the patient's urine often proved indispensable. According to early modern medical theory, only the *ephemera*, or one-day fever, was limited in its impact on the spirits. Most fevers stemmed from a spoiled, putrid pathological substance in the blood, that is, from a humoral cause which could be determined only from urine, since urine was a direct secretion of the blood.[188] At the same time, an examination of urine could shed light on the spirits and on the strength of a person's innate heat, which was crucial to the genesis of the spirits in the heart.

On top of its limited diagnostic scope, pulse diagnosis was also fraught with great practical difficulties. According to Da Monte, many had something to say on the subject of pulse diagnosis but they had no experience and no true knowledge to speak of. Even the basic differences between the various kinds of pulse were easily misjudged. Galen himself was quoted as admitting that he had worked for 20 years before he could identify the diastole, that is, the expansion of the chamber of the heart, and only God knew if Galen had ever recognized a systole.[189]

Paracelsian Uroscopy

The most important alternative to traditional uroscopy goes back to Paracelsus.[190] While he also claimed that all diseases in the body could be recognized by examining the urine, Paracelsus, in line with his new conception of the body and illness, attempted to put uroscopy on a new footing. He distinguished three kinds of urine: internal, external, and mixed urine. External urine resulted from the concoction and separation of ingested food in the stomach, liver, and kidneys. Its changes pointed to an incomplete separation of the three Paracelsian principles—sulfur, salt, and mercury. Internal urine resulted from Nature's excretory efforts and reflected the condition of the body and its individual parts. Mixed urine was a combination of external and internal urine. While some pathological changes of urine could be made out with the naked eye or gave off a characteristic smell, others, especially those that arose from tartaric diseases, were too subtle. They could be detected only by distillation and other chemical procedures.[191]

---

[188]　Da Monte, *Lectiones* (1552), no pagination; idem, *Tractatus* (sine anno), 3v.

[189]　Da Monte, *De excrementis* (1554), 6v.

[190]　The literature on Paracelsism is extensive; cf. Pagel, *Weltbild* (1962), with a discussion of Paracelsian uroscopy/urinalysis on pp. 190–200; Grell, *Paracelsus* (1998); Debus, *Chemical philosophy* (2002); Bernabeo, *Paracelso* (1966), though focusing specifically on Paracelsian uroscopy, remains superficial.

[191]　Paracelsus, *De urinarum* (1568); idem, *De urinis* (1931); idem, *Beurteilung* (1928); cf. Schmelzer, *Vergleich* (1943).

Based on Paracelsian principles, Johan Hayne, in the late sixteenth century, wrote an extensive treatise on "the rational basis on which to judge and recognize the urines of healthy as well as sick people in an artificial, spagyric way."[192] Modifying the Galenic three-stage model, he followed Paracelsus when describing the formation of (external) urine in three stages of digestion or concoction. During the first stage, the stomach, as "the first and largest pot," separated the sulfur. If this digestion reached completion, the urine was golden yellow, the color of amber, oil, or topaz. If the separation remained incomplete, the resulting urine was pale and cloudy. The liver, as the second "pot," separated and digested salt, thus producing luminous, transparent, fine-grained sediment of a beautiful yellow color that acted as a balsamic substance and preserved all body parts. Beneath the salt, tartar in *prima materia* was hidden. Finally, the kidneys, as the third "pot," separated mercury, which served growth and reproduction. Upon full completion of this separation, a thick layer of heavy sediment could be found in the bottom of the flask, and the urine would exhibit no foam on its surface and would be of a good color. Besides this "external urine" and the "external tartar" it contained, Hayne, like Paracelsus, assumed an "inner urine," which flowed from the individual body parts directly to the bladder. Hayne claimed that distinguishing it from external urine was not easy but important and could be learned by diligent practice.[193] The uroscopist had to take note not only of the amount and color of urine but also of its smell, and above all of the tartar, its shape, and the location in the flask where it presented itself. Using numerous small illustrations, Hayne gave the reader detailed instructions on how to interpret the different deposits in the matula based on these ideas.

One of the most successful representatives of Paracelsian uroscopy was Leonhard Thurneysser, an alchemist, astrologer, and personal physician of the elector of Brandenburg in Berlin.[194] In his *Protokatalepsis* of 1571 he presented to the public his new method of examining urine through distillation and illustrated the manifold and detailed insights that could be gained from it with exemplary analyses.[195] In a second work, entitled *Bebaiosis Agonismou*, which was published in 1576, he defended the new procedure against his critics.[196] An extensive, richly illustrated anatomical section of the book served to underline Thurneysser's erudition and his ability to delve into the secrets hidden inside the human body, especially as the images were purportedly created from

---

[192] Hayne, *Drey Tractätlein* (1620), 194–348.

[193] Ibid., 215.

[194] Moehsen, *Leben* (1783); Spitzer, *Leonhard Thurneysser* (1996).

[195] Thurneysser, *Prokatalepsis* (1571); cf. Bleker, *Von der Uroscopie* (1966); eadem, *Harndiagnostik* (1970); eadem, *Kunst* (1970); eadem, *Chemiatrische Vorstellungen* (1976).

[196] Thurneysser, *Bebaiosis* (1576).

the autopsy of two corpses—identified by name—which Thurneysser had dissected personally.[197]

Thurneysser's method of urinalysis was based on a fairly simple principle. Thurneysser heated a urine sample slowly in a distilling flask. The steam rose and condensed in different places in the receiving flask. According to Thurneysser, the place where the steam settled corresponded to the location of the disease in the patient's body, while the quality and the amount of the deposit in the urine reflected the urine's composition and could indicate pathological changes. His procedure thus advanced the traditional concept of an analogy between the different regions of the matula and the afflicted regions of the human body. This concept was particularly appealing to Paracelsians who, even more than Galenic doctors, sought to relate individual pathological processes to specific locations in the body.

Thurneysser claimed emphatically that urine distillation was superior to conventional uroscopy. While other uroscopists would diligently evaluate "the circles, clouds and sediments" in his urine, he told the sick count Jost von Barbey, "without a doubt no doctor [had] a consistent and true perception that one would call perfect, to draw on or to find something of essence or of certainty." Only with the help of distillation would urine reassume its "first nature." Only through separating its individual parts did a sure diagnosis become possible.[198] Or, as he phrased it in his *Prokatalepsis*, published in 1571, only if through "the art of resolving, separating and dividing the elements the urine's spirits and subtleties become segregated and pull away from one another, and therefore their respective inner forces and opposing parts each decide on their own," could the root and origin of the disease be learned.[199]

In printed works and manuscript letters, Thurneysser gave his patients extensive and complicated explanations of the disease processes occurring inside their body, painting in this way a vivid picture of the superior capabilities of his method. Within a very few years he managed to attract a large and lucrative clientele. Patients from the highest ranks of society sent him their urine, asking his advice and paying lordly fees for his judgment and his precious drugs. To his patients, who usually lived far apart from each other, it would have remained unknown that Thurneysser's explanations often resembled one another quite closely even in their wording—despite the many different disease processes he discussed. Like other Paracelsians, Thurneysser still borrowed many explanatory elements from traditional Galenic medicine, which were familiar to his educated clientele and therefore more meaningful. Only occasionally did he

---

[197] Ibid., 29r–41r.

[198] StB Berlin, Ms. germ. 106, 117r–132r, letter from Thurneysser to Jost Graf zu Barbey, May 1, 1575.

[199] Thurneysser, *Prokatalepsis* (1571).

bring Paracelsian elements to bear—and it is telling that the elements he chose were predominantly of the variety that were easily visualized, such as tartar with its imagery of a dense substance that settled like limescale.

He diagnosed one patient, for example, with an excessive, evil, flying heat and a poisoned heat of the heart. Compressed in a small space, he claimed, the heat scorched the blood and created more yellow bile. For this reason, the patient suffered from "choleric, burnt, poisonous blood," as well as from a "viscous, mucous, putrid flux lying in the stomach." This created "at times a sudden quick heart beat and trembling, but not very strong, with a burdensome anxiety, fear and sadness without knowing why, whereof or on what account." In addition, the patient felt feeble when the blood rushed to the heart and left his limbs. The greatest danger was a "tear of a great artery or blood vessel in the innermost parts of the liver," followed by "an accretion or tartaric accumulation in the inner vital organs, namely the brain, heart, liver, and especially the kidneys." The weakness of the patient's cold, mucous, and tartar-covered stomach was the main cause of his fainting and of a "palpatory trembling and slight movement, also a heavy and grieved heart." Further, a dangerous disease (*morbus*) was hiding near the spine, where the kidneys were attached.[200]

Thurneysser emphasized that his procedure was superior even in cases when he was able to speak to the patient and do a physical examination. He had seen the sick wife of Hieronymus Pflug and was able to "personally and in part *ex phisionomia* take note of [her] complexion, behavior and condition," Thurneysser told her husband. But the human eye was weak and, especially with female patients, a doctor easily got the wrong impression because "women, when strange men look at them too directly, become bashful and therefore not only turn red, but also the different kinds of spirits and their laudable powers hide and withdraw." Therefore he hastened to distill her urine and was able to make a diagnosis just in time: "It is only good that I was able to take a urine sample, so this woman had time to receive help. [Otherwise] it would have been too late and the woman would have been overcome [by her disease]."[201]

Apparently, many patients saw their trust in Thurneysser's diagnostic art fully confirmed. Their gratitude for his advice was effusive. We find phrases in their letters, such as "we have truly found in this judgment of the urine nothing but the truth."[202] Hans Christoff Brenner thanked Thurneysser for the summary of what the doctor had "found in the water" with the words: "So I have been telling my trusted noblemen that I feel just as you say in head and heart and

---

[200] StB Berlin, Ms. germ. fol. 106, 153r–159v, undated letter from Thurneysser to an unnamed patient, possibly Graf von Kanitz.

[201] Ibid., 43r–44v, letter from Thurneysser to Hieronymus Pflug, May 13, 1574.

[202] StB Berlin, Ms. germ. fol. 426, 100r–v, letter from Hans Albrecht Graf zu Mansfeld and Arnstein (around 1582).

all other respects."²⁰³ A medical practitioner himself, the Paracelsian Daniel Reinisch had a similarly positive experience with Thurneysser's diagnostic art. He told Thurneysser in a letter that he had treated a burgher of Leipzig two years earlier and this patient had secretly sent his urine to Thurneysser, "without my knowledge, so he didn't have to worry that I would babble [and perhaps tell you about] the patient's condition." This could easily have produced a contradiction, but Thurneysser's judgment had "hit the mark so precisely" that, from this point on, the patient believed Reinisch—who apparently had made the same diagnosis at the sickbed.²⁰⁴

Thurneysser's achievement also offers an early example of the successful introduction of a technical, apparatus-based diagnostic procedure in medicine. Patients and their relatives had trust in the procedure even though they usually did not get to see this equipment. Martini, in looking back, made a point of praising Thurneysser as the first proponent of a *mechanica ratio pronuntiandi*, a "mechanical" procedure of judgment.²⁰⁵

---

²⁰³ StB Berlin, Ms. germ. fol. 423a, 40r–41v, letter from the patient, February 20, 1580.

²⁰⁴ StB Berlin, Ms. germ. fol. 423b, 8r–9r, letter from Daniel Reinisch, June 10, 1581.

²⁰⁵ Martini, *Anatomia urinae* (1658), 285.

Chapter 3
Uroscopy and Popular Culture

As we have seen, uroscopy had a major place in early modern medical culture. Among ordinary people, it was incontestably recognized as the most important diagnostic procedure into the nineteenth century. Physicians became more skeptical about uroscopy as time went on, especially when it came to the exclusive reliance on uroscopy for diagnosis, but it retained a secure position even within the medical profession.

Such unshakable trust in uroscopy may surprise us today. We may wonder why intelligent and well educated people failed to recognize that uroscopy was hardly reliable. From today's perspective, we cannot help but assume that patients and their relatives should have realized that uroscopy was completely bogus. Taking a closer look at the place and function of uroscopy in premodern medical culture, however, makes it clear that this assumption is based on false premises. People's experience with uroscopy by no means offered proof that it was worthless. Quite to the contrary—and this is true for physicians and non-medical, irregular uroscopists alike—"daily experience," as Liessell put it in 1668, seemed to confirm the value of uroscopy for diagnosis and treatment over and over.[1]

The reason for this lay in the nature of the procedure. The uroscopic diagnosis was hard to falsify. After all, it was uroscopy's trademark that it offered a rare glimpse at the mysterious pathological processes deep inside the sick body, which were inaccessible, at least during the patient's lifetime, by other means. If a uroscopist diagnosed an overheated liver, for example, the patient had no way of testing this conclusion. At best, he or she could question whether the diagnosis made sense in the light of the symptoms. Prognosis was a different case. It could be spectacularly refuted by the further course of the disease. Yet, even grave errors need not call the value of uroscopy as such into question. It was only natural that individual uroscopists made mistakes, perhaps because they did not fully understand their craft or did not examine the urine thoroughly enough. It was precisely for this reason one tested the uroscopist's abilities by asking him to describe the patient's current complaints even though—indeed because—the complaints were well known, unlike the diagnosis and prognosis. It was not the validity of uroscopy as such but the trustworthiness of the particular uroscopist that was at issue in these instances.

What is more, a false prognosis could also be explained without calling into question the abilities of the uroscopist, let alone the validity of uroscopy as a whole.

---

[1]   Liessell, *Konste* (1668), 14.

Contemporary medical doctrine had various explanations at its disposal for sudden favorable or unfavorable changes in the course of the disease, changes that even the most experienced uroscopist could not foresee. The case of Anton Hirt's wife, who was a patient of the "doctress" of Schozach, illustrates this well. The 58-year-old man reported that his wife used to collect herbs and roots and sell them to the doctress. In this way she got to know her and "had great confidence in her." When his wife fell ill, the husband took her urine to Schozach. The "doctress," it was reported, looked at the urine and explained to him that "it is not yet a fatal illness," but the woman had at most a year to live. The married couple did not want to believe this. The next day Hirt brought more of his wife's urine but now the doctress had even worse news to report. She told him, it was now over, the "stroke" that had been lodged between his wife's shoulder and the nape of her neck had now moved to her bladder, and the *gichter* had moved to her small intestines, so that she would die in 48 hours. The term *gichter* generally referred to cramps and convulsions at the time.[2] For 12 *kreuzer*, she gave him 12 dark red drops for the sick woman to take. According to Hirt, they did not have much effect, but his answer may have been influenced by his awareness of the suspicion on the part of the interrogators that his wife's death had been caused by the doctress's drops. In fact, he reported, his wife had died two days later, hardly moving her limbs. She had "the dormant stroke of *gicht*," as the doctress of Schozach had called it. In other words, the fact that the doctress initially gave an all-too-favorable prognosis did not dissuade the husband from trusting in her abilities. For the doctress understood how to explain the sudden and drastic change in her prognosis on the basis of a bodily process that made sense and was plausible for the layperson of the day. As long as morbid matter or, as in this case, a "stroke" or *gichter* were sitting in the neck or back, in the body's periphery that is, there was no immediate danger, according to common belief. But when they suddenly moved inside, as the doctress later found, and fell back on the vital organs—the bowel and bladder in this case—then death was knocking at the door. And such "falling back" was hardly predictable.[3]

The concept of "dormant" *gichter* was not current in scholarly medical literature but was well known in popular medical culture. It served to underline the possibility of a sudden change.[4] In particular with infants, *gichter* accounted for many deaths. Thus a death from "dormant" *gicht*, which supposedly was not accompanied by any noticeable convulsions, appears to be a contradiction in terms. But the pieces begin to fit together when we consider how *gichter* were talked about in sources from the eighteenth and early nineteenth centuries. In popular medical culture, *gichter* were not simply cramps, that is, a symptom of illness. Similar to the sometimes

---

[2]   Höfler, *Krankheitsnamenbuch* (1899), 189–92.

[3]   HStA Stuttgart A 213 Bü. 6734, interrogation of Anton Hirt, March 3, 1780.

[4]   E.g. Scultetus, *Zeug-Hauß* (1666), 23, report about a farmer with head injuries; Tissot, *Abhandlung* (1781), 553f.

synonymously used *fraisen* (infant spasms), *gichter* were rather understood as independent morbid agents. They were endowed with a will of their own, were able to more or less arbitrarily throw themselves on one part of the body and then on another. As a rule they produced cramps, but the vernacular also knew inner *gichter*, without any visible movement. The claim that *gichter* (and the stroke, for which, however, the assumption of such an ontological nature is not proven to the same extent) had thrown themselves on the vital organs was plausible in this context and it was understandable that an inspection of the urine could hardly foresee the *gichters'* sudden "decision" to move to a different part of the body of their own volition. The claim that the *gichter* had, then, effectively lain down to rest opened up still further interpretive potential.

In some cases a false prognosis could ultimately even strengthen the uroscopist's reputation:[5] when the illness took an unexpected favorable turn, he could attribute this to his timely and vigorous intervention. On the other hand, if the disease followed a course more detrimental than predicted, the uroscopist would have to contend with skepticism and doubt on the part of the sick person and his or her relatives. Indeed, the ill-fated outcome might even be ascribed to the harmful effects of his treatment. It is no surprise then that experienced uroscopists seem to have preferred making judgments that were on the pessimistic side. In the case of the sick wife of Wirsing, the pastor of Sinbronn, the attending doctor Reysner skillfully left a back door open: "This person already is or will soon be bedridden unless something is done quickly. The jaundice has laid itself tightly around the heart, making the vapors (flatulence) rise and weaken all the limbs."[6] If the patient fared better, or if the disease took a more favorable course than Reysner assumed it would, and she did not become bedridden, he could claim that he had stalled the disease with his medicines. In Leonhard Thurneysser's epistolary consultations, such a preference for pessimistic findings and prognoses—which might be shockingly negative for patients—is striking. As he explained to his patient Christoph von Meyenburg, the mangy, scabietic morbid matter in his body might lead to innumerable symptoms or complaints, from heart pains and renal inflammation to memory loss and convulsions. The patient could not yet know anything of this because "the least part of it is visible at this time but is only [present] in the blood, like the flesh secretly still lies in the yolk of the egg before it generates itself and prepares to be born."[7] In another case, Thurneysser pointed the count Jost von Barbey to the multiplicity of ominous signs of illness in the urine of people who by all appearances were in splendid health. Although the tendency toward unconsciousness, vertigo, and memory loss was not "at the present moment perceptible" in Barbey's urine, it would "with time become

---

[5]   Cf. van Dueren, *Ontdekkinge* (1688), 128.

[6]   Wirsing, *Altfränkisches Pfarrleben* (1952), 38.

[7]   StB Berlin, Ms. germ. fol. 106, 45r–55v, uroscopic council for Christoph von Meyenburg, May 2, 1575.

more noticeable and increase drastically, like all symptoms." In addition, there was the threat of numerous other complaints which, although they were not present at the moment, certainly resided in the body as future illnesses, ranging from shortness of breath and angina pectoris to lumbago and kidney stones.[8]

This idea that the seed of some dangerous illness was lurking in the body of a patient, ready to sprout and grow, further buttressed Thurneysser's credibility and the esteem of his therapeutic successes. If he diagnosed disease processes and threats inside the body which were completely unknown to the sick person, Thurneysser could be assured of the gratitude of the patient—provided he or she believed Thurneysser—when the disease did not progress and the looming threat did not become a reality thanks to Thurneysser's drugs. Georg von Traupnitz thanked Thurneysser by saying that he had received Thurneysser's letter and "woefully noted the urgent matter and imminent danger." Yet, he appreciated that he had "learned of this thorough and truthful account of my condition." After all, he "was obliged to admit" that Thurneysser was "right about all circumstances to such a degree that I myself would not have been able to give a better account."[9]

Nevertheless, it would seem inevitable from today's perspective that patients and relatives would sometimes cast serious doubt, at least in all those cases where the uroscopist's treatment was to no avail. After all, it was very easy to judge whether the patient improved under the treatment that the uroscopist, based on his uroscopic judgment, recommended. Yet it is precisely on this point that the modern presumption is premature, that sooner or later the unreliability of uroscopy and the inefficacy of the treatment had to become manifest. It was in fact the very outcome of treatment that in many if not most cases appeared to prove the uroscopist right. Most patients did get better at some point, or showed at least a temporary improvement. Modern medicine may judge most therapies of those days to be ineffective or outright harmful, and especially the ubiquitous laxatives and emetics, bloodletting and cupping. But even modern medicine acknowledges that it is often very difficult to decide whether the treatment itself or other factors are responsible when a favorable outcome is observed.

One such factor is the so-called placebo effect. Simply taking a medication or being treated in some other way can boost the healing process significantly. Probably even more important in our context is a second factor: Many, if not most diseases tend to take a favorable course or at least show some improvement in between, no matter whether or how they are treated. This is especially true for acute infectious diseases, which were very common in the early modern period.

Some early modern authors explicitly allowed for such influences, especially when they discussed the apparent successes of their less learned competitors.

---

[8]   Ibid., 117r–132r, letter from Thurneysser to Jost Graf zu Barbey, May 1, 1575.

[9]   StB Berlin, Ms. germ. fol. 420a, 146r–147r, letter from the patient November 29, 1571.

Although he considered uroscopy alone very unreliable, K.B. Behrens in 1668 had to admit that some patients did become well again when treated on the sole basis of uroscopic findings. Occasionally, this was, according to Behrens, because the uroscopist, in spite of his almost inevitable misdiagnosis, would prescribe a medication that happened to be effective against the true illness. But sick people often simply recovered on their own without taking any effective medicines. This was because "Nature often does her best, even if we do not notice it, and attribute [it] to our art." And as Behrens added in a passage reminiscent of modern accounts of the placebo effect "opinion and conceit come into the picture too, and to great effect."[10]

Without a doubt there must have been many cases, especially with chronic diseases, when patients' hopes and expectations were nevertheless disappointed. They would spend a small fortune on the drugs that were prescribed to them on the basis of uroscopy, only to witness how their condition deteriorated, indeed perhaps even due to the drugs, as they may sometimes have believed. But even negative experiences did not call the value of uroscopy as such into question, nor the possibility of finding an effective treatment through an examination of urine. There were other explanations.

For one thing, many people, in an era in which the plague and other fatal diseases were a constant danger, were more aware of the finitude of human life and more willing than most people today to accept the limits of what was medically possible. Common sense told people that for some illnesses there simply was no cure. If God, in his inscrutable judgment, wanted to take a person, then even the best doctor, the best medicine, would not be able to make a difference. The widow of the shoemaker Adam Nägele recounted, for example, that her husband had complained over the course of months about his "lower back" and his "pain in the side." In the end, the man's 15-year-old son was sent to the "doctress" of Schozach with his father's urine. She explained that he had "taken a drink," meaning in all likelihood that he had imprudently drunk cold water when his body was hot, a widely accepted cause of illness at the time. She gave him red drops and a yellowish mixture he was to take every two hours. And indeed, the sick man said at first that "he felt better afterwards," but 14 days later he died. Apparently the man's widow saw no reason to reproach the "doctress" of Schozach in any way, especially considering that the remedies, which he had received from the apothecary shop following the doctress's treatment, did not have any effect either.[11] In another case, the "doctress" even predicted an impending death right from the beginning. As the patient's brother related, she examined the man's urine and said "she would soothe his pains, but he would certainly die in 24 hours." For 26 *kreuzer* she gave him some medicine, but

---

[10] Behrens, *Wasserbeschawen* (1688), 17; on the history of "placebo" see Kaptchuk, *Intentional ignorance* (1998); the term was originally used in a religious context.

[11] HStA Stuttgart A 213 Bü. 6734, Verhör der Margarita Nägele, March 4, 1780.

told him it would not save him from death. The brother indeed died the next day in his house while suffering *"gichter"*—in convulsions, we may presume.[12]

It was also clear that any particular uroscopist could err not only in his diagnostic judgment but also in selecting the proper medicines, without any implications for the credibility of uroscopy as such. For example, the vintner Johann Georg Krafft, as he reported himself, brought the urine of his 28-year-old consumptive wife to the doctress of Schozach upon his wife's request. He "had felt indebted and compelled to try anything that might save his wife's life." He was initially impressed with the healer's diagnostic abilities. She had examined the urine and "known from it all the circumstances of the disease, for instance that [my wife] had a disadvantageous first birth, from which ensued side pains and dizziness." Krafft was unsatisfied with her treatment, however. The doctress had given him a white-yellow mixture and black-red drops. Upon taking them, his wife experienced an intense heat. Her condition did not improve. The couple did not hesitate to draw their own conclusions. They no longer relied on the help of the "doctress," turning instead to physicians in Marbach and Heilbronn (who could not help her either at this point).[13] If the uroscopist's treatment met with no success—as this example illustrates very clearly—this did not necessarily mean that his or her uroscopic diagnosis was called into question. An unsuccessful treatment could also be explained by the healer having prescribed the wrong medicines or simply not knowing of remedies that were sufficiently strong, effective, or specific.

Practical Advantages

Uroscopy did not only appear tried, tested, and true. In comparison to other medical diagnostic practices of the time, it also had a number of practical advantages. For one thing, it was relatively inexpensive since the uroscopist did not have to make his way to the patient's house. According to the Württemberg tax ordinance of 1566, even a learned doctor was only allowed to ask the modest fee of a *batzen*—or four *kreuzer*—to "judge a person's urine" and give his "advice" based on such an examination.[14] If the doctor visited poorer patients in the same location and examined the urine at their residence, double the amount was due to him. If the sick person lived—like the great majority of the population—in one of the numerous villages and hamlets in the countryside, the doctor was permitted to charge 48 *kreuzer* if the distance was half a mile, and 60 *kreuzer* or a *gulden* if the

---

[12] Ibid., interrogation of Johannes Finkk, March 3, 1780.

[13] Ibid., interrogation of Johann Georg Krafft, March 4, 1780.

[14] HStA Stuttgart A 282 Bü. 1299, *Ordnung der Ärzte und Apotheker im Fürstentum Württemberg*, December 7, 1566; when patients also asked for a regimen or a prescription he could charge more, however.

distance was one to one and a half miles. In other words, even if the patient lived relatively close to a town, a house call cost 12 or 15 times more than having the doctor examine urine that was brought to him.

Occasionally the sources indicate the fees charged by non-academic uroscopists. The statements are usually quite general and can be compared with one another only to a limited extent due to the multitude of coins and currencies that existed even within the German language area. But the sums were never prodigious, it seems. Around 1600, Foreest spoke of one "nummus," Lange of one "tribulus,"[15] Kolreutter of a "Wassergroschen."[16] One Frankfurt Jew is reported to have charged one *weißpfennig* around 1620.[17] In England in the middle of the seventeenth century, the price was cited as six pence or one shilling.[18] In eighteenth-century Germany, the fee was regularly said to amount to six *groschen* or eighteen *kreuzer*. This was also the price that the "doctress" of Schozach asked for uroscopy.[19]

Physicians at the time saw the main reason why non-academic uroscopists "were in such high demand," in the fact that "these fellows" asked "a little less money than the real doctors."[20] And they questioned these apparent savings: even though the urine examination itself might be less expensive, the patients, they claimed, often had to spend a pretty penny on the drugs that the uroscopist gave or prescribed them.[21] Some uroscopists were even said to diagnose illnesses that did not even exist. Cordus, for instance, told the story of a female uroscopist who talked a "noble man" into believing that his liver had first become inflamed from excessive intercourse and then had disappeared and been expelled. She promised to make him a new one, and received 80 *gulden* to do so.[22] According to Rega, other healers likewise claimed that a patient's liver or spleen had been entirely consumed, or that the kidneys had been expelled through the bladder.[23] Doctors further accused some uroscopists of manipulating urine so as to be better able to impose their services. Thoner told of a uroscopist who showed a noble patient with mild catarrh his supposedly black urine—a well-known ominous sign—and received 1,000 gold pieces because he promised to cure his alleged life-threatening illness.[24]

---

[15] Neumann, *Geschichte* (1894), 60, note.
[16] Ibid., 66.
[17] Foreest, *Uromanteia* (1620), 170 (presumably added by the German translator).
[18] Turner, *Compleat bone-setter* (1656), 126.
[19] HStA Stuttgart A 213 Bü. 6734, interrogation of Johannes Schunz, March 3, 1780.
[20] Fries, *Spiegel* (1518), LXIIIv; see also Foreest, *Uromanteia* (1620), 170.
[21] Turner, *Compleat bone-setter* (1656), 129.
[22] Cordus, *De urinis* (1543), no pagination; van Dueren, *Ontdekkinge* (1688), 69, also told about a woman from his own experience who thought she was ill only because a certain uroscopist had persuaded her to that effect.
[23] Rega, *Tractatus* (1733), 1st treatise, 44.
[24] Thoner, *Observationum medicinalium* (1649), 341–6 (epistola 21)

Stories such as these were by all appearances pure fiction. True, some non-academic uroscopists seem to have lined their pockets quite handsomely. A certain Bergmann charged no less than 2 *gulden* and 45 *kreuzer*, promising Franziska Eichert to free her of the complaints she had allegedly brought upon herself by drinking cold water when she had been angry at her unfaithful fiancé.[25] This amount was equal to several days' income of a common worker. Probably we also need to distinguish between healers who traveled from town to town or, at least, had a large catchment area, and charged higher fees, and local healers who played an important role in the continuous medical care of the local population and expected a more modest remuneration. Franziska Eichert paid the barber-surgeon of Essingen 9 *batzen* or 36 *kreuzer* for two small flasks of medicine.[26] The blacksmith of Gnadenthal Monastery demanded 13 *batzen* for two flasks of medication to treat "the chill" in Maria Margaretha Weidner's blood, though, according to her account, her mother only gave him half the money.[27] The "doctress" of Schozach asked Johannes Schunz 24 *groschen* for medicine to treat his consumptive wife, but settled for 18 when he said he had brought no more money with him.[28] She asked the same amount of the weaver Gottlob Wagner for dark red drops that were to restore his wife's absent monthly bleedings.[29] Johannes Finkk was to pay her 26 *kreuzer*, almost half a *gulden*, for drugs that he was to take to his sick brother.[30] Anton Hirt paid 12 *kreuzer* for the drops that she gave him for his wife,[31] and the wealthy baker Konrad Nägeli paid 18 *kreuzer* for the drops upon whose ingestion he felt "a good effect."[32] The widow of shoemaker Adam Nägele paid 9 *batzen* at one occasion and 6 *batzen* at another—a total of one *gulden*—for his drugs.[33] Johann Georg Krafft paid 5 or 6 *batzen* for the white-yellow mixture and the red-black drops she gave him for his consumptive wife.[34]

The patients and their families thus often paid the unlicensed healers several times the uroscopy fee for medicines. This was by and large also true of the learned physicians' practice, however. For less affluent patients, treatment by an academically

---

[25]   Staatsarchiv Ludwigsburg, A 213 6734, interrogation of Franziska's mother, December 10, 1765.

[26]   Ibid.

[27]   Stadtarchiv Schwäbisch Hall, Bestand 11, 84, interrogation of Maria Margaretha Weidner.

[28]   HStA Stuttgart A 213 Bü. 6734, interrogation of Johannes Schunz, March 3, 1780.

[29]   Ibid., interrogation of Gottlob Wagner, March 4, 1780; during the interrogation he was advised to consult the physician in Laufen in the future; his medicines would in that case be paid for from the poor relief funds.

[30]   Ibid., interrogation of Johannes Finkk, March 3, 1780.

[31]   Ibid., interrogation of Anton Hirt, March 3, 1780.

[32]   Ibid., interrogation of Konrad Nägeli, March 4, 1780.

[33]   Ibid., interrogation of Margarita Nägele, March 4, 1780.

[34]   Ibid., interrogation of Johann Georg Krafft, March 4, 1780.

trained physician was difficult to afford not least because one needed to purchase the expensive drugs from the apothecary.[35] Thus obtaining a uroscopic judgment from one of the many unlicensed healers was still usually the less expensive alternative.

From the point of view of patients, uroscopy could also help to save money in other ways. When uroscopy led to an effective treatment, the patient could go back to work more quickly and knowing, from uroscopy, the unfavorable, or indeed fatal course the disease was likely to take could at least help avoid unnecessary expenditures for a futile treatment.

Apart from its low cost, uroscopy could also offer a welcome degree of anonymity. Those seeking advice did not have to call or visit a healer in person, something that could not go unnoticed especially in small village communities. They only needed to have a relative or confidant discreetly take the urine to the healer. As we will soon see in more detail, this was particularly attractive to unmarried women who feared they might be pregnant. But the same goes more or less for patients with shame-laden complaints such as sexually transmitted diseases or illnesses that were thought to be hereditary such as epilepsy, which could jeopardize marriage plans. In such cases, sending the urine to a distant urospocist made it possible to keep the suspected disease secret.

In the case of the doctress of Schozach, it was mainly relatives who set out with the urine: husbands, wives, brothers. As we have seen, the same was true for the Weinsbergs and the Wirsings. In the person of Sabina Bremerin, however, we encounter a figure who by all appearances was not unusual for her time. She served practically the whole village as a medical messenger. She recounted that she had been going to the barber-surgeon in Essingen for "many people" for 18 years. She would also pay him for the medicines, which he would give her right away. The necessary money, she reported, she would get ahead of time, "from the people, upon taking the urine."[36] Sometimes she also advanced the money, as in the case of the pregnant Franziska Eichert, whose mother she later approached "to ask for the money she had advanced for the daughter in Essingen."[37]

Such messengers seem to have existed in many places. Daniel de Superville in the early eighteenth century, for example, claimed that one would see "so many piss messengers" walking with "a great burden of urine glasses" to the sextons and farmers who practiced uroscopy.[38] In the Netherlands as well, there are reports of messengers who had made a profession of transporting urine.[39]

---

[35] See e.g. Valenti, *Medicina clerica* (1831), 115.

[36] Staatsarchiv Ludwigsburg, B 412 37, interrogation of Sabina Bremerin, December 10, 1765.

[37] Staatsarchiv Ludwigsburg, B 412 37, interrogation of Franziska's mother, December 10, 1765.

[38] Superville, *Nachricht* (around 1732), 9.

[39] Van Dueren, *Ontdekkinge* (1688), 86.

These messengers played an important role and carried significant responsibility as they communicated between sick people and uroscopists. To the extent that patients wanted the uroscopist to know more about their medical history, current complaints, physical condition, or lifestyle, they had to trust that the messengers would transmit the information as accurately as possible. If the messenger failed to do so, the diagnosis and subsequent treatment risked being based on erroneous premises. The dangers were even greater in the other direction. It was up to the messenger to remember the uroscopist's words precisely, to relay accurately the prescribed therapy. For this reason some uroscopists and patients resorted to writing on slips of paper in order to avoid incomplete or distorted information. Thus we find the German translator of Pieter van Foreest mentioning in 1620 the "wide slips of paper" sent along for the patients of the former village pastor Johann Almersbach, who was known as a uroscopist in the Frankfurt area. Alongside the numerous herbs that Almersbach prescribed in faulty Latin, the papers apparently also communicated his "statement from the waters."[40]

A written message did not only presuppose that the uroscopist was able to write, however. It also only made sense if the patient or someone close to the patient was able to read it. The blacksmith of Gnadenthal Monastery, by his own account, wrote his diagnosis on a slip of paper for the mother of the pregnant Weidnerin only "because she absolutely wanted that and [he] did not want to deny her."[41] Neither mother nor daughter were literate and, as the mother recalled, "because they were not able to read it," she gave it to "the baker of Gelbing to read"—that is, to precisely one of the two men suspected of having impregnated her daughter.[42] Lorenz Fries's account of a patient who "brought me urine and asked that I give him in writing what it indicated, which I did," also suggests that this was not common practice.[43]

With increasing literacy among the populace, written messages may have gained more significance over time. The barber-surgeon of Essingen, for instance, a popular uroscopist, was well known in the middle of the eighteenth century for giving "written slips of paper" to messengers.[44] Daniel de Superville, too, said about uroscopists: "And if you are only willing to give them a good number of *groschen*, they are quite happy to give you handwritten slips of paper."[45] Also, visual representations of the time show slips of paper in the hand of the uroscopist or the messenger, on which the uroscopist had apparently written something. There is always the possibility, however, that these were simply prescriptions for the apothecary (see Figure 3.1).

---

[40]   Foreest, *Uromanteia* (1620), 236–44.
[41]   Stadtarchiv Schwäbisch-Hall, Bestand 11, Nr. 84, interrogation of the blacksmith, September 18, 1784.
[42]   Ibid., interrogation of the mother, September 11, 1784.
[43]   Fries, *Spiegel* (1518), LXIIIv.
[44]   Staatsarchiv Ludwigsburg, B 412 37, interrogation of Sabina Bremerin, December 10, 1765.
[45]   Superville, *Nachricht* (around 1732), 28.

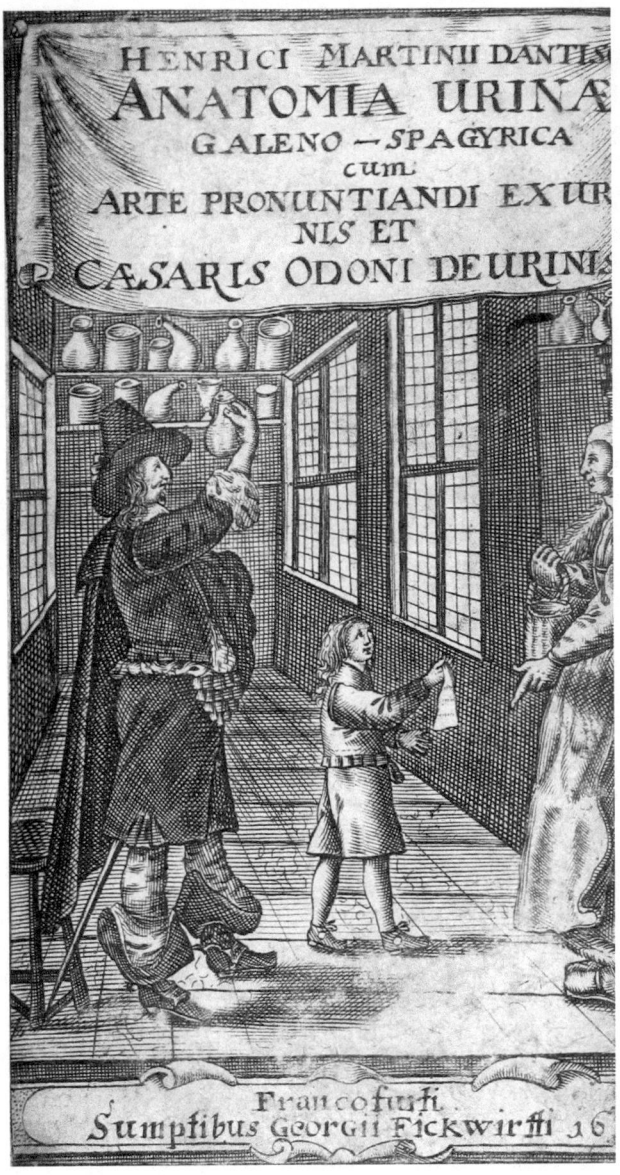

Figure 3.1   A uroscopist and his customers, in: Martini, *Anatomia urinae* (1658)

Diagnosing Pregnancy

The possibility of an anonymous diagnosis was of particular importance in confirming or ruling out pregnancy,[46] and by all accounts, demand was great. "I saw the urine of many women in Leipa who wanted to know, whether they were pregnant," the young Bohemian physician Georg Handsch, for example, reported about his visits in his native town around 1550. His own sister was among them, as was the daughter of the local ruling family Berka.[47] In medieval and early modern medical writings, various typical characteristics of the urine of pregnant women were described. The most important signs were patches of cloudiness forming in the pregnant woman's urine, with dust particles inside them that moved up and down.[48] This reference to a clouding of the urine and to a rather coarse and granular substance as a sign of pregnancy can be found in most uroscopy treatises. According to Jean Fernel, if you shook the urine of a pregnant woman lightly, little bubbles or granules formed on its surface. If you let it sit for a long time, a coarse, not very dense material would settle on the bottom or remain floating in the liquid. It looked not unlike plucked wool,[49] a comparison that is also found with other authors and was attributed to the Arabic tradition.[50] Rowland Watkyns went so far as to assert the presence of shells as a typical characteristic of pregnant women's urine: "When that a swimming cloud is found or known/ in womans urine driving up and down/ and mixt with shells; this symptom ne'r beguil'd,/ but plainly shews, that woman is with child."[51]

The color of pregnant women's urine was generally described as reddish. Ambroise Paré's explanation for this red coloration was that the menstrual period, suppressed during pregnancy, heated up the cervix of the uterus, which was located near the bladder's exit. Small particles of blood would enter the

---

[46] On uroscopic diagnosis of pregnancy see especially Vieillard, *Urologie* (1903), 90–94. Cheymol's *Le diagnostic* (1973) uses the medical knowledge of around 1970 as its yardstick and draws largely on the sources named by Vieillard.

[47] ÖNB Vienna, Cod. 11205, 76v; see also e.g. Primrose, *De vulgi erroribus* (1658), 102; Cordus, *De urinis* (1543), no pagination; Kolreutter, *Von rechten Gebreuchen* (1574), chapter 1.

[48] Cf. e.g. Fries, *Spiegel* (1518), LXVIIr; Apollinaris, *Tractätlein* (1663), 96; Apollinaris warns at the same time, however, that this sign can be deceiving and that its absence in no way means that pregnancy can be ruled out. Avicenna, *Canon* (1595), 51v, also mentions particles that move up and down as a sign of pregnancy.

[49] Fernel, *Universa medicina* (1644), 594; similarly e.g. Walaeus, *Medica* (1660), 77f; Rega, *Tractatus* (1733), 1st treatise, 124.

[50] Pfizerus, *Zwey sonderbare Bücher* (1673), 170; Kräutermann, *Curieuser und vernünfftiger Urin-Artzt* (1732), 114.

[51] Watkyns, *Flamma* (1662), 147.

neighboring bladder and were excreted with the urine.[52] According to a similar account, in Wood's *Epitomie*, if a woman was pregnant, her urine became clouded and reddish for the most part "as soon as the child is alive."[53] Some authors also considered gold-colored urine with a watery ring to be a sign of pregnancy but gold was often also described as "red" at the time.[54]

In the writing of some authors we encounter more specific clues and somewhat more unusual procedures. According to Fernel, if the urine of a pregnant woman was mixed with white wine, it resembled a broth of boiled beans.[55] If you looked at the urine—he probably meant in the patient's chamber pot—and saw your face, then this too was a sign that the woman was pregnant, if she did not suffer from a fever.[56] Other authors recommended letting the woman's urine sit for three days and then filter it through a linen cloth. If little animals or worms were visible in the cloth, the woman was pregnant. A further possibility was to put a clean needle in the woman's urine and leave it there for a night. If there were red spots on the needle the next morning, the woman was pregnant.[57]

An examination of the urine was also thought to indicate how advanced the pregnancy was. Valentin Kräutermann (aka Christoph von Hellwig), in his *Curieuser und vernünfftiger Urin-Artzt*, named the most important criteria, although he did warn that such changes could also occur in women with menstrual disorders. He claimed that in the first three months of pregnancy, the urine was more on the golden-yellow side and very cloudy, shot through with small particles that formed little balls. In the second and third months of pregnancy, there was "a lot of clear [urine] on top, but thick [urine] at the bottom, looking like yeast." Toward the seventh month, the urine would first become paler and resemble water in which knuckles of veal had been cooked. Toward delivery, the urine became red and cloudy.[58]

The urine was also thought to reveal whether the baby was a boy or a girl. If the characteristic cloudiness of the urine tended to move toward the bottom of the flask, a girl was expected, but if it ascended toward the surface, a boy. Following another tradition, the sex of the unborn child could be determined

---

[52]   Paré, *Oeuvres* (1633), 687.

[53]   Wood, *Epitomie* (1653), 233f.

[54]   Anonymous, *Judgment of all urynes* (around 1555): "Uryne of a woman red as gold with a watry cyrcle above, betokeneth that she is with chylde"; cf. Geyl, *Traité* (1909); Fernel's description of the urine of pregnant women as "lemon yellow" or moderately "livid" in color was unusual (Fernel, *Universa medicina* (1644), 594f.).

[55]   Fernel, *Universa medicina* (1644), 594f.

[56]   Anonymous, *Judgment of all urynes* (around 1555); Anonymous, *Key to unknowne knowledge* (1599).

[57]   According to a clearly skeptical Zacchia (*Quaestiones* (1651), 70), quoting Mizaldo and Wecher.

[58]   Kräutermann, *Curieuser und vernünfftiger Urin-Artzt* (1732), 114.

by the germination of grains of either wheat or barley soaked in the pregnant woman's urine.[59] His own mother, young Georg Handsch reported, had observed that her urine was turbid when she carried a girl and clear when it was a boy.[60]

Diagnosing pregnancy from urine was firmly rooted in the medical tradition. As with other aspects of uroscopy, some early modern physicians emphatically rejected this widespread practice, however. Thus K.B. Behrens, while admitting that urine changed during pregnancy, indeed that it had a different color in the first months of pregnancy than in the last, derided the belief that one could make a specific judgment on that basis. It seemed to him "as ludicrous as [the idea] that one could, as some believe, see tiny dogs' heads in the spittle of rabid dogs."[61] According to Laurent Joubert (1529–1583), if the urine of a pregnant woman changed at all, the change only showed that the menstrual period was absent, something the woman knew better than the doctor and without the help of uroscopy.[62] In Paolo Zacchia's view, pregnancy could be learned from the urine of a woman as much as her secret thoughts could be read from it.[63] Some physicians drew on personal experience as well. His wife had given birth to 10 children, said Thoner, and her urine had never shown the expected typical changes during her pregnancies.[64] To underscore his point, he told the story of two doctors from Ulm who examined the urine of the sick wife of a burgher on a daily basis. It happened that her maidservant feared she might be pregnant and secretly replaced the sick woman's urine with her own. The doctors noticed no changes in the urine and the maidservant felt relieved. But several months later, she gave birth to a child.[65]

Such learned criticism seems to have had very little effect on the widespread popular acceptance of uroscopy as a means of diagnosing pregnancy, however. The outstanding significance of uroscopy in diagnosing pregnancy in early modern lay medical culture thus also throws revealing light on the changing perception and experience of pregnancy. Barbara Duden, in particular, has sparked lively discussion with her assertion that since the early nineteenth century, the doctor's feeling for the child's movement and listening with a stethoscope increasingly took the place of the subjective experience and personal narrative of the pregnant woman.[66] In the twentieth century, according to Duden, the shift to laboratory diagnosis and the use of ultrasound gave this development further momentum: "Today pregnancy begins with a test." Duden describes this development as

---

59   Wood, *Epitomie* (1653), 233f.
60   ÖNB Vienna, Cod. 11205, 77v.
61   Henninger, *Theses* (1712), 2; Henninger was critical of this technique.
62   Behrens, *Wasserbeschawen* (1688), 11.
63   Joubert, *Erreurs* (1578), 273f.
64   Zacchia, *Quaestiones* (1651), 70.
65   Thoner, *Observationum* (1649), 344.
66   Ibid., 345.

the story of a "destruction of corporeal sense." The "perception of pregnancy as the unique, intimately personal state of an 'expectant' mother" has been lost, argues Duden.[67]

Without a doubt Duden has made an important point. Especially due to the visualization of the fetus via ultrasound, the experience of pregnancy and the perception of the unborn child as an independent person have changed in the past decades. If we are to trust the early modern sources on the subject, ordinary women only began to experience the fetus as a real, ensouled child when they felt it move. The English term "quickening" is, in fact, said to be derived from the original meaning of "quick," that is, "alive." Women today, by contrast, experience the fetus within days and weeks as a "baby," one that might seem to be "waving" at them in the first ultrasound image. This has serious consequences when it comes to the trauma of a miscarriage and a massive impact on the social and political discussion of abortion.

The great significance of uroscopy as a means of diagnosing pregnancy in premodern medical culture sets Duden's thesis of "the former precedence of somatic over learned knowledge" in a rather different light, however.[68] Clearly, early modern women did not necessarily prefer to rely on their subjective, bodily perception to confirm or rule out pregnancy. Quite to the contrary: they hoped that an examination of their urine would allow them to know as quickly as possible whether they were pregnant or not, at a time when their own bodily sensations were ambiguous. Possible signs of pregnancy, especially the missing of a menstrual period, were considered rather unreliable at the time, especially in women who had not yet given birth. As mentioned above, women (and for a long time doctors as well) understood their periods as a monthly purification. With the help of menstruation, the female body regularly freed itself of harmful, corrupted, or at least superfluous matter, which, if it were allowed to remain in the body, could cause a vast array of serious diseases.[69] If a woman missed a period, this therefore by no means provided a clear indication that she was pregnant. It was just as likely that her monthly bleeding was suppressed or had slowed down; and if she began to put on weight, this could just as well be due to an increasing accumulation of retained menstrual blood or other morbid humors in the lower abdomen.[70] Sometimes the initial suspicion of a pregnancy due to a missing period was somewhat corroborated a few weeks later by the vomiting typical of pregnancy and by strange food cravings. But these signs were often missing, and when present they could equally be interpreted as the consequence

---

[67] Duden, *"Geheimnisse"* (1992).
[68] Duden, *Wissen* (2002), 11f; cf. eadem, *Frauenleib* (1994).
[69] Cf. Stolberg, *A woman's hell?* (1999); idem, *Erfahrungen* (2004).
[70] Duden, *Wissen* (2002), 12.

of a disturbed menstruation.[71] Thus there was often a fair share of uncertainty, until the woman finally felt the first movements of her child.

By the same token, early knowledge of pregnancy was of great importance when it came to the woman's health. If pregnancy was not the cause of the missing menstrual period, the woman was well advised to take remedies that would bring back her period or would empty her body of the morbid matter in another way. If she failed to do so, the corrupted menstrual blood would accumulate in her body, with potentially fatal effects. However, if the woman was pregnant, medicines which were given to promote menstruation could cause a miscarriage. In light of this situation, an unambiguous confirmation or ruling out of pregnancy was essential. And this was exactly what many women hoped to get from uroscopists—who, for their part, were most responsive to this demand. In a way then, the lines of conflict were exactly the opposite of what recent historical research has presumed. Women preferred the "objective" diagnosis based on urine, based on criteria that had been established by tradition over hundreds of years, to merely relying on their subjective sensations. Physicians like Laurent Joubert, on the other hand, were quite happy to rely on the women's narrative. Joubert had great appreciation for what experienced women, in particular, the mothers of several children, had to tell: "you have to believe what they have experienced many times, [namely] the change in herself that the woman feels due to her pregnancy, in both her belly and her breasts."[72]

While even learned doctors had to admit that their less educated competitors were occasionally remarkably accurate, they believed this was just luck. They might just as well have tossed a coin, they argued.[73] Savoring the moment, Thoner recounted the case of a woman whom he had diagnosed as pregnant judging from various signs. Yet she had had her urine examined by a famous uroscopist who ruled out a pregnancy. He was so sure of himself that he vowed to provide for the child's sustenance and education if indeed she were pregnant. Following birth, Thoner added with praise, he had at least honored his word.[74]

However, there were some uroscopists who were renowned for diagnosing pregnancy with remarkable accuracy. The vintner Kizler, for example, recounted how his sick wife had "not really known what ailed her [...] and therefore asked him to take her water to the woman in Schozach." The healer had then explained that his wife was pregnant—and indeed she was.[75] Misdiagnosis—above all an incorrect ruling out of a pregnancy—could have fatal consequences, however. Such was the lamentable experience of the newlywed wife of the farmhand

---

[71]   On early modern notions of menstruation and its role in the female body see Stolberg, *A woman's hell?* (1999) and idem, *Erfahrungen* (2004).

[72]   Joubert, *Erreurs* (1578), 281–3.

[73]   Ibid., 281.

[74]   Ibid., 280.

[75]   Thoner, *Observationum* (1649), 344f.

Jonas Stoffer from Bahlen when, a few months after the wedding, her "head, feet and everything [became] extraordinarily swollen."[76] According to an official report, she "was given the opinion" by an itinerant drug peddler (*Laborant*) "that she was not pregnant" after the man had been shown "the woman's urine, salvo respectu." Rather, she was said to be "very obstructed and tending toward dropsy." When her husband brought her urine to the Wittenburg apothecary soon after, the apothecary "agreed with the above opinion" telling him "if he wanted to preserve the woman, he would have to take some medicines with him." The husband, it was said, feared that she "might be harmed by them" if she were pregnant, saying that "it [was] a matter of conscience." But the apothecary replied that he, the apothecary, "really ought to know, [and that she was] not pregnant." So the woman took the remedies, which did not, as the apothecary had announced, stimulate the flow of sweat, but "had a purgative effect." The following night, the woman gave birth to a child. According to the midwife and other women who were standing by, the child was "premature" and died following the emergency baptism, as did the mother two days later. The midwife stated that the child was still moving in its mother's body the day before the birth. She was convinced that "if the mother had not used the drugs, the child would not have come so early."[77]

Sometimes the wish for an early confirmation of pregnancy was motivated by a desire for pregnancy. Women were eager to know as soon as possible when they had conceived so they could take precautions that might prevent the loss of the child. They could stop breastfeeding their previous child, as was popular custom, according to Georg Handsch, in sixteenth-century Bohemia.[78] They could adopt a healthier lifestyle, for instance, or have a prophylactic bloodletting done, which was common practice. But for unmarried women, too, knowing early about a pregnancy was a matter of urgency, although for very different reasons. For them, much was at stake. Pregnancies out of wedlock may not have been uncommon in early modern society, but the consequences were often grave for the affected women and could jeopardize their existence. In many places they were subject to drastic reactions and dishonoring punishment. Parents and employers might cast the woman out. If the father of the child did not marry her, she would probably never be able to live a "normal" life as a married wife and mother.[79] Knowing as soon as possible about the pregnancy allowed her to try to get married before the pregnancy showed, or else, if she wanted to disregard the commands of the Church, to take "expelling" medicines so as to

---

[76]   HStA Stuttgart A 213 Bü. 6734, interrogation of Johannes Kizler, March 4, 1780

[77]   Landesarchiv Schwerin, Altes Archiv 2.12–2/3, 178, report to the Duke, November 15, 1702.

[78]   ÖNB Vienna, Cod. 11205, 93v, "why they want to know, whether they are pregnant."

[79]   Landesarchiv Schwerin, Altes Archiv 2.12–2/3, 178, interrogation of the midwife, November 25, 1702.

effect a miscarriage. The latter was strictly forbidden, but naturally it was very hard to prove if it was done in the early stages of pregnancy. Since many women seem to have understood the life of the child to begin only when they felt the first movements, they may have found it none too difficult to reconcile with their conscience.

As we have seen, uroscopy promised in these cases in particular a welcome degree of anonymity in a society in which word of who consulted which healer got around quickly. It was not necessary to visit the uroscopist in person; it was enough if he looked at the urine which he had discreetly received from relatives, friends, or paid messengers. In certain cases, women even feigned a different identity. Karin Stukenbrock has found a case in which the mother of a pregnant woman sent a maidservant to a midwife with her daughter's urine and asked the maid to pretend the urine came from the daughter of a *Bauernvogt* (peasant reeve) from a different village. She wanted to know if the daughter was pregnant and, if she was, how far along she was. The midwife diagnosed a pregnancy of 11 weeks and refused to give her an abortifacient. And indeed, the woman gave birth around six months later, in other words at the end of the nine months after the date of conception the midwife had identified.[80]

The outstanding importance of uroscopic diagnosis when pregnancy out of wedlock was feared is nicely illustrated, together with the various, sometimes strategic, functions it could assume, by the records of the detailed interrogations carried out as part of official inquests into suspected cases of abortion or child murder. One such case was that of Franziska Eichert from the Stuttgart area, who was unmarried and around 38 years old.[81] She had given birth to a dead child. It was her conviction that it was "her great rage" at the father of the child, Private Josef Heydelberger, that caused the death. Strong affects were recognized by both doctors and laypeople as an important cause of illness.[82] Heydelberger, she said, had had a close and ongoing "association" with the former maid of an innkeeper who had allegedly even become pregnant by him. A certain man or "doctor" from the woods, to whom her daughter had sent her urine, also thought that "in a rage, she had had a quick drink, which harmed her more than if she had drunk poison." What was meant here was presumably the hasty consumption of cold water, a recognized cause of stagnation and obstruction in the body. Later, a witness, Anna Maria Mettmännin, confirmed that Franziska's mother had called her, as her daughter lay wailing in bed, to ask if she could take her urine to a certain Bergmann, who indeed explained that "the person had had a great rage" and that "the bile had gone into the blood." For two or three *gulden* he promised to help, but Franziska did not have the money. At that point he advised her to

---

80   Stukenbrock, *Abtreibung* (1993); Labouvie, *Andere Umstände* (1998).
81   Staatsarchiv Ludwigsburg, B 412 37.
82   Stolberg, *Zorn* (2005).

"send her urine to a local doctor," in which case the medicine would be paid for by authorities if she "asked for it."

Since she had sought the advice of a barber-surgeon in Essingen earlier in her pregnancy and received medication from him, and because the child had died in the end, Franziska fell under suspicion of abortion. All that Franziska's mother could remember at the beginning of the interrogation was that her daughter "was always sick" during her pregnancy. Which is why she, the mother, had sent the urine to the doctor, in order to see "whether or not she was pregnant, having missed her monthly cleansing this whole time." She claimed that they did not consult the barber-surgeon of Essingen but had only asked him two years earlier for his advice, although it would have been better if she had sent someone to him "because he would surely have known her state and could have told her whether or not her daughter [was] pregnant" since the barber-surgeon knew everything. Two years before that her daughter was also doing poorly due to her "time of the month" and the barber-surgeon rejected the idea of pregnancy, saying that she had upset her stomach with a piece of liverwurst. Yet Sabine Bremerin, who had brought the urine of various people to the barber-surgeon, stated that Franziska had commissioned her to take her urine several years earlier and "had not given any message so the barber-surgeon would see what ailed her and would send her suitable medicine." And because he had "helped her back then" she "gave her the urine again" this time telling her not to say anything more about her condition. The barber-surgeon excluded a pregnancy, saying her stomach was "quite slimy [and with] bile in it; she is also languid in her limbs" and gave her two small jars of medicine. Confronted with the account of Bremerin, the mother was suddenly able to recall that indeed, this had taken place, right at the beginning of the pregnancy, soon after "her monthly time was missing" and thus long before they had known about her pregnancy. But the barber-surgeon had said that "he could not see that the person was with child."

The mother's initial denial suggests that it was entirely clear to her that a consultation with the barber-surgeon could easily be construed as an attempt to determine pregnancy as early as possible so as to be able to secretly end it. But as soon as the consultation came to light through the messenger's statement, the barber-surgeon's diagnosis brought welcome relief: When the daughter, trusting the barber-surgeon's proven diagnostic abilities, ingested a bile-expelling remedy, one could hardly hold this against her.

Another case illustrates even more clearly the strategic, legitimizing function uroscopy could take on when used to rule out pregnancy: the case of Maria Margaretha Weidner who was investigated in Schwäbisch Hall in 1784 on suspicion of attempted abortion.[83] The 28-year-old maid, now detained, confessed during her interrogation that she had "mingled in the flesh" first with her married master, a baker, and then twice with his servant in the following three weeks. "Eight days after

---

[83]　Stadtarchiv Schwäbisch-Hall, Bestand 11 (Kriminalakten), Nr. 84.

she had lain with the baker's servant"—this is how it is stated in the interrogation record—"she expected her time according to her female condition, but such a time was missing." However, since her periods were "often disorderly she still doubted that she was pregnant." Her mother, whom she had told about her worry, "wanted to know for certain" and went to a blacksmith in the nearby Gnadenthal Monastery. She had heard that he was "used by many people" and was able to "identify diseases from the urine." They did not, according to the mother, "have any evil intentions in going to him." She was met by the blacksmith's wife, to whom she gave the urine without saying anything further and without letting on what she wanted to know. The blacksmith examined the urine and concluded that the female person in question must have "hurt herself with snow-water" and that her disease stemmed from "chilling" her blood. In the end she only spoke with the blacksmith's wife, saying that if the person in question were pregnant, she did not want any medicine. The woman said, however, that there was no pregnancy in this case, and when the mother explained "that the body of this woman rose toward the heart," that her belly was swollen, in other words, the wife replied that "it was simply due to flatulence" and gave her drugs for 10 *batzen*. For his part, the blacksmith confirmed in an interrogation before local authorities that indeed an old woman had come to him at the time, giving him the urine and telling him nothing more. He claimed, however, that she had asked him if it was a case of pregnancy, to which he replied that he could not judge this from the urine and, responding to her request, gave her a few lines saying "that he [had] found right away that she could possibly be pregnant." His statement, however, clearly contradicted what he had written on a piece of paper, which the mother had saved and which said nothing of a possible pregnancy (cf. Figure 3.2). It seems that the mother had asked for his diagnosis in writing with a precise goal in mind: She wanted to be able to prove that the uroscopist had seen no signs of pregnancy and thus that her daughter would not be guilty of abortion if she took his remedies. A judicial assessment of the case came to the conclusion that the blacksmith had "hidden the pregnancy" from the mother. Despite these precautions, however, the daughter visited the blacksmith a week later, if only, as she claimed, because she felt unwell, and after she had told her sister and others that she was pregnant.

In the end, the blacksmith's remedies caused heavy vomiting but no abortion. The daughter, despite the exonerating circumstances, was ultimately handed down the punishment of sweeping the town square three times in public disgrace and was banned from the Hall area for four years. Her mother was reprimanded, the baker's servant was sentenced to 14 days in prison, and his master went without punishment.

Making Sense of the Body

Another reason why uroscopy enjoyed immense popularity and lasting trust is buried still deeper in the medical culture of the day. As the example of menstrual disorders and their explanation shows, the uroscopists' diagnostic judgments simply made sense in the eyes of patients and relatives. They fit seamlessly into their ideas about the body and its diseases. The physicians' epistolary council presented above has already provided some illustration of this. In the course of the seventeenth century, physicians began to part company with the traditional doctrine of humors which was familiar to and understood by ordinary people. Among the vast majority of the population, however, the old ideas, images, and terms continued to dominate—and to make uroscopy an obvious choice—well into the nineteenth century. "People for the most part derive their knowledge of the nature and causes of illness from humoral pathology," a doctor in Swabian Mindelheim related as late as 1860: "The changes in the liquid or the deviations in the body's humors from their natural quantities and constitution occasion the various diseases. Thus the cure must be begun from the inside out and the quack etc. charlatan or old woman must be given a sample of the sick person's expelled liquid (urine) for the purpose of inspecting, judging and recognizing the disease and its prognosis."[84] The numerous unlicensed healers continued to express their diagnostic judgment in the language of traditional humoral medicine—originally promulgated by physicians—and to adapt the diagnosis to the medical world of patients and their families.

When they examined the urine in the presence of patients or those around them, skilled uroscopists also seem to have pointed out and explained the visible changes in the urine to support their diagnosis, just as barber-surgeons were eager to show sick people and their relatives the blood from a bloodletting to demonstrate how the blood was, for instance, burnt or phlegmy. As late as the end of the eighteenth century, F.X. Rehmann described this as follows: "The common people believe that the barber-surgeon can recognize all possible, imminent, or already present diseases in the blood let from a vein and collected in a pot, or pregnancy, and with the latter, whether the woman is carrying a boy or a girl in her womb. The barber-surgeons do everything they can to encourage this erroneous belief of the rural population because it is profitable for them, just as is making prophesies from urine."[85] In the same manner, uroscopy could satisfy the patient, as Glen P. Jenkins put it, by providing "the tangible evidence of what ailed him."[86] He could see with his own eyes the morbid matter which had been expelled with the urine.

A relatively early source affords a particularly rich view of the way in which the uroscopic judgment could be integrated into widely accepted lay ideas about the

---

[84] BSB Munich, Cgm 6874 111, medical topography of Mindelheim, 1861.
[85] Ackermann, *Glaubens-Bekenntniß* (1783), 72.
[86] Jenkins, *Diagnosis by diagram* (1989), 439f.

body and its diseases and derived plausibility from them. It is a handwritten guide to uroscopy ascribed to a "plebanus," that is, a priest, by the name of Doct. Micha Braun from Krems—by all appearances the author was the physician Michael Braun who moved to Krems in 1526 to serve as a priest but continued to practice medicine and seems to have died two years later.[87] The manuscript has survived in the *Bayerische Staatsbibliothek* in Munich under the title *Modus iudicandae urinae*.[88] Of particular note for our discussion is the section entitled *De formula loquendi vulgariter in iudicio urinali*. As the title suggests, it offers formulae, so to speak, from which uroscopists could put together their *judicium*, depending on the case and written in "vulgar speech" so as to be comprehensible to ordinary lay people: "Dear friend, as the urine shows me, the person's disease comes above all from and is based in the stomach, where a lot of slime has accumulated and settled in the folds. This is why the stomach is upset and cannot digest or turn food into nutrition for the body. [The person has] not much appetite and what appetite there is, it is not natural. Also, food is not turned into good humors but only into slime and waste."[89]

In this, from the contemporary perspective, familiar and plausible diagnosis, we encounter once again the old doctrine of the cold, phlegmy stomach. It no longer had enough heat to concoct food sufficiently and thus accumulated morbid matter. It was precisely this morbid, wet, cold phlegm that patients and healers thought they were looking at in the watery, slimy vomit that was produced when a patient was given one of the widely available emetics.

Furthermore, the reader was advised to say that he found in the urine "several fluxes from the head," which, however, had "their origin in the stomach." This was because there was "a lot of slime and dirt in the stomach, which sends its vapors to the head and there causes the flux." Again we are dealing with a very versatile interpretive pattern. "Fluxes" counted among the central disease categories in traditional humoralism and played a key role in lay medical culture well into the nineteenth century.[90] They referred to morbid, unnatural humors, which moved in a more or less unrestrained manner within the body and could accumulate in various places. Joint complaints, for instance, were often ascribed to "fluxes," especially to those whose substance was particularly "acrimonious," which helped explain the burning, cutting, or stabbing pain. According to traditional humoral doctrine, the most important source of "fluxes" was the brain, which was characterized mainly by phlegm, and was thus moist and cold. The majority of "fluxes" were thus "fluxes from the head." In many cases, the diagnosis of a flux from the head was confirmed by a perceptible "catarrh." The mucous matter that flowed out from the nose or down the throat was

---

[87]   Wiedemann, *Geschichte* (1882), 60.

[88]   BSB Munich, Clm 25087.

[89]   Ibid., 5v–6r; the meaning of the German term *feld*, translated here as "folds" (for *Falten*), is not entirely certain.

[90]   Cf. Stolberg, *Experiencing illness* (2011), 95–100.

taken to offer tangible proof that morbid or at least excessively abundant phlegm was collecting in the brain. The older academic medicine as well had assumed that this phlegm could flow directly from the brain downward.

This overarching concept of the flux from the head was to be linked to the well-established notion of *vapores*: under the influence of the concoctive heat in the stomach or due to heat arising from its putrefaction or fermentation, subtle, vaporous morbid matter was released and rose from the belly upward.[91] The manuscript advised the uroscopist to illustrate these processes to those seeking advice ("so that you understand correctly") by comparing them with the familiar image of a steaming dung heap: "Every day, when the sun shines on the dung heap pile, the dung heap emits steam, because the sun moves it to; it is the same way with the stomach." The ascending vapors cooled down and liquefied again, much in the way of the vapors in a distilling flask. Depending on where this happened, in the chest or only in the head under the skullcap, different symptoms resulted.

If the urine had come from a woman, a third diagnosis could be added to the *judicium*. The uroscopist could identify "some impurity of the uterus," which had collected over a long time. Around 1600, the majority of learned physicians had parted company with the traditional conception of menstruation as serving primarily to cleanse the female body of all those impurities which built up in it every month.[92] Among the population, however, the interpretation of menstruation as a beneficial, life-preserving "purification" of the body dominated well into the nineteenth century. The wife of Gottlob Wagner, for example, who sought uroscopic counsel from the "doctress" of Schozach because of her bloated body, shortness of breath, and pain in her side, was convinced that her complaints stemmed from the fact that she had not had her period in 26 weeks.[93] Women from the upper classes as well took great care in noting down every little irregularity of their period, recording the slightest change in the amount and consistency of their "monthly flux." To them such changes could indicate grave danger for their bodies and lives. A reduced or absent menstrual flow almost inevitably meant—except in the case of pregnancy—that the impure, corruptible matter which the body usually freed itself of now remained in the body, and in the uterus in particular, and was most likely to decay further. Thus the manuscript suggested that one say of the female patient and her "flower" "that she did not have it at the right time or else had little and it was colored differently" than corresponded to her nature and when "such mucus" became rampant, what followed were "headaches, fainting, weakness of the whole body; and her breath is such that she feels she is suffocating and all her limbs are without strength."

A dreaded consequence of disturbed menstruation and the accumulation of morbid matter in the uterus—suggested here by the symptoms of fainting, physical

---

[91] Ibid., 165–7.

[92] Stolberg, *Erfahrungen* (2004); Stolberg, *Monthly malady* (2000).

[93] HStA Stuttgart A 213 Bü. 6734, interrogation of Gottlob Wagner, March 4, 1780.

weakness, and shortness of breath—was the "suffocation of the mother" or "hysteria," a disease that was still attributed to the uterus by many early modern physicians and only gradually came to be reframed as a "nervous" disease that could affect both sexes.

There was a further diagnostic possibility for the uroscopist, one that was independent of gender, which centered on whether the urine was cold (i.e. pale and bright according to traditional criteria) or warm (i.e. dark, with a more intense yellow color). In the case of "cold" urine, the uroscopist could conclude that there was an "obstruction" of the vessels and bowels and thus deduce "weight loss and weakness of the whole body." The idea behind this reasoning was probably that cold made the mucus—as, in fact, it did any morbid matter—particularly viscous. The resulting obstruction of the vessels and bowels hindered the vital flow of humors in the body and the excretion of morbid matter. In addition—though this is not elaborated in the manuscript—the obstruction of the vessels was often associated with decomposition and decay in the body. In the same way that water left to stagnate in ponds or pools became foul, the humors in the body, it was feared, would putrefy if not kept in motion.

If, on the other hand, the uroscopist found "warm" urine, he was to explain that the patient's urine showed "a great heat of the whole body from which comes weakness, fainting, obstruction of the bowels, thirst, headaches and the like." Patients were to be warned that if they did not follow a careful regimen of good eating and drinking, a "consumption" of the body might come to pass. Here as well, the cause of such a condition is not explained, but it can be easily deduced from the imagery used in the overarching explanatory model of humoral medicine. Strong heat made the liquid components of the humors evaporate, so it thickened the humors and ultimately this too led to an obstruction of the bowels and vessels. But, different from cold, heat also threatened to consume the substance of the body itself. "Consumption" was the obvious consequence.

Finally, a formula was offered to the uroscopist, which served to make provisions for misdiagnosis and misprognosis. He was to say: "For the time being, this is what the urine shows me." Whether there were other changes in the urine which could not be discerned because other material was mixed in, he could not say.

These terms, concepts, and images have become foreign to us. They seem to come from a very different, strange world. Yet this was the world, the medical cosmology in which ordinary people lived and moved and which they took for a granted. No patient today would ask his physician, for example, as the Austrian Archduke Ferdinand did, whether his urine was "digested."[94] What is more, when we study these humoral concepts in more detail it is striking how closely many of them were linked to what patients perceived as naturally given bodily experience, to their subjective sensations and perceptions, which were taken, in turn, to constantly corroborate these concepts.

---

[94]   ÖNB Vienna, Cod. 11206, 20v.

We do not know the degree to which this diagnostic guide found practical application. Regrettably only very few of the actual uroscopic diagnoses of irregular uroscopists are extant. The few that have been preserved suggest, however, that unlicensed uroscopists used terms and concepts that corresponded to those known and trusted by the population at large. Thus the aforementioned note written by a uroscopist near Schwäbisch Hall at the end of the eighteenth century at the request of the mother of the sick/pregnant woman reads (see Figure 3.2): "We have seen here a cooling of the blood, with putrefaction of the humors and accumulating mucus in the kidneys as well as acrimony in the bladder and obstruction in the spine. Also, lower back pain and flying heat in the head, fitful sleep, swollen stomach and intestines, with a tearing in the nerves." We find a whole range of concepts here which were central to the lay medical culture of the day and which also had their place in scholarly medicine, from "cooling," "putrefaction," and "mucous obstruction" to "flying heat" and a "tearing in the nerves."

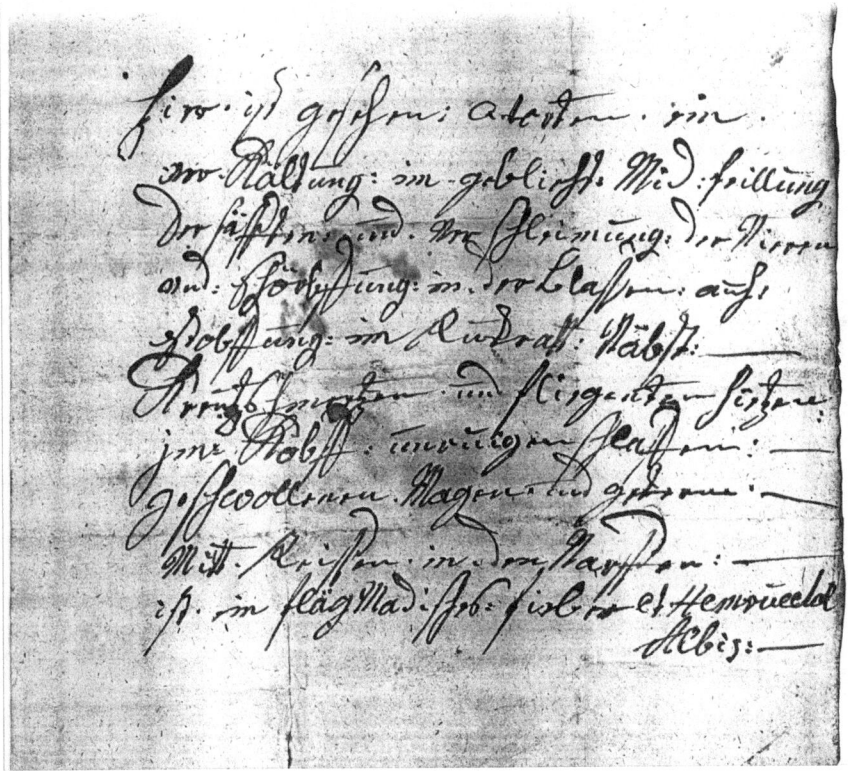

Figure 3.2   Uroscopy note of a blacksmith, 1784 (Schwäbisch Hall, Stadtarchiv, Best. 11, 84)

A similar note by a Parisian uroscopist from 1820, published by François Victor Mérat, draws primarily on two familiar concepts which resonated with popular notions: "winds" and the accumulation of "mucus." Mérat had a 64-year-old hypochondriacal patient from his practice in Paris to thank for the note. She had secretly had a gardener take her urine to a uroscopist in the *Quartier des Halles* but after she had taken the uroscopist's remedy, she suffered intense stomach pains. "According to the patient's urine," Mérat quoted from the uroscopist's note, "it seems to me that the regular functioning of the chest is inhibited by phlegm and a fatty plethora, which makes breathing difficult. Walking is disrupted, presence of fever, lack of sleep, which provokes winds, which leads to bloating. Appetite varies. The stomach is full of morbid mucus and is hardly emptied. The back and limbs are tired." Mérat saw this as an example of the "incomprehensible phrases" and "commonplaces" which uroscopists made use of, when they were not able to gain additional information about the patient. As Mérat pointed out, the healer had learned from the gardener only that the patient was an overweight, 64-year-old woman. His presumption of disturbed sleep, Mérat thought, would have seemed obvious for someone of her age, and any person who is sick generally feels weak. Finding a phlegmy stomach, he thought, was enough to make some Parisian physicians rich since people had an incredible fear of morbid mucus. The notion that the lungs or stomach were phlegmy seemed all too often confirmed by experience—by the slimy sputum that was expelled during respiratory tract infections or by the mucous vomit sometimes produced with the help of emetics. The same was true of the "winds" which, according to Mérat, were held responsible for any number of diseases and which were widely attributed to an accumulation of insufficiently concocted food whence the "winds" ascended like the fumes from dung heaps.[95]

A 1782 urine consultation of a Swabian hangman, published by Josef Xaver Rehmann, was also composed mainly of such familiar elements: "Concerning the patient's illness, I find from the—salva venia—urine that he has much feverish bile in the stomach, which impedes the power of digestion and goes into the blood in great amounts with the chyle, making the blood thick and heavy, so that it cannot complete its round in 4 to 5 times 24 hours; the liver is heated and dry, and the spleen obstructed, and while the bile is supposed to be separated from the blood in the spleen, the black and heavy blood moves mostly to the golden vein [hemorrhoids, M.S.], and this is the whole cause of most of the complaints; this is why a strong heat rises in the body, with feverish changes showing on the outside, frequent blockage of the chest, with changing axudit [accidentia (= symptoms)?, M.S.] and since most of the complaints come from the golden vein, a burning and tearing in the lower back occurs often, [a sense of] running and pain in the feet and the like. The illness itself, judging

---

[95]   Mérat, *Uromancie* (1821), 346.

from what the urine looks like, would not be that fatal, but such circumstances are often followed by apoplexy, which often causes death or otherwise palsy, therefore it would be advisable to lift the bilious raw matter from the stomach, attenuate the blood and keep the lower belly open properly." [96]

Again the *judicium* was based on widely recognized ideas. A hot "feverish" bile in the stomach together with an excessively hot and dry liver produced overheated, black (burnt), and viscous blood, which heated the entire body, brought forth pain, and collected near the hemorrhoids, so as to leave the body. The consultation also reveals that irregular healers were prepared to adopt new theories or explanatory models, as, in this case, the doctrine of blood circulation which, according to the hangman, was significantly slowed by the patient's viscous blood. [97]

Uroscopy as Ritual

We have seen how uroscopic diagnosis, using the familiar terms and concepts of humoralism, offered meaning and orientation to patients. Often underappreciated in their complexity and adaptability today, these concepts were readily understood in the context of the dominant ideas about the body and its illnesses and they generally accorded with patients' own—culturally framed—bodily experience. In the face of frightening and potentially fatal symptoms, uroscopy thus inspired a sense of control. Children already grew up with the knowledge that if one's relatives or neighbors fell ill, the best thing to do was to have their urine examined. And in a circular, self-fulfilling process, the daily practice of uroscopy strengthened people's belief in its significance and validity time and again. Quite rightly, physicians attributed people's unshakable trust in uroscopic diagnosis to the fact that patients witnessed again and again how their doctors examined the urine and then prescribed a treatment under which the patient got better. [98]

Uroscopy had even more to offer, however. It was not just a particularly popular diagnostic method among others, with a scope that was incomparably wider than that of nineteenth-century chemical urinalysis. Far more than most practices in modern medicine, uroscopy can be understood in cultural-

---

[96] Ackermann, *Glaubens-Bekenntniß* (1783), 83f; according to Ackermann (i.e. Rehmann) the patient suffered from a venereal disease. "Salva venia" was an expression commonly added to apologize for mentioning shameful substances or parts of the body.

[97] On the medical activities of early modern hangmen see Nowosadtko, *Wer Leben nimmt* (1993); eadem, *Scharfrichter und Abdecker* (1994), 162–78; Herzog, *Scharfrichterliche Medizin* (1994).

[98] Cf. e.g. Liphimeus, *Warnung* (1626), 64.

anthropological terms as a ritual.[99] It is true that some cultural anthropologists have argued that the term "ritual" ought to be essentially restricted to the domain of the occult and supernatural but this has remained controversial even within cultural anthropology. For early modern culture, at any rate, as for many non-Western cultures, it is virtually impossible to draw a clear-cut dividing line between the realms of the natural and the supernatural. Many contemporaries took sympathy and magic and even witchcraft and "inflicted" illnesses as part of the given natural order. For the purpose of historical analysis, a semiotic definition of "ritual" thus appears more helpful. From this perspective, uroscopic diagnosis, like other rituals, can be seen, to borrow from Stanley J. Tambiah's performative theory of the ritual, as "a medium for transmitting meanings, for the construction of social reality or, for that matter, for the creation and bringing to life of the cosmological scheme itself."[100] From this perspective, uroscopy, like other rituals, truly embodied "episodes of a repeated and simplified cultural communication in which the direct partners to a social interaction, and those observing it, share a mutual belief in the descriptive and prescriptive validity of the communication's symbolic contents and accept the authenticity of one another's intentions."[101]

This may seem rather abstract at first glance, but understanding uroscopy in this way as a ritual helps us to understand and explain the enduring validity of uroscopy in premodern lay medical culture. As soon as we see rituals not on a purely formal level as a predetermined sequence of different actions, but rather as a way of communicating meanings, it becomes clear that the cultural function and the success of uroscopy cannot be adequately explained based on the standards of modern scientific rationality. As "symbolic practices,"[102] as "constitutive and convincing acts,"[103] rituals cannot be falsified in the way a scientific theory can. A diagnostic practice or ritual that is so deeply anchored in culture and daily life needs no justification to begin with. It is by and large self-confirming and only begins to lose significance when the cultural context as such begins to change fundamentally, when new conceptions of man and nature, body and disease take hold. When this happens, as it did, in the case of uroscopy, gradually in the nineteenth century, new diagnostic procedures find their way into medicine and are accepted as appearing significantly superior to the previous methods.

---

[99] See for instance Winn's definition of "ritual" as a "standardized, repetitive, interpersonal symbolic act, that is formed according to social habits, retains a constant form over a long period of time, and influences or orients human affairs" (Winn, *Rechtsrituale* (1998), 449).

[100] Tambiah, *Performative approach* (1981), 120.

[101] Alexander, *Cultural pragmatics* (2006), 29.

[102] Alexander/Giesen/Mast, *Symbolic action* (2006).

[103] Tambiah, *Performative approach* (1981), 127.

The interpretation of early modern uroscopy as a ritual thus highlights dimensions to which justice is hardly done when uroscopy is treated merely as a "diagnostic procedure." In a sense, early modern physicians seem to have been quite aware of this. They tried to distinguish between their own approach to uroscopy, which they considered serious-minded, rational, and scientific, and "divination" from the urine, or "uromancy." They attributed the latter to the many popular uroscopists who, following the requests of their clientele, set out to identify diseases based on an inspection of the urine alone.[104] They compared such uroscopists with an "oracle"[105] or used terms such as "casting the urine,"[106] "urine prophets,"[107] "uromancy,"[108] or "urine prophesy."[109]

Such language was meant to be critical, even polemical. It was to unmask the uroscopic practice of their competitors as superstitious, rendering the physicians the sole representatives of a medicine that was rational and God-pleasing. Yet comparing uroscopy with an oracle actually hit the mark in several respects. The concentration in the uroscopist's face as he raised the matula—as recommended in uroscopy treatises—the delicate manner in which he shook the flask, held it into the light, perhaps making the liquid shimmer in a golden glow, all this helped lend the practice of uroscopy an aura of mystery. Even the physicians' disdainful accounts evidence how skillfully many uroscopists created a powerful aura with more than "double-tongued and stilted"[110] words alone. Ananius Horer launched a strident complaint against "empirical urine prophets, urine examiners, and seers," who "properly thumb their nose at the ignorant common folk, performing all kinds of strange ceremonies and gesticulations, holding the matula close to a mirror, measuring it with a compass, walking to and fro with it in their room, shaking and swirling the urine in the flask, pouring several drops of it on the floor, weighing the flask in their hand, smelling it, even tasting it (in which case they truly deserve the malmsey) [...] Several of these bamboozlers

---

[104] Zwinger/Staegerus, *De uromantias usu* (1705); presumably the work was written by Zwinger himself and merely defended by the doctoral candidate. Rega (Rega, *Tractatus* (1733), 2nd treatise, 1) by contrast distinguished between *uroscopia*, the viewing of the urine, and *ouromantia*, the uroscopist's judgment based on the inspection.

[105] Hechstetter, *Rararum observationum*, vol. 2 (1627), preface; Saltzmann, *De uromantia* (1651), no pagination; Turner, *Modern quack* (1718), 127.

[106] Turner, *Modern quack* (1718), dedication.

[107] Horer, *Artzney-Teuffel* (1634), 59; van Dueren, *Ontdekkinge* (1688), 34 ("pis-profeet").

[108] Saltzmann, *De uromantia* (1651); Schmidt, *Uromanticus castratus* (1697).

[109] Stahl, *Gründliche Abhandlung* (1739).

[110] Hygiander, *Regeln* (1744), 3r.

first distill or boil the urine, so that they may cause wonder with their antics, come into great demand and make a lot of money."[111]

Foreest, in Holland, also wrote about many uroscopists "who, in their inspection of urine, follow the superstitious Jews, using many odd ceremonies, walking around in their chamber now in this corner and now in that, making use of burning lights even in broad daylight, or even stepping outside into the air, or turning toward the sun, and finally going back into their chamber always holding the urine, swinging it back and forth, commonly smelling it too and pouring it out in drops or weighing it on scales and performing more of this kind of trickery, all to deceive the people, to cover up their lies, and gain a greater reputation with the rabble."[112] Indeed, to further their "authority and reputation" and "to cause wonder in the foolish rabble" many held the urine up to a "bright and clear mirror."[113] This use of mirrors is mentioned by various authors.[114] Others claimed that people favored taking the urine to the uroscopist on Sundays, "out of a certain superstition," because this was the day dedicated to holy things.[115]

With all its caustic sarcasm, the following description of the uroscopic practice of a "doctress" in Zottishofen around 1800—probably written by a physician—offers a particularly striking account of the healer's ability to stage the ritual of uroscopy: "Inspecting urine; strong bloodletting; even stronger purging; herbal potions that clear you out completely and fill many of her rooms—these are the mainstay of her medical miracle cures. She has learned most of them, as she says, from a thick medicine book she inherited from her grandfather, which we now see lying open every day—like a Sibylline book of oracles—before the bustling miracle doctress *in officio*, and from which she sometimes announces with prophetic power the pathological condition and its cure to the patients who come running to her. Much of her indeed wondrous renown, unshakable with the common pack, is however owed to the circumstance that she usually gives out her prescriptions in a state of heightened brandy enthusiasm, while expressing herself in ambiguous oracular language."[116]

---

[111] Horer, *Artzney-Teuffel* (1634), 59; a very similar description can be found in Hörnigk, *Politia medica* (1636), 177f.

[112] Foreest, *Uromanteia* (1620), 204; in similar terms, Behrens, *Wasserbeschawen* (1688), 31, scornfully commented on "all kinds of superstitious and ridiculous ceremonies."

[113] Foreest, *Uromanteia* (1620), 196,

[114] Hörnigk, *Politia medica* (1636), 177; Saltzmann, *De uromantia* (1651), no pagination; in addition, the German editor of Stahl's diatribe against popular uroscopists (Stahl, *Gründliche Abhandlung* (1739), preface, no pagination) and Hygiander, *Regeln* (1744), 3r, also mention the use of crystals.

[115] Seidel, *Liber* (1662), 115; a more obvious explanation would be their weekly work schedule.

[116] *Allgemeine deutsche Justiz- und Polizei-Fama* 1805, 599.

As much as they poured scorn over the "urine-prophets," learned physicians, too, seem to have pulled a rabbit or two out of their hat to satisfy their patients' expectations and so as not to be "taken for or decried as, albeit undeservedly so, someone unlearned and inexperienced in the art," as Nicolaus Pfizerus put it. He complained with a slight sneer, that more than one physician, "clasps the matula, turns it this way and that, craning his neck all the while, but then, after having cleared his throat several times, gives in a somewhat lofty voice his usually high-flown answer: which is readily accepted as a Delphic oracle."[117]

With good reason, the announcement of the uroscopic diagnosis was often referred to as a *judicium*, that is, a "judgment" or "sentence." Thanks to their esoteric knowledge, the uroscopist seemed able to gain insights that were not accessible to ordinary people. And the prognostic judgment of the future course of the disease which patients and relatives routinely expected brought uroscopy even closer to divinatory, prophetic practices. It comes as no surprise that it was combined at times with other, similar practices. Whether a patient would die or not, for example, could be foretold by adding a few drops of breast milk to the urine. If the milk floated on the surface of the urine, the sick person would survive; if it sank, he or she would die. In Germany, submerging a stalk of burning nettle in the patient's urine served the same purpose. If the plant changed color and wilted after a time, the patient would die. If it remained green, he or she would recover.[118]

The desire for a *judicium* about the past, present, and future that was founded on more or less esoteric knowledge emerges as a salient feature of early modern popular culture in general. There existed at the time a wide spectrum of "divinatory," oracular practices, whereby particularly gifted and clairvoyant individuals interpreted the most varied kinds of signs, took a reading of the past and future on this basis, or sought out lost things, treasures, and evildoers. The spectrum ranged from divination with the help of crystal balls to chiromancy (palmistry), and physiognomy (interpretation of facial features). Even more than these, astrological prognosis had a well-established place even in medieval academic medicine and continued to be practiced by some learned physicians far into the seventeenth century.[119] A number of authors wrote works that combined uroscopy and astrology.[120] Painters occasionally staged uroscopy and astrology alongside one another. In Franz Christoph Janneck's (1703–1761) painting *The Medical Alchemist*, an astrological book lies on the table in front of what is doubtless not an alchemist but a uroscopist (see Plate 15).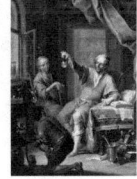

117 Pfizerus, *Zwey sonderbare Bücher* (1673), 169f.

118 Homblé, *Uromantie* (1974), 56.

119 Traister, *Simon Forman* (2001).

120 Schylander, *Medicina astrologica* (1577); Culpeper, *Urinalia* (1655).

Uroscopy and Witchcraft

The uroscopists' ability to unravel the mysterious and hidden extended to the supernatural, to diseases caused by witchcraft.[121] Even in academic medicine the notion of "inflicted" illnesses was taken very seriously in the sixteenth and seventeenth centuries.[122] Among the rural population it was widely shared until well into the second half of the nineteenth century and even then it was slow to die out. Suspicion would be aroused in particular if an illness began suddenly or was characterized by unusual or dramatic symptoms such as convulsions, paralysis, lunacy, or acute pain as with lumbago, which to this day is tellingly called "Hexenschuss" in German, that is, literally, "witch's shot."[123]

Non-physician uroscopists seem to have resorted to this type of diagnosis quite frequently: "They also recognize all kinds of witchcraft in the urine, especially when they realize that they are unable to help the patient," complained Euricius Cordus.[124] If they found that a person had been ill for a long time, Foreest recounted in the same vein, they said that "the person had been attacked by evil people and bewitched and had much strange and unnatural things in his body." He claimed that he personally knew a uroscopist whose habit it was to proclaim that "people had been bewitched or robbed of their manliness by evil people."[125] The belief in the effectiveness of love magic and the possibility of rendering men impotent through magical means was widespread at the time.[126] Foreest claimed that even the wife of a relative of his was advised by a uroscopist to have an exorcism performed.[127] Lorenz Fries's description of an old woman who poured the urine into a bowl "and tells much witchcraft from it," suggests that some uroscopists not only specialized in supernatural illnesses but also developed peculiar rituals of their own.[128]

Unfortunately, we very rarely have access to more detailed information about common ways of dealing with "inflicted," "cast-upon" illnesses and about the role of uroscopy in diagnosing them. For this reason, one of the few relatively well documented cases will be presented here in some depth.[129] Despite the

---

[121] In individual cases, Leonhard Thurneysser, too, judged from a patient's urine sample that "something had also been done to her by ways of magic," as a husband relayed Thurneysser's diagnosis of his wife's condition (StB Berlin, Ms. germ. fol. 421a, 164r, letter from Barttel Kimmel, November 1, [1576]).

[122] Clark, *Thinking with demons* (1997).

[123] Stolberg, *Experiencing illness* (2011), 36–9.

[124] Cordus, *De urinis* (1543), no pagination.

[125] Foreest, *Uromanteia* (1620), 200.

[126] Hacke, *Liebeszauberpraktiken* (2001).

[127] Foreest, *Uromanteia* (1620), 214–17.

[128] Fries, *Spiegel* (1518), LXXIIIIr.

[129] HStA Stuttgart A 213 Bü. 8416.

limitations of using court records as historical sources—they reflect the unique situation of an interrogation—a picture of the use of uroscopy in the fight against "evil powers" and "evil people" emerges that is much more complex than that offered by the physicians' polemical accounts.

When Anna Maria Schittenhelm died on November 15, 1748, her death prompted an official inquiry. This was because the daughter of the dead woman, according to the report of the court clerk, had "been wholly convinced," "influenced by several people," but in particular due to the judgment of a healer she consulted, that her mother's death "had been caused by sorcery alone." Others, however, identified a different culprit. They were convinced that the sick woman had been harmed by the "remedies of incompetent doctors."[130] As the questioning of relatives shows, Anna Maria Schittenhelm had returned from harvest work in Alsace three months earlier and had fallen ill soon after. She felt languid, had no appetite, and suffered from shortness of breath. Four weeks before her death her feet and her abdomen began to swell. At first she tried some household remedies, but when these failed, her brother, about three weeks before her death, asked the hangman Carl of the neighboring Oberndorf for help. He paid him 27 *kreuzer* for a white emetic powder, which did not, however, produce the desired effect. He went back to the hangman who said "it might be a stomach fever." The hangman handed the woman's brother a laxative and a "stomach elixir." The sick woman, upon taking the remedies, began suffering from severe diarrhea which "got worse and worse," at which point her brother, it seems, lost faith in the hangman. Instead, the sick woman's daughter went to the hangman, who, however, refused to give any further medications, saying "it is an evil disease, there is nothing one can do." This was also, according to the daughter's testimony, the general conviction of the community. "Everyone in the village said it was an evil disease, and if it had come from evil people, then she ought to go to the wife of the Schindlen Hannßen in Reuthen, who could help in such a case." So the daughter went to Reuthenr. As she herself had heard from her previous master that woman had "helped his livestock, which had been attacked by evil people." The healer examined the patient's urine and concluded that it was "something evil." The urine looked "white, milky" and she proclaimed that the patient had been "attacked by evil people; she got it through her food. But she wanted to help." She gave the daugher a powder for her the sick mother which the woman was to ingest all at once. It did not help, however. The mother only became "more wretched and weak."

A few days later the daughter returned to the healer, upon which the healer spent a night in the patient's house. According to the family she used "this trick of saying at first that she would not ask for any money until the sick woman was healed." The healer asked for half a pint of wine, into which she grated roots,

---

[130] Ibid., report and interrogation protocols, November 16, 1748.

then cooked all of it and gave it to the sick woman to drink. But the remedy had a poor effect and the woman became weaker and weaker. The healer also "hung a small bundle of herbs" on the mother. And to fight the "evil people," she took the sick woman's urine and stool on Tuesday, cooked them in the kitchen in a new pot and then, the following morning, buried the excrements in the barn. She claimed that the witch would soon enter the house and ask for something, but should not be given anything. No one came, however. The mother had not really believed her in the first place, saying the illness had come from her harvest work. Upon leaving, the woman also said, "The person who attacked your mother will have to die." She claimed as well "that she killed the woman who attacked Conrad Mayer's livestock." And indeed, it was reported that around that time a sudden death in the shoemaker's family had prompted a flurry of rumors.

Carl the hangman's diagnosis of a "stomach fever" was not explicitly attributed to uroscopy. The female healer, however, drew her conclusion that it was a "cast-upon illness" from "evil people" from the changes she perceived in the urine and which were described in some detail. The villagers already harbored the suspicion that Anna Maria Schittenhelm was suffering from an inflicted illness. But it was only through uroscopy that the suspicion was confirmed. Even supernatural forces and evil powers, then, could be exposed with the help of uroscopy.

Chapter 4

Revealing Images: Uroscopy in Early Modern Genre Painting

My account of the place and role of uroscopy in early modern medical culture has so far been based almost exclusively on textual sources, printed and handwritten ones. Like few other aspects of early modern medicine, however, uroscopy was also the object of numerous visual representations. Early modern genre painting, in particular, offers valuable insights into how early modern laypeople perceived uroscopy and its ritualized nature.[1] Dozens of paintings on this subject are known, especially from the Netherlands.[2] Nearly all famous Dutch genre painters, from Gerard Dou (1613–1675) to Jan Steen (ca 1626–1679), from Gerard ter Borch (1617–1681)[3] to Caspar Netscher (1639–1684), depicted uroscopy, and several of them even more than once. To a limited extent the tradition was carried on into the eighteenth century.

At first sight it may strike us as surprising that a rather unsavory topic like uroscopy should be so popular. After all, urine was perceived as repulsive in those days too. At closer analysis, however, the topic of uroscopy did provide some attraction of its own, and for various reasons: It offered a variation on the popular theme of ordinary, everyday life, in the private, even intimate setting of the burghers' houses and made it possible to combine the representation of a dramatic event with elements of still life. From the perspective of the artists, uroscopy also allowed them to demonstrate their exquisite skills. Painting the characteristic urine baskets made of fine wickerwork and, even more so, the matula with its subtle color nuances and reflections demanded a great command of the high art of light distribution that was the mark of the leading genre painters. Celeste Brusati's account of the contemporary ideal of a "reflexy-const" as exemplified by the depiction of wine glasses, applies similarly to that of the filled urine flask: "Light focused on partly filled wine glasses projects upon them the images of unseen windows and shines through their reflected transparent

---

[1] Aalkjaer, *Uroscopia* (1973), 9–11.

[2] Good overview in Franits, *Dutch seventeenth-century genre painting* (2004).

[3] Ter Borch (also: Terborch) devoted his first (signed) painting to the topic, *The consultation* (1635); cf. Hellens, *Terborch* (1911), 29f; Gudlaugsson, *Ter Borch* (1959), 30; Netscher made a copy of the painting; on Netscher see Wiesemann, *Caspar Netscher* (2002).

contents to generate colored reflexes of reflected light, which in turn stain walls and table-cloths with the red and golden of the liquids they contain."[4]

For the historian today, these painted representations of uroscopy are not only of artistic and esthetic interest. They also prove to be valuable sources in their own right. They reveal how artists, as medical laypeople of their time, perceived and experienced uroscopy and/or what they inferred about the view of the wealthy burghers to whom they hoped to sell the paintings and to whose expectations they were catering.

The Doctor's Visit

Most depictions of uroscopy found in early modern genre paintings can roughly be put into one of two categories. Paintings of the first kind show a uroscopist—usually one with an artisanal or rural background and only rarely identified as a physician—inspecting in his own home the urine brought to him by a messenger. Paintings of the second kind—often with titles like "The Doctor's Visit"—show us the uroscopist in the patient's home, in the sick chamber. Here the uroscopist is usually a learned physician and the patients are living in affluent, even luxurious circumstances.

Art historians have so far focused almost entirely on paintings of the second type that treat "the doctor's visit." We usually see a doctor who examines urine next to a young, pretty, and well-dressed woman. Many paintings show the woman seated in an arm chair, and she would not easily be recognized as ill were it not for the presence of the doctor who examines her urine and frequently also feels her pulse. The women may have an air of melancholy, seemingly looking into the distance, sometimes holding a letter, or there is a letter lying on the table or floor. There are a number of recurring props in different combinations: pictures or statues of Venus or Cupid, small coal stoves, dogs or cats.

Dutch genre painting is widely praised today for its fascinating naturalistic reproduction of even minute details, a sense of perfection which sometimes approaches modern photorealism. Artists took pride in it and tried to outdo one another.[5] However, as art historians have clarified over the last decades, the paintings' often strikingly "realistic," even illusionist facture must not lead us to conclude that those painters actually aspired to depict the reality of everyday life as if in a photographic manner. There are various layers of meaning to be discerned.[6]

---

[4]   Brusati, *Natural artifice* (1997), 153.

[5]   On the relationship to contemporary natural history see Alpers, *Art* (1985).

[6]   Cf. e.g. Meige, *Les médecins* (1900); for a different assessment see Franits, *Dutch seventeenth-century genre painting* (2004), 1f.

The so-called iconological method, associated in particular with the work of Aby Warburg and Erwin Panofsky, has been criticized for its tendency to assign a hidden meaning to nearly every single pictorial element, with the help of contemporary textual sources such as emblem books, plays, scientific treatises and writings on art theory. In the case of Dutch genre painting, however, this method serves very well to show that these works are anything but the snapshots of everyday bourgeois or peasant life that they might appear at first glance. Not uncommonly, we do find that a painting was modeled on a contemporary epigraph or proverb or that the artist drew on an emblem book or literary work. Animals such as birds or cats, for example, or objects such as closed or open bird cages point to well-defined iconographic traditions. For early modern contemporaries, such props bore a meaning that was more or less evident, such as sexual desire and infidelity in the case of a cat, and virginity in the case of the bird cage.

Paintings which feature uroscopic diagnosis in the sick chamber of a beautiful young woman are apt examples of this type of symbolically laden iconography in painting. Figures and objects are often painted in a very "realistic" manner and we can learn, for example, what the wicker-baskets looked like in which the urine flasks were carried. Yet these paintings were much more than that. As historians of art and medicine argued already around 1900, many of the paintings were dedicated to a subject that was fairly widespread in the literature and medicine of the day: lovesickness. The notion goes back to classical accounts by Soran, Plutarch, and others. According to Soran, Hippocrates was once called to the sick and emaciated King Perdicca of Macedonia, where he observed that the patient's pulse changed every time Phyle, the wife of Perdicca's deceased father, came to the sickbed: Perdicca had fallen in love with her but did not confess his love. Thanks to her caresses, he soon got better.[7] More widely known still was a similar tale about King Seleucus's son Antiochus, who had fallen in love with his beautiful stepmother Stratonice. He became increasingly ill but was not able to confess his passion. The famous physician Erasistratos finally identified the true cause of the disease, noticing a change in the patient's complexion and pulse whenever his beautiful stepmother entered the room. Seleucus then gave his young wife to his son and his son got well again.[8]

The concept of "lovesickness" accompanied by strong physical symptoms was well known and taken seriously in the early modern period. Medical textbooks such as Johann van Beverwijk's *Schat der Ongesontheydt* discussed it in considerable detail.[9] Far into the eighteenth century, allusions to lovesickness

---

[7]   Beverwijk, *Schat der ongesontheyt* (1672), part 2, 50.

[8]   Crohns, *Geschichte* (1905).

[9]   Beverwijk, *Schat der ongesontheyt* (1672), part 2, 48–53.

can be found, particularly in Dutch genre painting.[10] Jan Steen, who initiated this tradition, alone left at least 18 such paintings to posterity.[11] There is the pale, melancholy face, the hand of the sick woman reaching for her heart, her clothing loosened and opened around her chest and heart, a letter—presumably from her lover—in her hand, on the table, or on the floor. She is surrounded by numerous allusions to female sexual desire, such as pictures with erotic subjects on the walls, sculptures of Cupid, cats, and so on, which all can be read as clues to both the cause of the disease and the best, most effective cure, as expressed in the motto of the contemporary emblem "Amans amanti medicus," "the lover is the lover's doctor."[12]

Sometimes the painter made the meaning even more explicit by adding words to his painting. In three of Jan Steen's paintings we read: "There is no cure for it if it is lovesickness."[13] However, most of these paintings do not convey their subject this clearly, even if they have many of the characteristic elements that point in this direction. In fact, as we will see in more detail later on, some of the paintings may also be understood as depicting the diagnosis of a pregnancy. The two subjects were closely linked: A young woman might become lovesick—as staged in contemporary plays, too—because her father did not accept her lover, and becoming pregnant would then have been a way of leaving her father little choice but to consent.[14]

Some paintings can also be understood as depictions of chlorosis, hysteria, or other diseases that were considered typical women's diseases.[15] Like lovesickness, these diseases were thought to be caused amongst others by unfulfilled erotic desire and to be curable, in that case, by sexual fulfillment. Hysteria, at the time, was often still equated with *furor uterinus* which might in turn result from lovesickness.

The small pans or stoves holding glowing embers that can be found in many of Jan Steen's paintings may be taken to point in the direction of hysteria, though their use or meaning remains subject to debate. It has been suggested that they served to heat urine and some passages in contemporary literary texts support this view. A doctor in Petrus Baardt's *Deughden-Spoor*, for example, asks for a "choffoor," a small heating stove, to warm up urine.[16] The scholarly uroscopy

---

10   Meige, *Le mal d'amour* (1899); Petterson, *Amans amanti* (2000).

11   On Steen cf. Jansen, *Jan Steen* (1996); on his uroscopy paintings in particular see Meige, *Les médecins* (1900).

12   Petterson, *Ikonologie* (1984); idem, *Amans amanti* (2000).

13   According to Naumann, *Mieris* (1981), 99 (note); "Daer baet geen medesyn, want het is minne pyn" viz. "Hyr baet geen medisijn, waar het is soete pijn"; "soete pijn" was a synonym for "minne pijn" or "minne-koorts."

14   Cf. Petterson, *Ikonologie* (1984).

15   This has been affirmed, above all, by Laurinda Dixon (Dixon, *Perilous chastity*, 1995).

16   According to Gils, *De dokter* (1917), 75f.

treatises of the day, however, cautioned that reheating urine might corrupt it, and I know of no painting that hints at this practice.[17] Considering that we see women resting their feet on these stoves in some paintings, it might simply be the case that they served to warm the feet. That the women often seem quite warmly dressed would be a further point in favor of this interpretation. After all, grief, as a central symptom of lovesickness, was understood to cause the warm vital spirits to withdraw from the body's periphery to the inside. This interpretation is also underscored by the sick—and by all appearances already elderly—woman in Dou's *The Dropsical Woman* (see Plate 2), who has one foot resting on a small stove of this type; dropsy was commonly associated with cold. Then again, cold hands and cold feet were also seen as symptoms of hysteria, and Gils has pointed out that in many, if not all of those paintings, we see a smoldering ribbon lying on the embers. As Gils has found in contemporary medical texts, blue linen ribbons in particular were commonly burnt for their repulsive odor, which would make the patient come to after fainting. Most of the women depicted in these paintings show no sign of having fainted but Laurinda Dixon has found the related advice in the gynecological literature of the time to use offensive odors on hysterical women. A uterus that had risen up toward the chest and throat—the central cause of hysteria—was to be spurred to move back to the abdomen by the quite literally repulsive odors. Most doctors no longer accepted the traditional notion of a mobile, wandering uterus.[18] Among the population, however, it persisted into the twentieth century,[19] and there were women as late as the eighteenth century who described how they literally felt the uterus rising into their chest and throat and threatening to take their breath away.[20]

---

[17]   Gils, *Een detail* (1920); idem, *De dokter* (1917).

[18]   In medical literature, by contrast, hysteria was primarily linked to pathological vapors and fumes, the *vapores*, which rose upward from the uterus, and only gradually became reinterpreted as a nervous illness. Occasionally *vapores* might arise from an accumulation of female seminal fluid; in the Galenic tradition, women also possessed semen. Widowed women who previously had had regular intercourse were therefore particularly at risk. However, unnatural abstinence could lead to an accumulation and putrefaction of semen even in younger women, similarly giving rise to pathological *vapores*. We have here a possible connection to the way in which the unsatisfied desire of lovesick patients was viewed. Mainly, however, *vapores* emanated from spoiled menstrual blood that accumulated in and around the uterus, especially in the case of a disturbed menstruation.

[19]   Berg, *Krankheitskomplex* (1935).

[20]   Stolberg, *Experiencing illness* (2011), 168–70. The small stoves might also be understood as a clue to pregnancy diagnosis. According to the contemporary conception, the cervix of the pregnant women closed up so tightly that not even a needle would go through (Fernel, *Universa medicina*, 1644, 594). It was believed that a pregnant woman did not smell any smoke or fumes wafting up into her genitals, as they were prevented from rising upward through the uterus. In this case, however, we would expect the woman's body and head to be wrapped up so that the smell of the smoke would not reach her nose from the outside.

The example of the small stoves goes to show how difficult it can be to assign meaning even to the smallest, seemingly inconspicuous details in genre paintings. For our purpose, however, the question of which "pathology" contemporary viewers were to read into these paintings is of secondary importance. In fact, it is precisely this "diagnostic" ambiguity that allows us to draw the conclusion that the painters were not so much interested in showing a specific illness. It seems they wanted to paint, above all, a dramatic, emotional situation in which a young pretty woman and uroscopy (and similarly in some paintings, pulse diagnosis) played a key role.

The Image of the Uroscopist in Genre Painting

Especially in respect to paintings about lovesickness, art historians have long taken the view that genre painters intended to ridicule doctors in their practice of uroscopy and to attack uroscopy as a long outdated procedure. They have corroborated this interpretation by pointing at the critical and often polemical writings of physicians about uroscopy.[21] As we have seen, this criticism was primarily aimed at the dominant practice of diagnosing illness based on uroscopy exclusively, however, and not at the examination of urine done at the sickbed. The latter remained an important feature also of learned medical practice. From the same time period, the seventeenth century, we also have depictions of "Christus medicus," which, far from intending to ridicule, show Jesus, surrounded by a halo, yet acting as a worldly healer with a matula in his raised hand (see Figure 4.1).[22] Clearly then, the claim that doctors and uroscopy were depicted in largely critical ways in genre paintings of "The Doctor's Visit" can by and large not be substantiated.

Certain paintings undoubtedly did mock the learned physician who relied on uroscopy and pulse diagnosis to arrive at a diagnosis—unrequited desire—that was obvious to any common observer, or, worse still, missed that diagnosis. Such critical and satirical elements, which seem to reflect contemporary theatrical representations,[23] can be found in some paintings by Jan Steen in particular.[24] Erotic paintings within the painting, women's gestures of longing and obvious sexual innuendos—a raised fish, an obscene gesture of the thumb—these were elements that at times were combined with the depiction of an old-fashioned

---

[21]   Westermann, *Amusements* (1997), 111–15.

[22]   Krafft, *Christus* (2001); on the great popularity of this motif in contemporary prints see Homblé, *Uromantie* (1974), 60–62.

[23]   Gudlaugsson, *Ikonographische Studien* (1938); idem, *Comedians* (1975).

[24]   Meige, *Les médecins* (1900), 190; Meige also underlines, however, that even Steen's attacks were more subtle than those of Molière and did not aim as much at ridiculing the physicians.

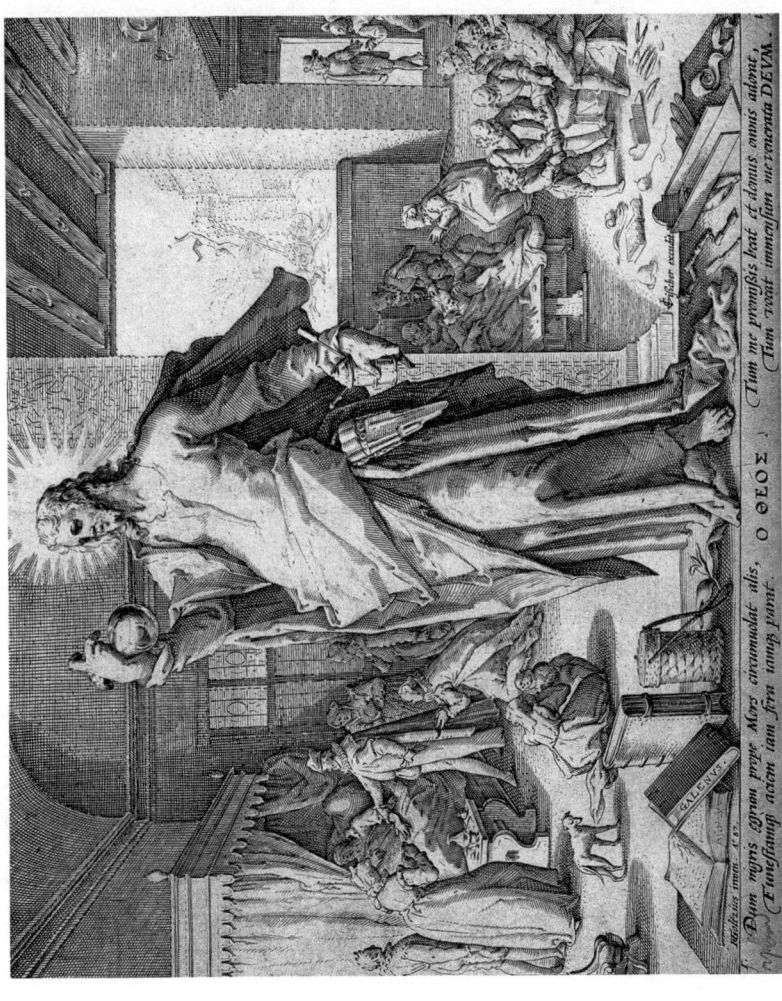

Figure 4.1   C.J. Visscher (after H. Goltzius), *Christus medicus* (Wellcome Library, London)

doctor—his outlandish dress sometimes modeled on the *Dottore* in the *Commedia dell'Arte*—who can tell neither the disease nor the cure suggested by the painter. Some of Steen's paintings even seem to be picture versions of a contemporary joke: The doctor feels the pulse of a lovesick girl, whereupon the servant says that he is feeling the wrong place—he ought rather to put his hand on her belly.[25]

In this light, Steen's (and Brakenburgh's) doctors have been compared to those that Molière put on stage in his comedies. But even Steen's depictions, which are more farcical than those of most other painters, cannot simply be taken to mock the medical profession and their trust in uroscopy in general. What was being denounced and satirized here was the individual learned doctor's inability to practice what was otherwise a valuable art.[26] Compared to other paintings by Steen, his depiction of uroscopists was in fact rather mild. Steen tended to caricature and ridicule virtually everyone, even the biblical Tamar who was raped by her half-brother Amnon and then cast out.[27] Yet even among Steen's uroscopy paintings, we find some that do not suggest caricature and mockery. Instead they present an elderly, dignified doctor, and this goes even more for painters like Caspar Netscher or Adriaen Ostade.[28] There is little in these paintings, if anything, to suggest that the viewer of the day was being invited to join in the fun of mocking the doctor or patient.

When trying to assess the degree to which the painters intended to deride uroscopy, we also have to take into account that it often played only a secondary role in their paintings, especially in the most widespread type devoted to lovesickness. The key to diagnosing lovesickness was feeling the pulse, a method that had been firmly established in medical tradition since antiquity. The patient's "pulse quickened" when his or her loved one was mentioned or else entered the room, and this permitted a much more exact diagnosis than uroscopy allowed: The racing pulse not only defined the patient's condition as an illness, it also pointed directly to its cause. Uroscopy, by contrast, identified only the general changes that lovesickness produced, in the long run, in the female body, without indicating its actual source. In particular, urine of an intense, even reddish tint was seen as typical for lovesickness. A Spanish poem quoted by Beverwijk put it succinctly: "Her pulse is racing stupendously, her water is very red. How can this mean anything but lovesickness?"[29]

---

[25] Westermann, *Amusements* (1997), esp. 101–5;

[26] Cf. Brant, *Ship of fools* (1944), 96f (ch. 55): "A fool is he, of little skill/ Who tests the urine of the ill/ And says: 'Wait, sir, and be so kind,/ The answer in my books I'll find.'/ And while he thumbs the folios/ The patient to the bone yard goes."

[27] Formerly Wallraf-Richartz Museum, Cologne; cf. Samuel 2:13, 1–21.

[28] See also Dixon, *Together in misery* (2003), 247.

[29] Beverwijk, *Schat der ongesontheyt* (1672), part 2, 51.

Some paintings show a doctor performing both uroscopy and pulse diagnosis at the same time. Clearly this was an artistic device which compressed consecutive practices in one picture. Doctors were urged to practice both methods with great care and would hardly have been able to perform them simultaneously.[30] Other paintings—this is especially true of Jan Steen's work—merely hinted at uroscopy by showing the typical wicker basket that was used to carry matulae, disregarding the fact that this made little sense when the doctor was making a house call. Still others omitted such indications altogether, as for example Frans Mieris in his two paintings on the subject.[31] Thus, even if we choose to see some of Jan Steen's paintings as medical satire and not simply as depictions of individual, particularly incapable members of the profession, a criticism of uroscopy cannot be understood as their primary concern.

Another group of paintings show doctors inspecting the urine of severely ill or dying patients. They give even less of an indication that they sought to deride and criticize the use of uroscopy. An early eighteenth-century painting by Egbert van Heemskerk shows a man surrounded by lamenting relatives, a physician, a clergyman, and what appears to be a lawyer taking the dying patient's will (see Plate 22). Again the physician is feeling the pulse and examining the patient's urine at the same time. By all appearances, uroscopy here does not serve to diagnose the illness but to confirm that the sick man will die. There is no hint that the physician is ignorant of what is obvious to everyone else.

The most famous example of uroscopic diagnosis of a severely ill patient is the abovementioned work *The Dropsical Woman* by Gérard Dou (1613–1675), held by the *Musée du Louvre* in Paris (see Plate 2). In several respects the painting still raises questions today. It was given its title only in the eighteenth century and there is, in fact, little to suggest that Dou meant to show a dropsical woman. The typical features of dropsy are missing, such as a bloated abdomen typical of ascites (abdominal dropsy), or a swollen face and feet. We might simply regard the painting as a sophisticated artistic portrayal of the examination of an older female patient's urine. But genre painting is known for its innuendos and hidden messages. The two wings that were added later to Dou's painting and could be used to cover it may be helpful here. They show a pitcher and a bowl of the kind that were used for washing oneself. Ella Snoep-Reitsma has interpreted the pitcher and bowl as hinting at a moral message. She has presented historical

---

[30]   Dixon, *Perilous chastity* (1995), 80; Dixon's claim that the simultaneous use of both procedures was recommended in particular with lovesickness is not corroborated by the sources; Dixon refers to Horine, *Epitome* (1941), who, however, writes nothing of the sort; presumably, Dixon misunderstood Horine's reference to Paracelsus (ibid., 227) who recommended—depending on the case—feeling the pulse if the urine seemed healthy.

[31]   Unless we concur with Buvelot, who interprets a flask on the table filled with something yellow-brown as a matula, though it is very uncharacteristic in shape; Buvelot, *Mieris* (2005), 107–11.

evidence that jugs and bowls of this kind were often used to refer to moral purity, which the depicted person was supposed to preserve or attain. Seen in this light, Dou's painting might have conveyed the idea that it was not the doctor, not medicine, that was crucial in deciding the fate of the seriously ill, possibly dying woman, but rather pure, virtuous conduct. Indeed, if she had lived a virtuous life, the tears shed by the child at her side were inappropriate as she could expect a better life in the world to come.[32]

However, this raises the question of why Dou did not employ more familiar and overt motifs of vanitas and death, such as candles or withering plants. Their absence suggests that the pitcher and the water shown in the wings may quite simply be understood as visual references to urine—commonly called "water"—which is being examined in the center piece. This does not exclude a moralizing component. The message could be that, beyond the physical purification with the laxative or emetic that seems to be administered to the patient, the purity of her soul and piety—hinted at by the bible—were also required for God, or the doctor with God's help, to return the patient to good health.

The Uroscopist as a Truth-Seeker

We have so far considered depictions of uroscopy in the home of the patient. A second type of genre painting presents the examination of urine in the home of the uroscopist rather than that of the patient. So far, this type has attracted little attention among art historians and insufficient thought has been given to the ways in which it differs from the first type. Yet in crucial respects, this second type follows a different set of conventions. Not only is the place where the urine examination is carried out different, in most of these paintings we also encounter different actors. Usually the uroscopist is not presented as a learned physician and is sometimes easily recognized as a barber or village healer. And in marked contrast to the richly attired young women in the first type, those coming for advice are most often dressed in simple attire. They do not appear sick either. Indeed, since they are usually women carrying the characteristic wicker basket, contemporary viewers could readily identify them as messengers.

Again, there is little indication that the painters intended to criticize or poke fun at uroscopy. Quite to the contrary, the uroscopist is depicted as a man to whom people turn trustingly, as someone who knows how to unlock the secrets of nature and the human body thanks to his art. These paintings convey some of the ritualistic, oracular quality of uroscopy—its ability to probe into natural

---

[32] Snoep-Reitsma, *Waterzuchtige vrouw* (1973). Dropsy was one of the most fear-inspiring diseases of the time, usually considered as incurable and ultimately fatal.

and human secrets—which we find in contemporary written descriptions. The paintings by Balthasar van den Bossche (1681–1715) and Gerard Thomas (1663–1720) are particularly illustrative examples (see Plates 23 and 24).[33] Sharply focused, spellbound gazes are directed at the matula, whose central significance in this diagnostic ritual is often emphasized by an artful distribution of light.

Though they have frequently come down to us with titles such as "The Quack Doctor," books that we find placed in front of the uroscopist in many of these paintings convey to the viewer that the healer is by no means an uneducated charlatan. In some paintings, his special knowledge is further underlined by an often chaotic assembly of objects of scientific inquiry scattered on the table and floor, such as chemical vessels, a terrestrial globe, or a skull. Like the books, these objects suggest wisdom and sometimes act as symbols of transience as well. Some of the paintings in their seemingly careless arrangement of such objects are reminiscent of contemporary depictions of Saint Jerome, thus alluding to a personal access to knowledge that cannot be reduced to academic book learning. They liken the uroscopist to the *magus*, who enjoys direct access to the supernatural and divine. His wisdom also encompasses the knowledge that man cannot escape death, which is conveyed with various vanitas symbols such as skulls and hour glasses.

This reading is supported by a striking parallel pictorial tradition that was alive in genre painting in the early modern period, but which art history has usually not considered in this context,[34] namely paintings of alchemists and alchemical laboratories.[35] Significantly, a great number of these paintings were created by the same painters who also depicted uroscopy, such as Steen, Teniers, Ostade, Mieris, and Metsu. The most important distinguishing feature compared to their representations of uroscopy is that of the alembic and similar vessels used for chemical processes and the stove or burner needed to perform them.[36] Otherwise, the two kinds of paintings share many similarities. The central gesture—the scrutinizing gaze at a glass flask that is filled with a liquid—was common to both traditions. In both, we often find a more or less chaotic array of different utensils that bespeak erudition, the exploration of nature, and the transience of human endeavors: books, sometimes carelessly dropped on the floor; glassware of all kinds; human and animal skulls; hour glasses; and terrestrial globes.

---

[33]   Cf. Bautier, *Les petits maîtres* (1924).

[34]   See, however, the recent work by Schummer/Spector, *Visual image* (2007).

[35]   Lennep, *Alchimiste* (1966); idem, *Alchimie* (1985); Principe/DeWitt, *Transmutations* (2002).

[36]   Brinkman, *Brueghel's "Alchemist"* (1974).

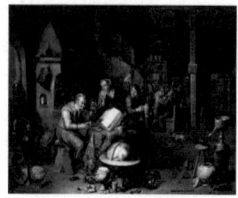Sometimes the line between representations of alchemists and of uroscopists is blurred beyond recognition. It is not surprising then that some paintings carry titles—they were often assigned only later—that seem arbitrary or downright incorrect. In a painting by Balthasar van den Bossche (1681–1715), known today by the title *The Iatrochemist* (see Plate 23), the central figure examines urine, which the woman next to him has brought, with a medical book by Galen open before him. In the background, we see that dental treatment is taking place, with shelves that seem to be filled with medicinal containers as a backdrop. There is no hint whatsoever at alchemy or iatrochemistry. Very similar elements can be found in another painting by van den Bossche, known under the title "The Doctor's Visit" in which the typical urine basket hanging from the woman's arm leaves even less doubt that we are witnessing a urine examination—despite the assistant at the stove, the glass vessel on the floor, and the various indications of naturalist learning.[37]

The same can be said of paintings of "alchemists" by Richard Brakenburg (1650–1702) and Justus Juncker (1703–1767) (see Plates 16 and 27). Again there is no indication of any chemical processes in the proper sense of the word, no test tubes, no distilling flask, and no furnace. Instead the purported alchemist holds a glass flask with a yellow liquid up to the light, and in the Brakenburg painting we find once more the familiar wicker basket for the matula.

Several reasons for the convergence of these two painterly traditions—the uroscopy painting and the depiction of an alchemist—can be identified. In artistic terms, both themes allowed the painter to show various objects and apparatuses in the manner of a still life. On a more practical level, painters may well have been aware of the decidedly medical and therapeutic side of alchemy. As an important variety of alchemy, iatrochemistry set its focus on the production of powerful drugs. Also, the parallels we find in the portrayal of uroscopists and alchemists appear to correspond with a generally very positive perception of both professions by the lay public, to which the artist and his clients or projected buyers belonged. To be sure, as with artists whose paintings show uroscopists, there were those who ridiculed alchemists—again, Jan Steen serves as a prime example. They represented them as crazy men who indulged in a pointless dream and put the wellbeing of their families on the line, or even their own life. This was certainly the message of Brueghel's famous painting of an alchemist, which would have served as a powerful model for these paintings.[38]

---

[37] Until a few years ago, the painting was part of the collection of the Nordwürttembergische Ärztekammer, Stuttgart (cf. Zimmermann ([1969]), 35). Its current owner is not known.

[38] Lennep, *Alchimiste* (1966), 149f; Principe/DeWitt, *Transmutations* (2002), 11f.

But as early as the seventeenth century, genre painters frequently portrayed the alchemist as a seeker of truth, as a researcher and sage who attempts to uncover nature's deepest secrets.[39] He, too, relies on scholarly books but, compared to first-hand experience and personal inspection, they are ultimately given secondary importance.[40]

The Secrets of Women

Just as the alchemist is taken seriously as a truth-seeker in many paintings, the uroscopist is presented not as a simple quack in most genre paintings but as a person with esoteric knowledge and a privileged access to truth. This may well be the major reason for the popularity that both subjects enjoyed. The viewer witnessed how a secret was unveiled, a truth discovered, or a riddle solved—with the significant difference that the alchemist concerned himself with secrets of inanimate matter, while the uroscopist probed the secrets of the living body.

In pictorial representations of uroscopy in the patient's home, this air of revelation is linked quite consistently to a gendered division of roles. Almost without exception, the uroscopist is male and the person seeking advice female. This was not, however, out of historical necessity. Going by the classical topos, lovesickness was, for example, a typically male complaint. It was Antiochus who fell in love with his young stepmother, not she with him. And there certainly were a number of "secret" male diseases that could have been staged in paintings to similar effect, for example impotence, which was greatly feared because it was seen as dishonoring.[41] Like lovesickness, it would have allowed for a more or less subtle play with many different visual innuendos. The widespread venereal diseases conveniently could have been used to spread moral messages. However, we find nothing of the sort in Dutch genre painting.

This was no coincidence. Presumably the male creators of such paintings, just as much as their potential buyers, would have approached depictions of implied male impotence or male venereal diseases with reservation, to put it mildly. Depicting a female patient, on the other hand, allowed them to put a young, attractivewoman on the stage. At the same time, the gendered role allocation that we find with very few exceptions in paintings of "The Doctor's Visit" points to the importance of gender in contemporary society at large and in medicine in particular. To the authors of medical books and their predominantly male readership, as well as to potential buyers of paintings, the desirable, desirous, and

---

[39]   Principe/DeWitt, *Transmutations* (2002), 31.

[40]   Similarly, with particular reference to David Teniers: Brinkman, *Brueghel's "Alchemist"* (1974).

[41]   Darmon, *Tribunal de l'impuissance* (1979); Ründal, *Impotenz* (2011).

fertile female body was the epitome of a secret waiting to be unveiled. Popular medical books about the *Secreta mulierum*, the "secrets" of the female body, had a long tradition.[42] And public anatomies of female corpses, which promised to reveal these secrets in a different way, were apparently greatly welcomed not only by doctors and medical students but also by a broader, male public.[43] According to a widespread topos, the female body—within which the uterus led something of an independent life—possessed a more fervent sexual desire than the male body; from a male viewpoint, the female body was the strange, mysterious Other.

Another commonplace was that a woman's word, or anything she revealed of her own accord, was unreliable, not to be trusted in the same way that it would be coming from a man. However, with the aid of uroscopy (and pulse diagnosis) male doctors were able to discover the truth behind the lies—and this is what the genre paintings vividly reiterated for the contemporary viewer. Doctors were able to decipher the mysterious processes taking place in the female body, even if the woman did not want to reveal her secrets.

Male desire to unveil the secrets of the female body also found expression in contemporary treatises on uroscopy, especially those that were written in the vernacular and addressed a broader readership. Some even offered advice that might be helpful to the male reader in his personal dealings with the opposite sex. A woman's urine might, for example, reveal that she had a desire and was only hiding it coyly. "Urine that is bright as gold indicates desire or the wish to get married," Wood informed the reader of his *Epitomie*.[44]

This motif of the secret that uroscopy brings to light is further underlined in many of the paintings by symbolic elements: half-opened doors, enfilades, half-parted curtains. As Steen's depictions of lovesickness illustrate particularly well, the painter in a given case might nonetheless give this gesture of revelation an ironic spin: The mystery lay only in the eyes of the physician, who could not see what was obvious to everyone else. If my interpretation is correct, this ambivalence merely reflects, however, what we also find documented in a number of other sources on the medical practice of this period: Confidence in the diagnostic capabilities of uroscopy as such went hand in hand with considerable distrust in the abilities (and honesty) of individual uroscopists.

This motif of the exposure of hidden truths is brought to bear particularly well in paintings that show examination of the urine of a pregnant woman. As we have seen, both unmarried and married women valued uroscopy highly as a means of determining whether or not they were with child, especially in the early stages of a (possible) pregnancy. Since physicians and laypeople alike believed that a missed period alone was not a reliable sign, otherwise only quickening brought

---

[42]   (Pseudo-)Albertus Magnus, *Secreta mulierum* (1485).

[43]   Park, *Secrets* (2006).

[44]   Wood, *Epitomie* (1653), 234.

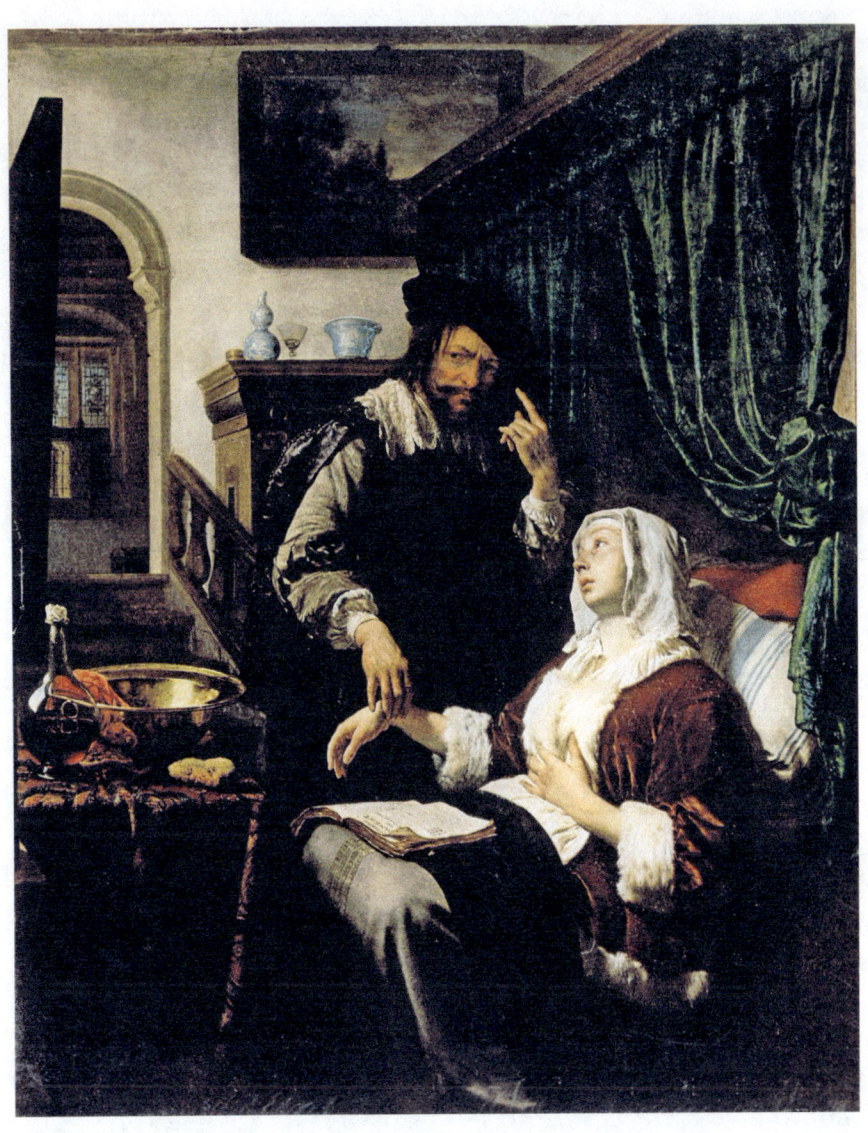

Plate 17   Color photolithograph after F. van Mieris (1635–1681), Physician
feeling the pulse (London, Wellcome Library)

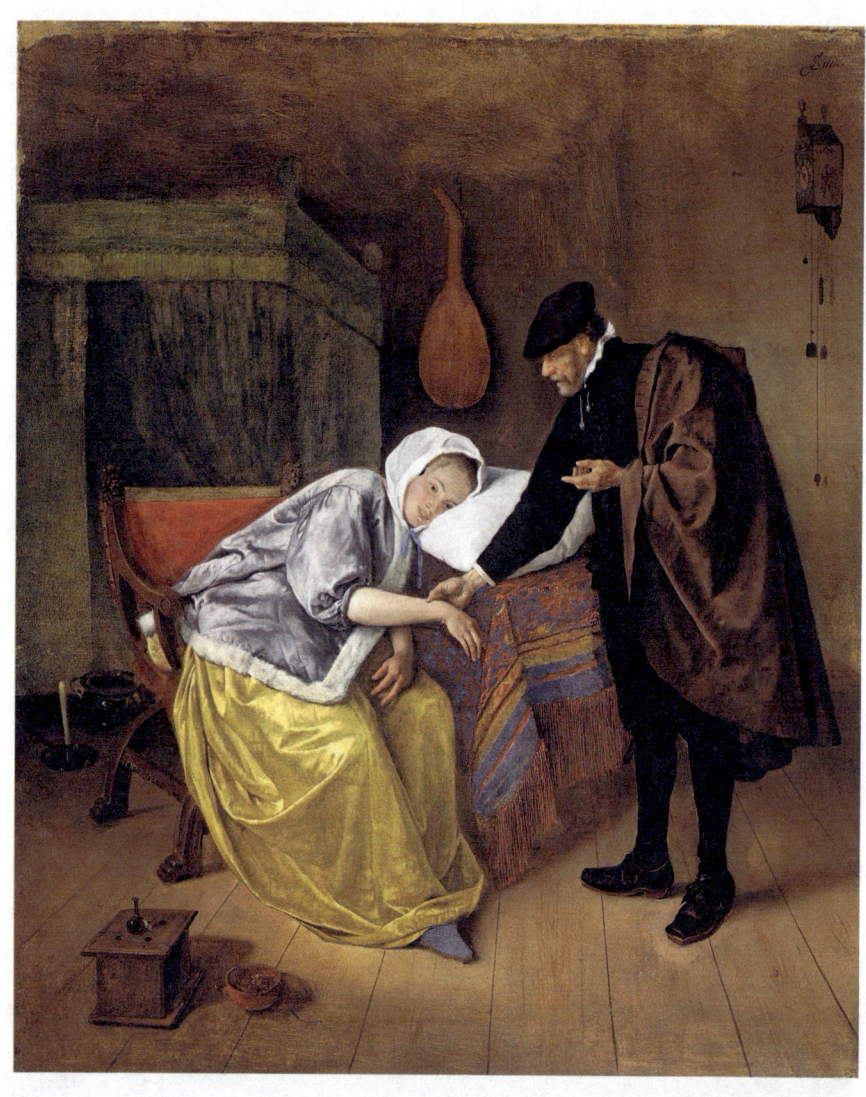

Plate 18   Jan Steen (ca 1626–1679), *The Doctor's Visit* (Amsterdam, Rijksmuseum)

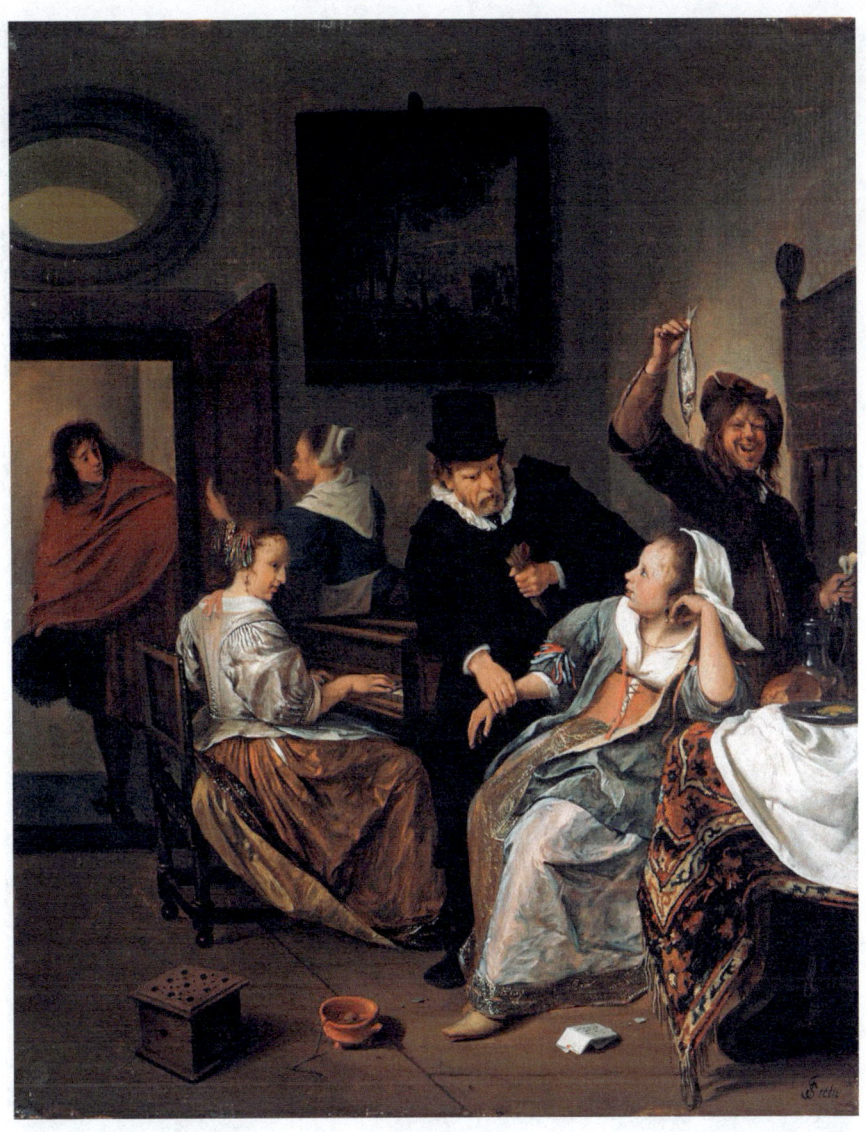

Plate 19   Jan Steen (ca 1626–1679), *The Doctor's Visit* (Philadelphia, Philadelphia Museum of Art)

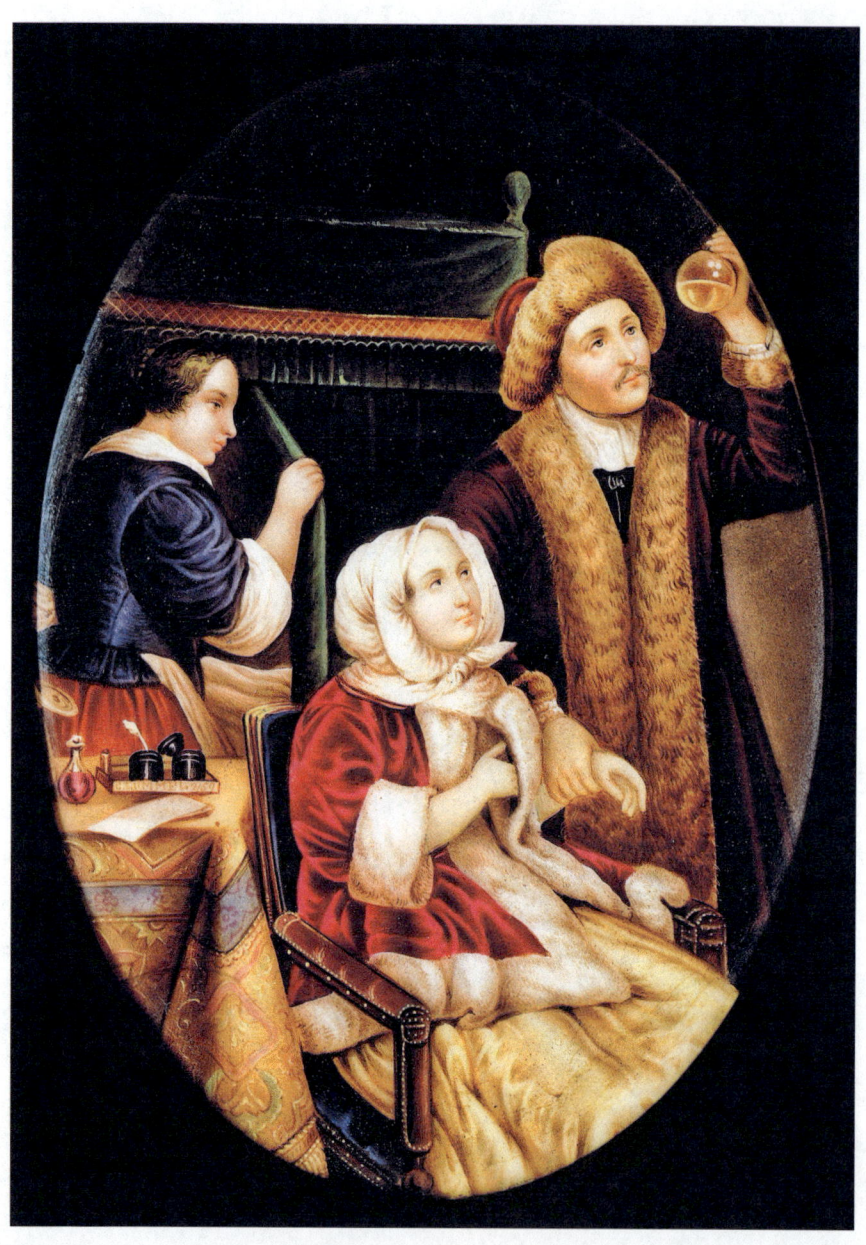

Plate 20   Enamel after Caspar Netscher (1639–1684), *The Doctor's Visit* (London, Wellcome Library)

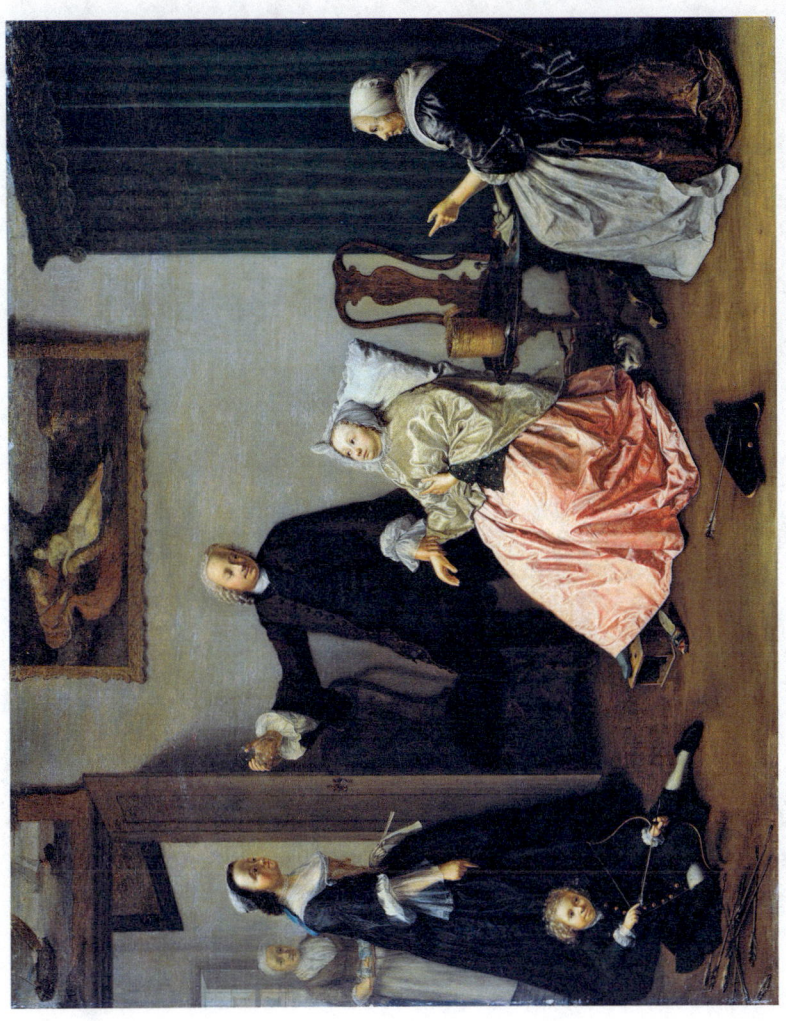

Plate 21   Elisabet Geertruida Wassenbergh (1729–1781), Physician feeling the pulse of a lovesick girl (Amsterdam, Rijksmuseum)

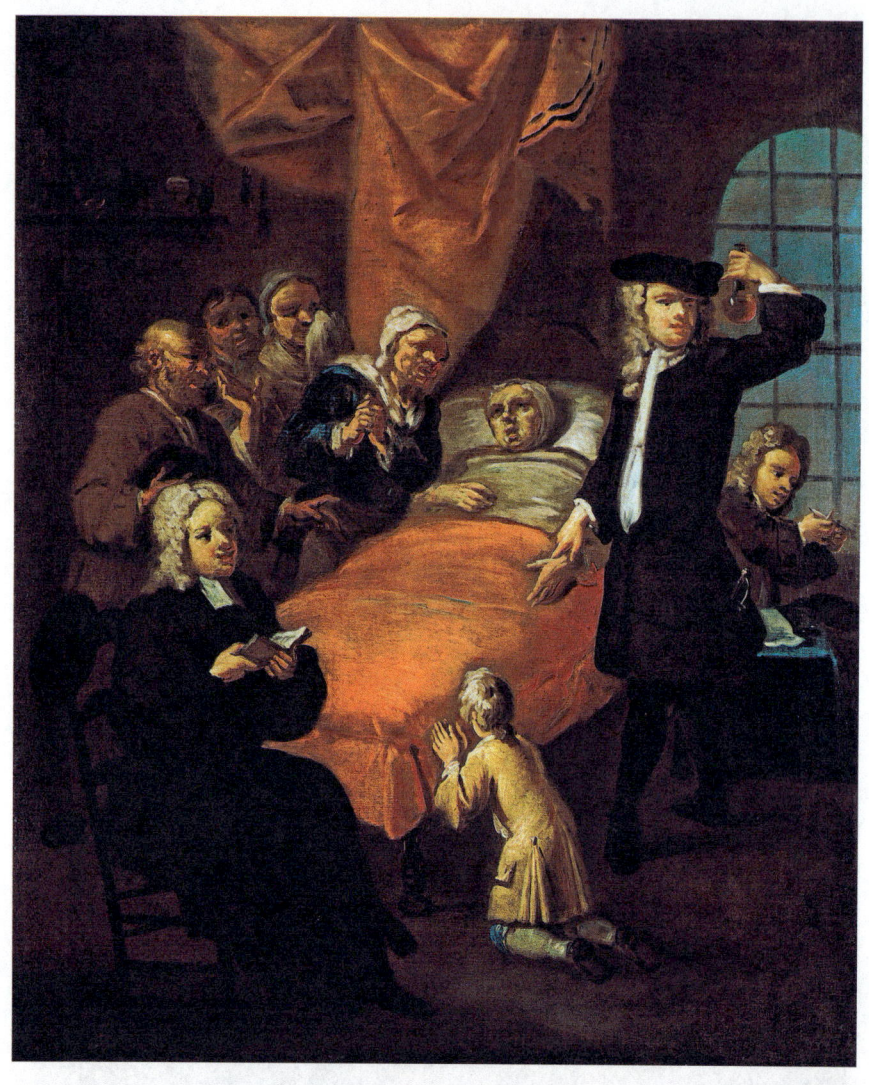

Plate 22   Egbert van Heemskerk (ca 1700–1744), Physician at a patient's death-bed (London, Tate Gallery)

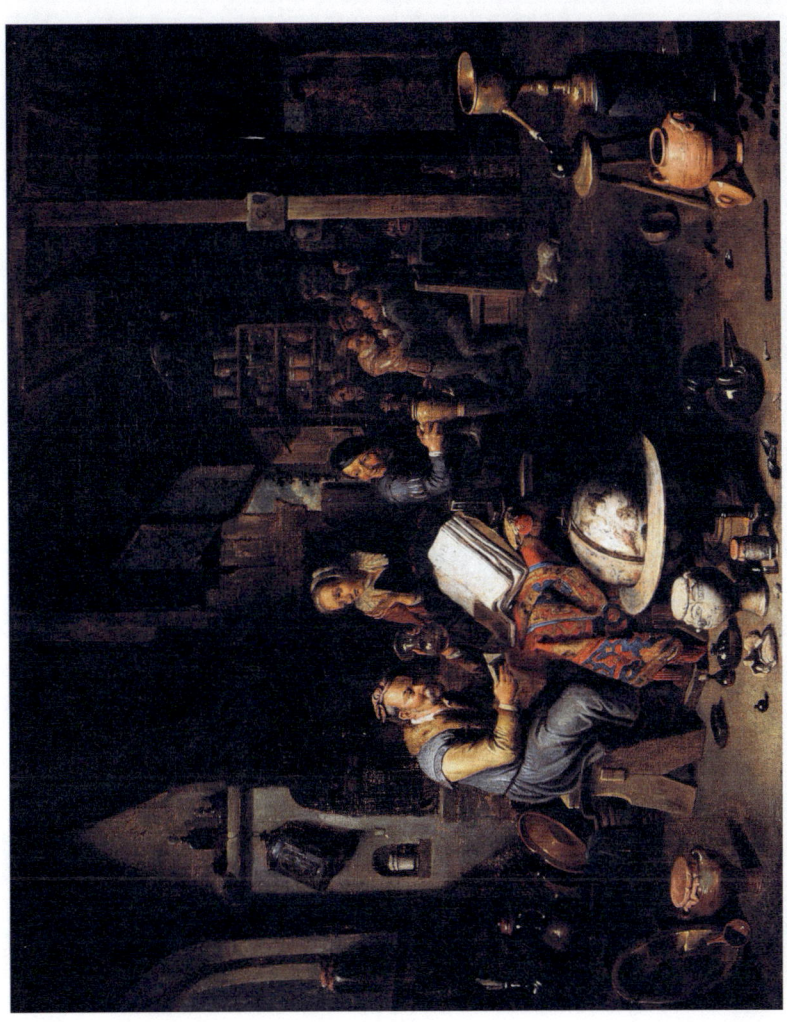

Plate 23   Balthasar van den Bossche (1681–1715), *The Iatrochemist* (Philadelphia, Museum of the Chemical Heritage Foundation, Eddleman Collection)

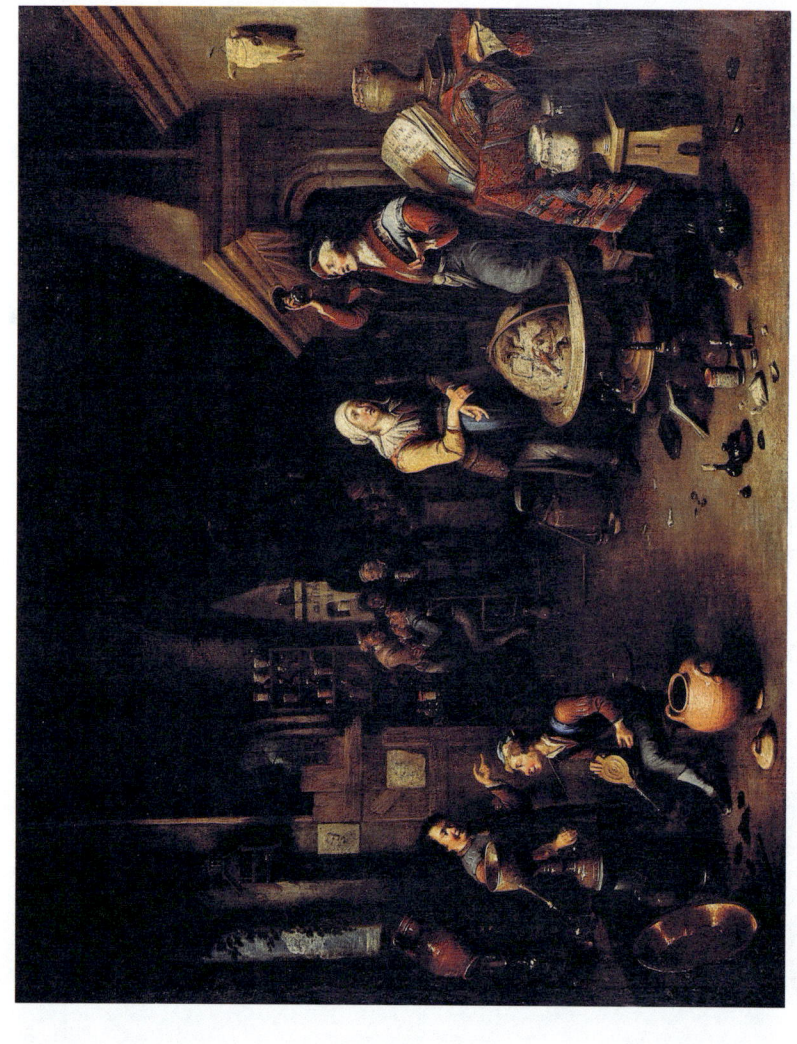

Plate 24   Gerard Thomas (1663–1721), Physician examining a urine flask (London, Wellcome Library)

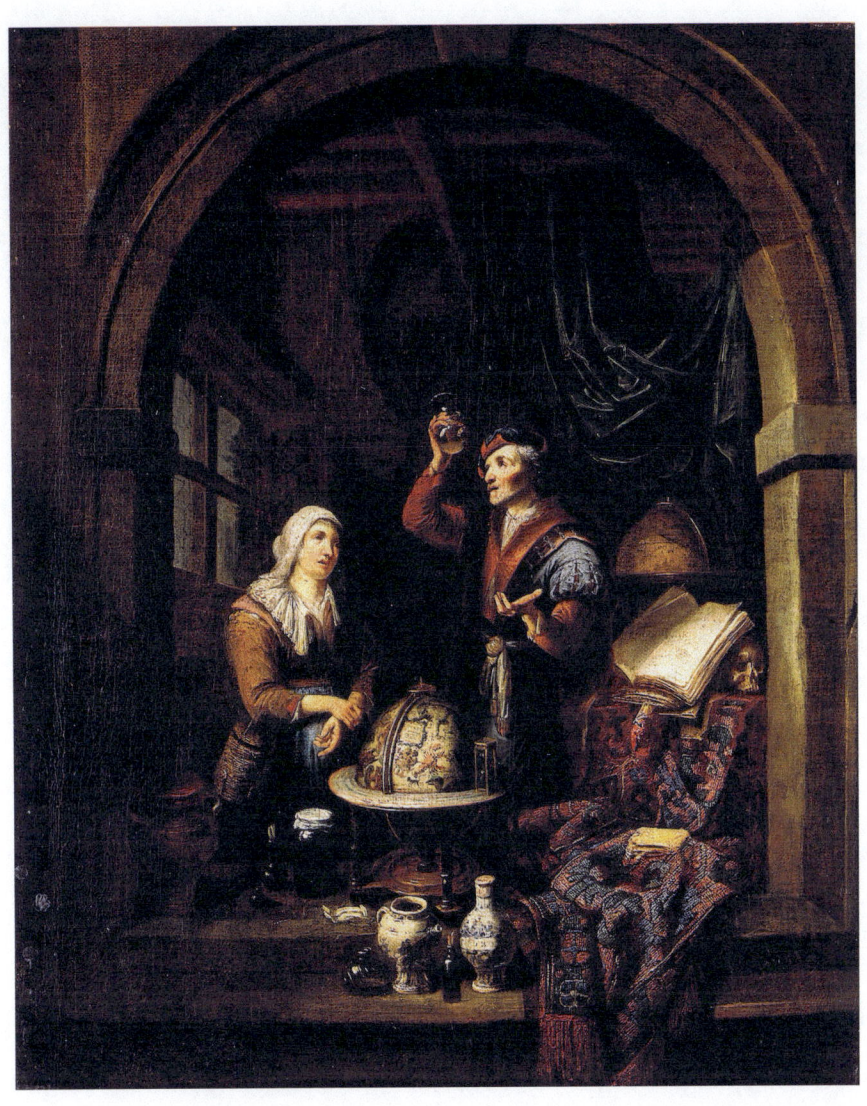

Plate 25   Gerard Thomas (1663–1721), Physician examining a urine flask (variation on Plate 24) (London, Wellcome Library)

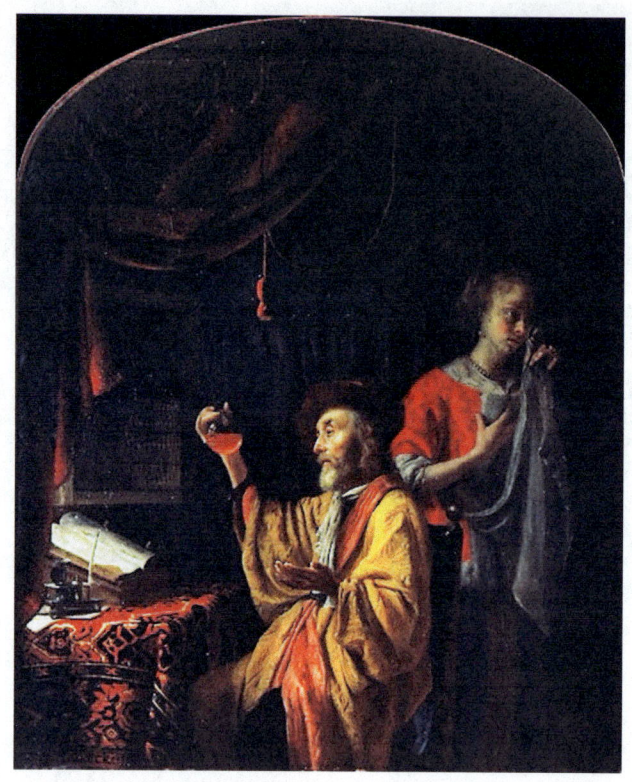

Plate 26   Godfried Schalcken (1643–1706), Uroscopic pregnancy diagnosis
(formerly Cologne, Wallraf-Richartz Museum, Dep. 530, current
owner unknown)

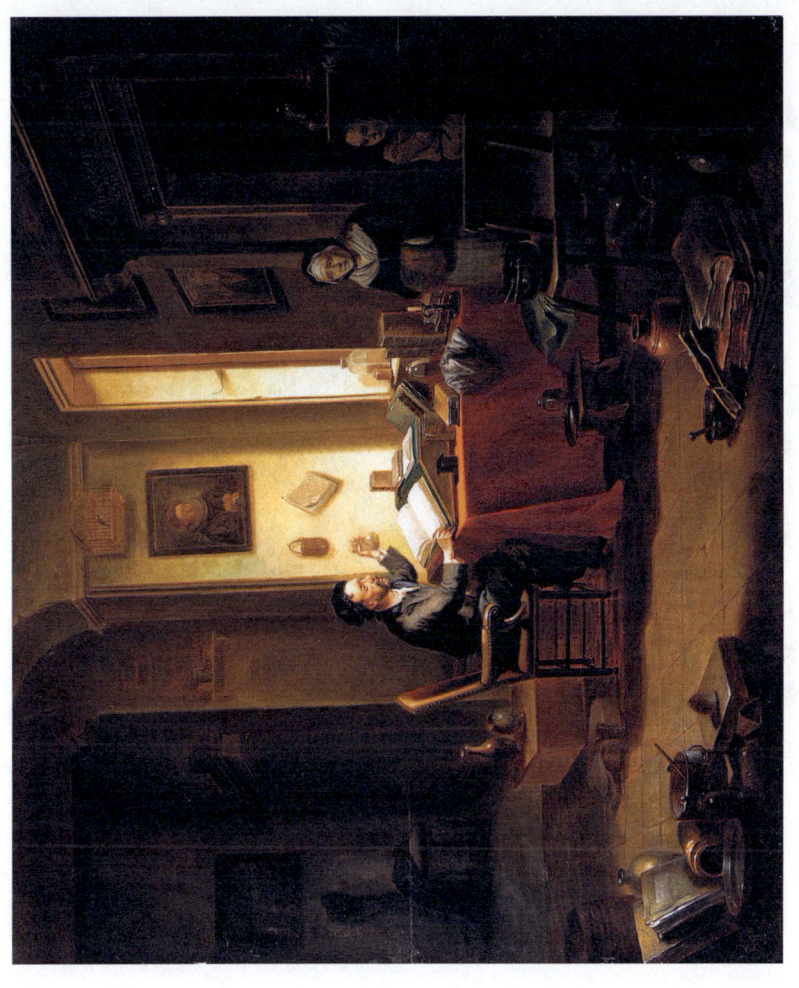

Plate 27 Justus Juncker (1703–1763), Physician examining a urine flask (London, Wellcome Library)

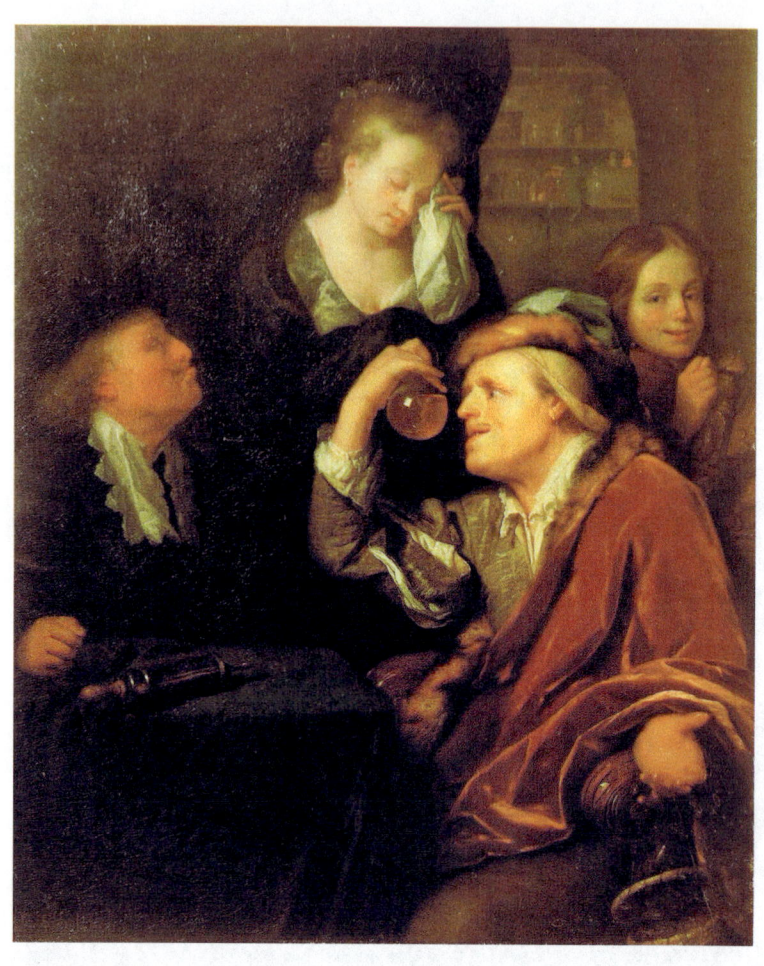

Plate 28   Godfried Schalcken (1643–1706), *Het onderzoek van de dokter*
(The Hague, Mauritshuis)

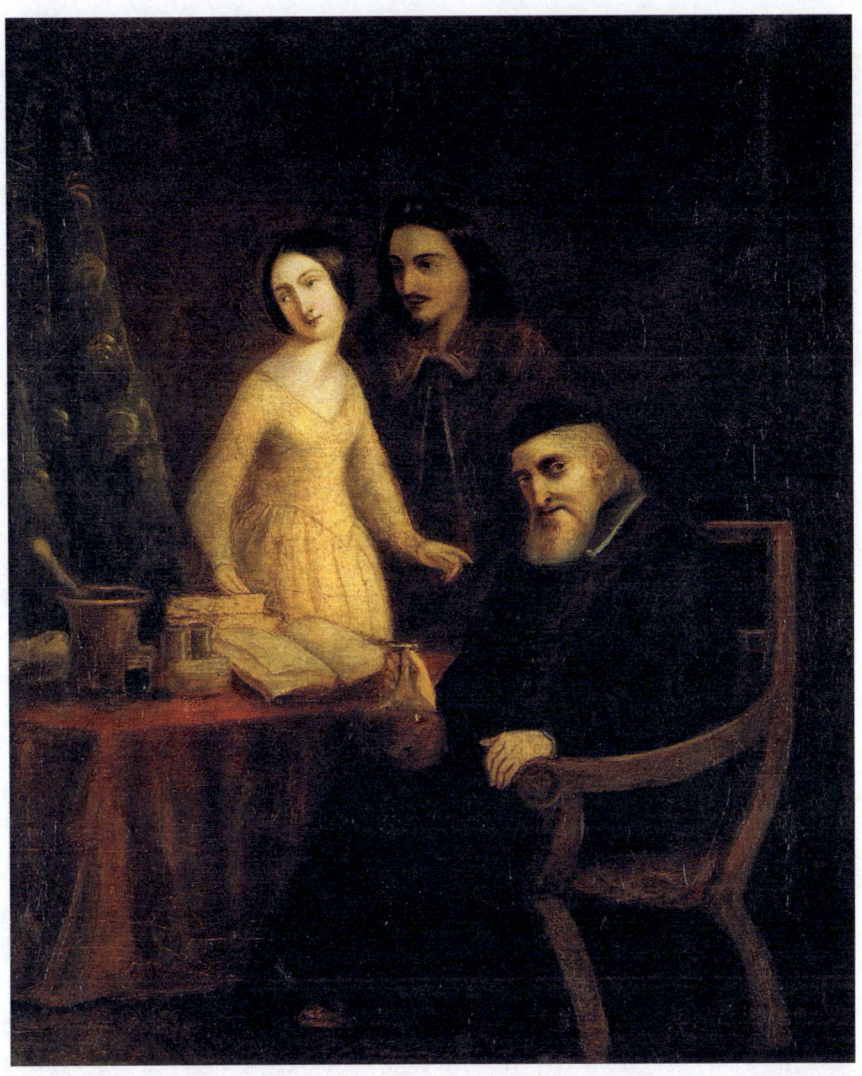

Plate 29   Oil painting by an unknown artist (around 1700?), Physician
examining a urine flask in the presence of a young couple (London,
Wellcome Library)

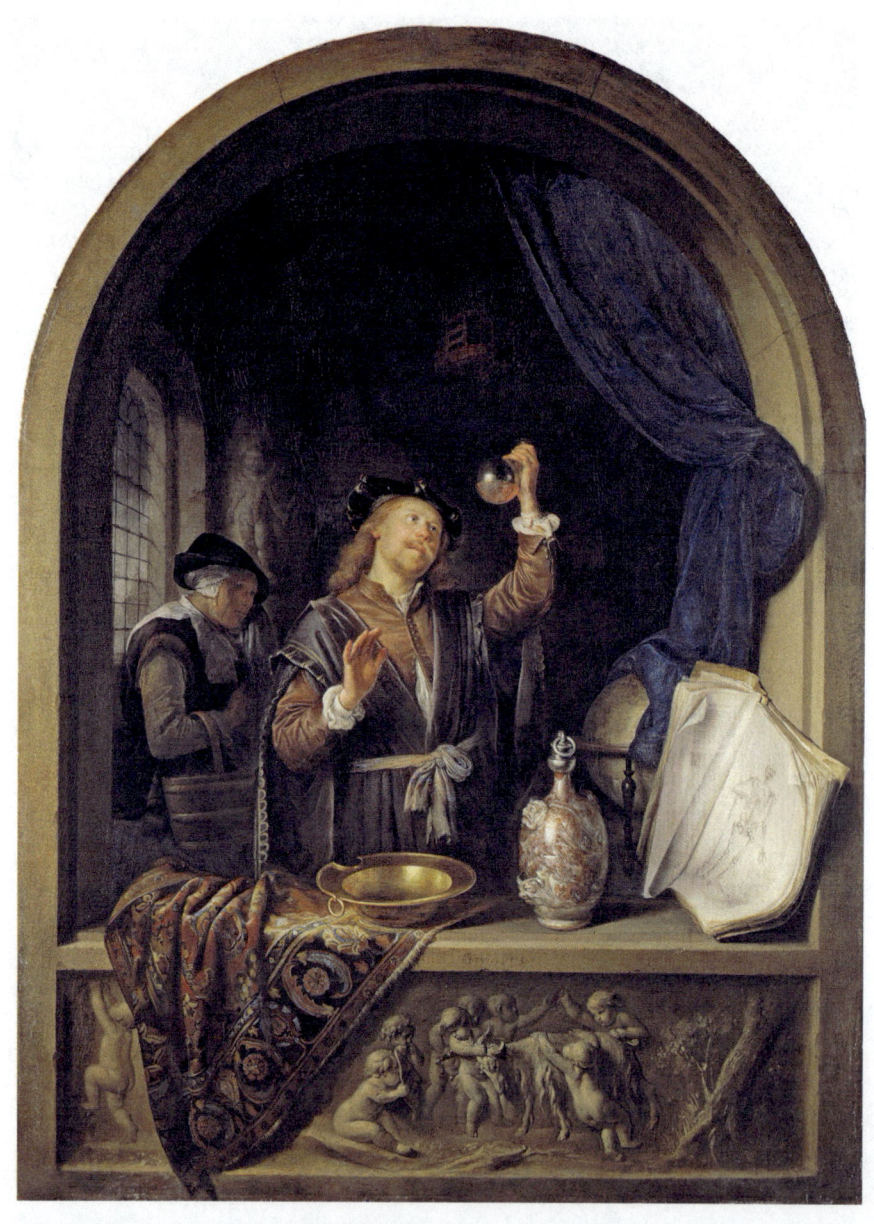

Plate 30   Gerard Dou (1613–1675), Uroscopist (Vienna, Kunst-historisches Museum)

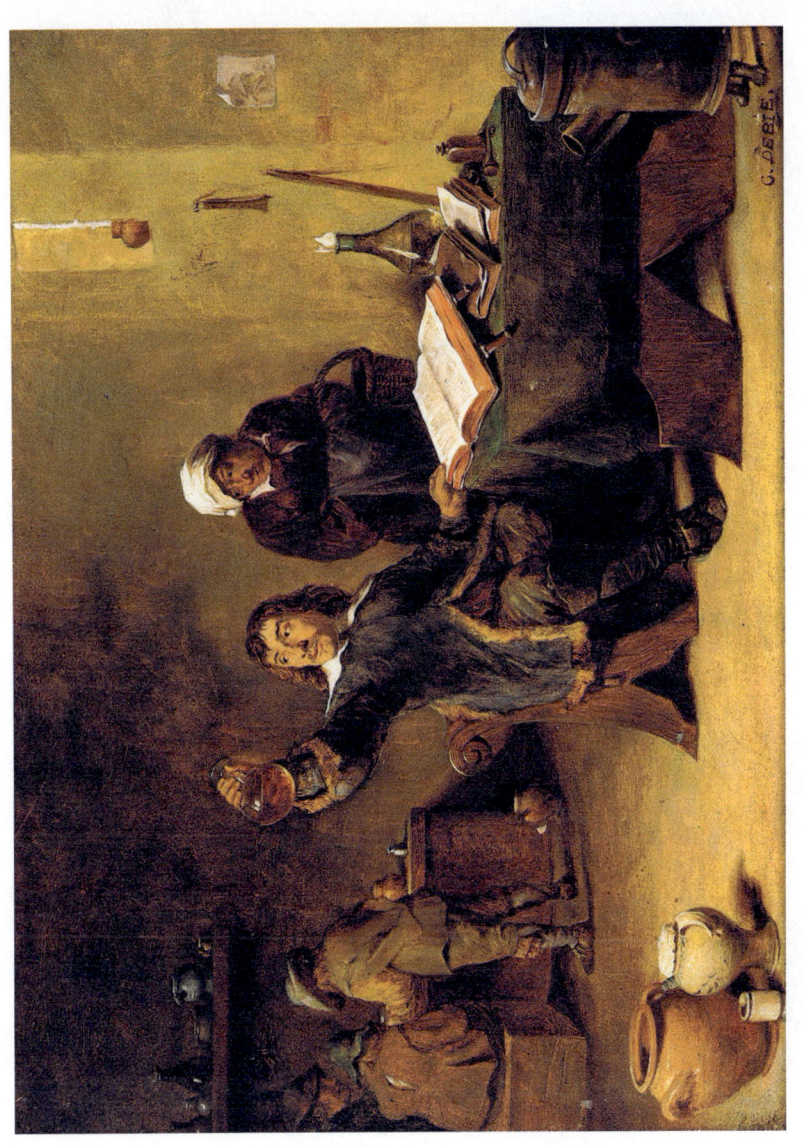

Plate 31   Oil painting by C. de Bie (?) after David Teniers (1610–1690), Village uroscopist (London, Wellcome Library)

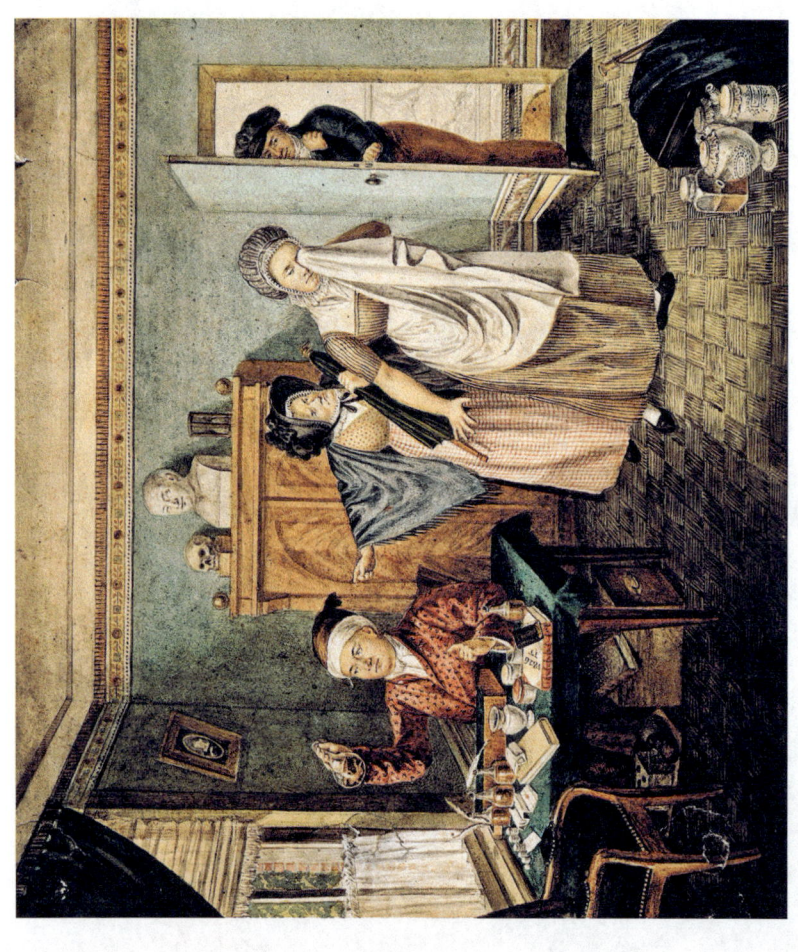

Plate 32   I.T., Pregnancy diagnosis (1826), (London, Wellcome Library)

the desired certainty. From the male perspective, however, uroscopy was useful for more than an early diagnosis of pregnancy. It offered a chance of drawing out a truth from the female body, which unmarried women, in particular, were intent on keeping to themselves.

Not all paintings addressing the uroscopic diagnosis of the secret sufferings of young women are easily classed as referring to pregnancy. A good example is the painting on the cover of this book, Samuel van Hoogstraten's *La femme chlorotique,* that is, *The Chlorotic Woman.* Chlorosis was well known and described as a disease entity in the medical literature of the day.[45] It was attributed to a disturbed menstruation and could be accompanied by a multitude of different symptoms, but it was characterized above all by a pale complexion, a disturbed appetite, and general weakness. Contemporary writings on uroscopy—including simple, practical health guides that would have been accessible to artists and other laypeople—described the urine of chlorotic women as watery and thin. The urine in Hoogstraten's painting, by comparison, has a tint that is even darker than the patient's yellow garment. The diagnosis of a "chlorosis" also can hardly be reconciled with the unmistakable sexual clues: the erotic paintings on the wall and the cat—a well-known symbol of infidelity—lying at the woman's feet. Rather than chlorosis all might seem to indicate lovesickness, an interpretation that is supported by the woman's pale complexion, sunken eyes, and melancholic mood. However, there is no hint at pulse diagnosis, which was deemed far more important than uroscopy, even indispensable, for the diagnosis of lovesickness. With all likelihood, the painting represents a diagnosis of pregnancy. Like chlorosis, pregnancy was accompanied by suppressed periods. Deprived of this "monthly cleansing," the woman's body accumulated impure, spoiled humors. Though pregnant women were supposedly capable of somehow sequestering the accumulating fluid inside their bodies until it finally found its way outside with the lochia, suppressed periods and pregnancy could have very similar consequences, including swelling of the belly, depraved appetite, nausea, and vomiting. Hoogstraten's intention to paint a suspected pregnancy would also best explain the presence of the man standing behind the suffering woman and his apprehensive facial expression. He could be seen as the lover, or more likely still as the cuckold who is about to see through his wife's game thanks to uroscopy.

It should be mentioned that Laurinda Dixon has rejected the interpretation of Hoogstraten's painting as a depiction of a pregnancy diagnosis. In fact, she has doubted generally that an illegitimate pregnancy could have served as a subject of art at that time, even in the relatively progressive Netherlands.[46] This assumption, however, is clearly at odds with some artworks of the period, which leave no doubt

---

[45]   Since the nineteenth century, the term has increasingly become synonymous with *anemia.* On Hoogstraten's medical subjects see Meige, *Les peintres* (1895).

[46]   Dixon, *Together in misery* (2003), 247.

whatsoever as to the subject of the painting and which, as we will see in a moment, sometimes even provide explicit written reference to illegitimate pregnancy. I also find it difficult to agree with Dixon's observation—which she uses to support her assumption that the genre paintings depict uterine complaints—that the urine is "usually colorless and translucent."[47] We predominantly find saturated golden yellow or reddish tints, which allowed the artist to bring out the play of light in the liquid.

In no uncertain terms, Godfried Schalcken's (1643–1706) *The Doctor's Visit* from 1669 makes reference to a pregnancy diagnosis (see Plate 26). A young woman dabs at her tears with a kerchief, while the dignified elderly uroscopist is examining a matula with red-colored urine. As mentioned, the urine of pregnant women was usually described as having a reddish tint, and considering the importance of pregnancy diagnosis, we may assume that this had become common knowledge among laypeople. The young woman's emotional turmoil, along with the absence of the typical urine basket, strongly suggests that she herself came for advice. However, it would be interesting to learn the significance of the small book she holds in her left hand.

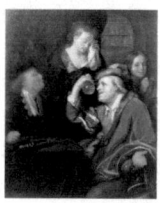

Schalcken is even more explicit in a similar, somewhat later painting, which today can be viewed at the *Mauritshuis* in The Hague (see Plate 28).[48] Here too, a young woman, crying, stands next to the doctor who examines her urine. But in this painting a boy near the right-hand margin makes an unmistakably obscene gesture with his finger. By pushing his thumb up between his middle and index finger, he signals to the viewer that fornication has taken place. The man depicted on the left is likely the less-than-pleased father. When we take a close look at the matula, we can even make out the silhouette of a fetus in the urine.

A painting ascribed to Jan Steen even bore the explicit inscription: "If I am not mistaken, this maiden is with child."[49] Unfortunately, we know this only from a surviving description of the painting. The painting itself has been lost, which is all the more regrettable as it would be instructive to compare it with other paintings by Steen which may erroneously have been taken for representations of lovesickness.

There is a similarly explicit but likewise missing painting by Jan Josef Horemans, but in this case at least a printed version is extant.[50] It shows a physician in his

---

[47]   Ibid., 79.

[48]   Cf. also Meige, *Urologues* (1900), 762f, who refers to an earlier painting by David Ryckaert (1612–1661) showing a uroscopist (or alchemist) who holds a glass in which a small homunculus can be seen.

[49]   Naumann, *Mieris* (1981), 101 (note): "Als ik my niet verzind, is deze Meid met kind."

[50]   Cf. Rubin, *Young woman* (1981); it is unclear, so far, whether the painter was Jan Josef Horemans the elder (1682–1759) or the younger (1714–1790).

working parlor, sitting on a chair in front of a well-stocked book cabinet. He looks at a matula with urine inside, which is clearly that of a young woman standing silently at the center of attention. She looks down at the floor shyly, tilting her head to one side. The doctor, another man—possibly a famulus—and two women all look at the young woman. Just outside the open door we see a man about to leave, dressed in simple attire and holding a cane. What the painting itself already suggests is further explained by the commentaries written below it, in German, Latin, and French. The viewer learns that the young woman's body does not yet reveal any signs of pregnancy and that she does not want to confess her sinful act. "Her words will not come out and her belly is silent still," the situation is described in German rhymes. "Her mother, the doctor, and the urine ultimately worm out the truth from her: Soon she will give birth to a child."

In a watercolor only signed "I.T." from the year 1826 we encounter a very similar scene—possibly borrowed from Horemans's painting—without an accompanying text. Again we find a young woman and what seems to be her angry mother (see Plate 32). Any remaining doubts are resolved here by closer scrutiny of the matula itself. As in Schalcken's painting, it contains a minuscule yet perfectly formed child—presumably something like a virtual reflection of the real child in the woman's womb.

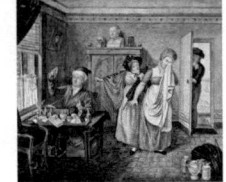

Under the title *The Doctor Diviner*, an English print, which carries a French and a German caption, approached the topic with milder humor (see Figure 4.2). According to the (slightly more detailed) German text, the physician, gazing at a urine glass in the presence of a woman whose hands touch her own belly, declares: "My child, I see from the urine, believe me, as truly as I am a doctor, that this itching, this pain, swelling and frequent vomiting will not cease until nine months are over."

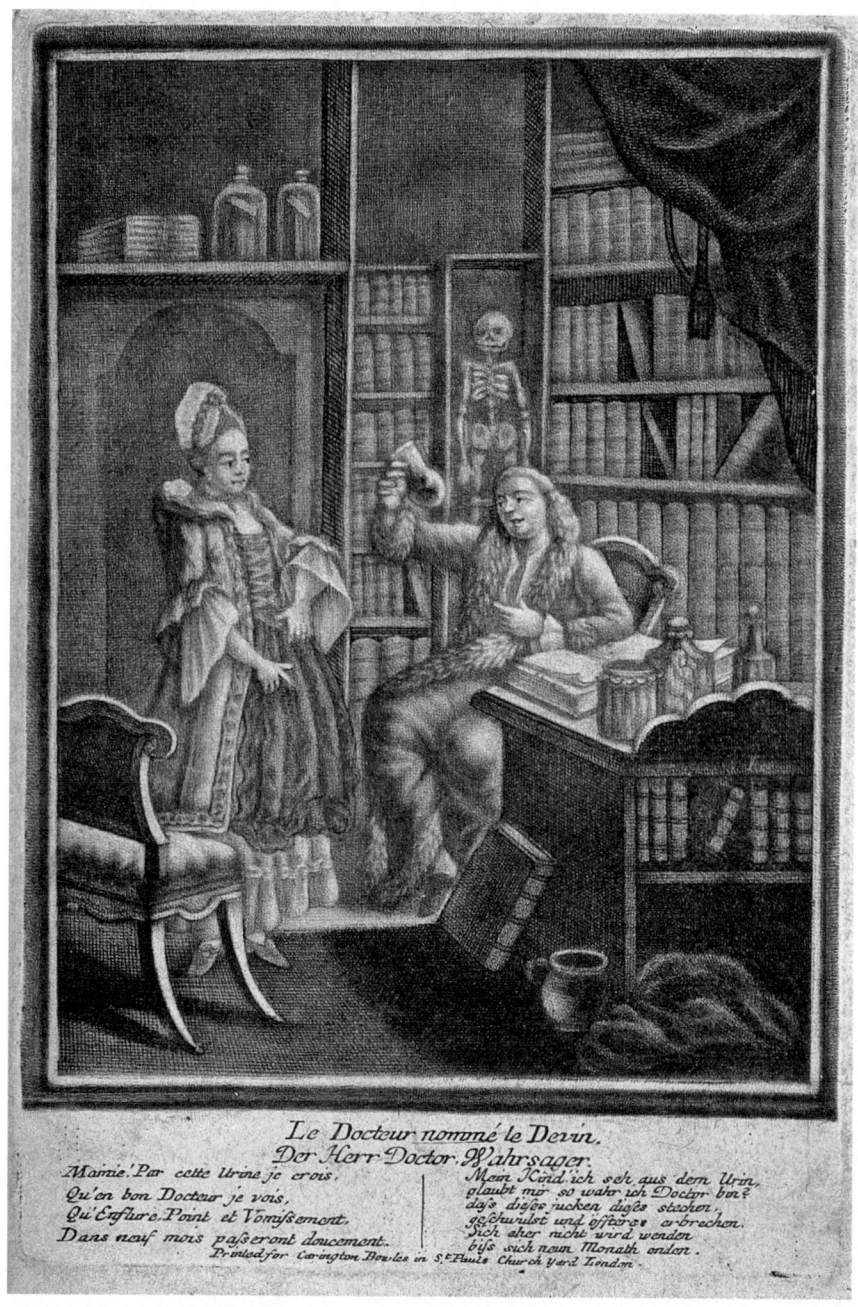

Figure 4.2   Unknown artist, *Le docteur nommé le devin*, printed for Carrington Bowles, London (Wellcome Library, London)

Chapter 5
The Gradual Decline of Uroscopy

As we have seen in the previous chapters, uroscopy retained its overarching significance in the medical life of the population at large well into the nineteenth century. To most laypeople, uroscopy remained more than just one of many diagnostic options: It was *the* key that opened the door to the secrets of the sick person's body, to the mysterious processes within it. Uroscopy enjoyed a secure place in the diagnostic practice of physicians as well. But by the seventeenth and eighteenth centuries this place had changed significantly, as is evidenced by medical writings. Leading medical writers now also emphasized the limitations of uroscopic diagnosis and cautioned their readers against placing too much trust in it.[1]

This critique was directed in particular at diagnosis based on the sole use of uroscopy, but there are also signs that uroscopy as a whole gradually lost significance among learned physicians. The tradition of great uroscopy treatises basically ended with the last comprehensive synthesis by the Byzantine Johannes Actuarius.[2] Physicians who wanted to attain renown in the medical republic of letters came to favor other subjects. A formidable number of medical publications on uroscopy continued to appear but most of them no longer aimed primarily at presenting the principles of uroscopy.[3] Instead they fulminated against its widespread "misuse"[4] and fiercely attacked as "uromancers" those among their learned colleagues who continued to take uroscopy seriously.[5]

Uroscopic diagnosis also had a remarkably modest place in the countless medical case histories that early modern physicians published. This cannot necessarily be taken to imply that doctors no longer performed uroscopy. Descriptions of urinary changes are conspicuously more common in hand-

---

[1]   This chapter is based in part on my analysis of this development in Stolberg, *Decline of uroscopy* (2007).

[2]   Actuarius, *De urinis* (1519); Actuarius, *De urinis* (1670); Gesnerus, *Compendium* ([around 1541]); Joannes Zacharias Actuarius lived in the thirteenth century and became a leading uroscopic authority upon the publication of his treatise on uroscopy in Latin.

[3]   E.g. Bertrand, *Nova philosophandi ratio* (1630) and, in spite of the promising title, Odone, *De urinarum differentiis* (1658).

[4]   Starck, *Harmspiegel* (1597); Hornung, *Uroscopia fraudulenta* (1611); Stahl, *Gründliche Abhandlung* (1739).

[5]   Cf. Munnicks, *De urinis* (1674) and the massive attack in Schmidt, *Uromanticus castratus* (1697).

written case histories and similar records that were not intended for publication. Rather, the virtual absence of uroscopic diagnosis in published case histories supports the impression that doctors were apprehensive about being connected too closely with uroscopy in the wider medical community.

What had happened? How could a diagnostic procedure to which learned medical practice had lent paramount importance over the course of hundreds of years and which it had lauded as the most certain means of learning about diseases of the body lose significance to such an extent? The question is all the more intriguing as historians have come to the almost unanimous conclusion that before 1800 patients enjoyed a powerful position in the doctor-patient relationship, and even a dominant one in the case of the minority of affluent patients. Physicians had to bend to their ideas and wishes if they did not want to lose them and ultimately their livelihood with them.[6] How could doctors reject uroscopy in such a situation when their patients had such trust in it and expected it as a matter of course?

Theoretical Contradictions

Critics had sound theoretical arguments for why uroscopy was often uncertain and unreliable. A first major objection was that some illnesses did not change the urine. The doctor risked pronouncing the patient healthy while he or she was, in fact, seriously ill and might soon die. Even within the medical community, this argument did not meet with unanimous approval, however. There was considerable debate on how reliable uroscopy was in different types of diseases. No physician seriously contested that uroscopy could indicate diseases in those parts of the body that were directly involved in the excretion of urine: the kidneys, the ureters, the bladder, and the urethra. Insofar as the majority of doctors acknowledged that urine was a by-product of the concoction of food in the stomach and liver, there was also little doubt that pathological change in these organs, too, would have an impact on the urine. Especially before Harvey's new theory of blood circulation became widely accepted, it was somewhat more difficult to explain how diseases in the remaining body parts could change the urine. After all, according to the traditional Galenic account, blood flowed very slowly and only in one direction through the veins, from the center—from the liver—to the periphery. There it was assimilated by the various body parts and the superfluities were expelled through perspiration. As the blood, according to this time-honored model, did not return to the center and, in particular, to the kidneys, the question arose how the blood, and with it, eventually, the urine, could be changed by diseases in the various parts of the body. Some leading

---

[6]   See the seminal work by Jewson, *Medical knowledge* (1974).

late medieval physicians did take Galen's *caveat* to heart that urine in the case of lung diseases could be deceptive. The well-known Italian doctor Michele Savonarola (ca. 1365 to ca. 1466) warned that if a disease did not affect the liver or the urinary tract, diagnosis on the sole basis of urine was unreliable and that the physician had to rely also on other diagnostic evidence.[7] According to Alessandro Massaria (1510–1598), urine shed light primarily on the liver, kidneys, and bladder and only indirectly, *per accidens*, on the remaining parts, namely to the degree to which the quality of the urine reflected the power of the body's natural heat, which was essential for "concocting" food and fighting morbid matter.[8] Along similar lines, Guillaume Rondelet (1507–1566) declared uroscopy to be "less certain" when it came to diseases of the head or chest or to those caused by morbid matter located outside the veins.[9] In the early seventeenth century, Ananius Horer went so far as to present a whole list of common diseases that could not be recognized in the urine, such as consumption and dropsy, chest illnesses, coughing, expectoration, pneumonia, white and red dysentery, apoplexy, cramps, contracture of the nerves, palsy, podagra (gout), arthritis, muscle diseases, tumors, the French disease, wounds and broken bones.[10]

This critique was based on controversial assumptions, however. Early modern medicine disposed of various explanatory concepts that did allow for urine to undergo characteristic changes even in the case of diseases outside the stomach, liver, and efferent urinary tract. We have already encountered one such model: According to Paracelsus, in addition to the "external urine," which was produced in the process of concoction, there was also "internal urine," which flowed to the bladder from the whole body and could thus reflect the body's changes.[11] Most doctors rejected Paracelsian theories,[12] though they acknowledged the effectiveness of certain chemical drugs.[13] Yet, Paracelsus probably derived his notion of an "internal urine" from ideas that had wide currency also in mainstream medicine. Medieval and early modern physicians described the body as highly permeable. Natural and pathological humors like atter could

---

[7]   Savonarola, *De urinis* (1561), 94r; similarly Salvianus, *De urinarum differentiis* (1587), 5f.

[8]   Massaria, *Tractatus* (1608), 165.

[9]   Rondelet, *Praelectiones* (sine anno), 3.

[10]   Horer, *Artzney-Teuffel* (1634), 63.

[11]   Paracelsus, *De urinis* (1931), 632–5.

[12]   In Wittenberg, Andreas Tentzelius (*De urinis,* 1609) discussed in a public disputation "whether the uromancy of the spagyric doctors with its separation and dissolution of mercury, sulfur, and salt must be acknowledged true"; his answers are not documented but the accompanying note "N. cum D." (instead of "A." for "affirmatio") suggests a negation with differentiation, that is, a (qualified) rejection of the thesis.

[13]   On the necessity of a nuanced understanding of anti-Paracelsianism cf. Walter, *New light* (2012).

move freely through it, independently of the blood vessels, almost at their own discretion. In the form of "fluxes," they could collect in a certain body part for some time and eventually move to another. So the movement of blood and of the humors in general was not only from the liver to the periphery but also back toward the center. If this was the case, changes in the blood and the humors could, in turn, easily cause changes in the urine on the way from the site of its production, the liver, to its exit from the body.[14]

When William Harvey's new theory of circulation became accepted in the course of the seventeenth century,[15] the argument that urine reflected only the state of the liver, kidneys, and efferent urinary tract lost even more of its persuasiveness. If the blood, from which the urine emanated, first flowed through the entire body before reaching the kidneys, where it would be strained, it could easily come into direct contact with morbid matter in any part of the body. As I. Fletcher emphatically put it in 1641, the urine gave "the most manifeste certaine and generall signification of all diseases; because with the blood it is conveyed into all parts of the body, and from thence returneth backe againe in the veines to the liver and vessels of urin, bringing with it some note of the state and disposition of all those parts from whence it commeth."[16] Late seventeenth-century authors elaborated on how the urine initially mixed with the blood and flowed through the whole body, and only after it had done so separated from the blood in the delicate, progressively narrowing renal tubules.[17] Even authors who cautioned against overvaluing uroscopy now described typical changes in the urine as caused by diseases which according to earlier critics left no traces in the urine.[18]

Less controversial was a second criticism against the practice of diagnosing illness on the sole basis of uroscopy: It was widely agreed that without detailed knowledge of the patient's age, temperament, lifestyle, and current complaints, uroscopy was inevitably unreliable. In 1518, one of the earliest "uroskeptics," Lorenz Fries, acknowledged that among all fluid evacuations the urine offered the most important diagnostic clues, yet "it is not sufficient to divine from it." It was also necessary to know the possible causes and circumstances of the disease.[19] In Italy, Leonardo Botalli, too, declared such additional information an indispensable prerequisite for a reliable diagnosis. Whoever claimed that he

---

[14]   Cf. e.g. Savonarola, *De urinis* (1561), 94r.

[15]   Harvey, *Exercitatio anatomica* (1628); Beverwijk, *Schat der ongesontheyt* (1672), 8; by contrast, Brooke, *Hygieine* (1650), 194–8, resorted only to pre-Harveyan arguments.

[16]   Fletcher, *Differences* (1641), preface; similarly Willis, *Five treatises* (1681), 18, who, however, further qualified that illnesses of certain parts of the body did not change the urine.

[17]   Liessell, *Konste* (1668), 14; Beverwijk, *Schat der ongesontheyt* (1672), 8; Behrens, *Wasserbeschawen* (1688), 3–5.

[18]   Rübel, *Gebrauch* (1762), 103.

[19]   Fries, *Spiegel* (1518), LXXXr.

could identify diseases or determine a pregnancy simply by looking at a patient's urine was on par with someone who claimed he could predict the outcome of dice rolls. Occasionally he would be right, but most often he would err.[20] "On the mere basis of urine that has been brought to him, a physician may not make a judgment"—was one of the basic rules of uroscopic practice which, around 1700, Friedrich Hoffmann sought to impress upon his students.[21] Even if the patient resided elsewhere and could not be questioned and examined, the doctor should at least be informed about the patient's sex and age and whether he or she was bedridden. Otherwise he should refuse to express a *judicium*.[22]

For understandable reasons, this rejection of the common practice of diagnosing diseases from urine alone was widely shared in the medical community. This practice ultimately challenged a central feature of early modern physicians' professional identity. Learned physicians sought to distinguish themselves from their less learned competitors above all by their ability to tailor the diagnosis and treatment to the individual patient, taking into account a wide range of potential influences and interpreting them correctly in the light of their extensive learning. From this perspective, if the uroscopist did not know whether the urine came from a woman or a man, a child or an elderly person, whether the sick person tended toward a phlegmatic, sanguine, choleric, or melancholic temperament, whether he or she ate well or poorly, or took certain medicines or foods that changed the urine, it would be utterly impossible to make a sure diagnosis. If a woman, for instance, produced somewhat cloudy, pale urine, this was no cause for concern because women, due to their weakaer vital heat, did not possess the same ability as men to concoct food and humors to completion, without residues. So urine of this kind was natural in women. But if the very same urine came from a young man, these characteristics might indicate a weakness of the stomach or liver which required treatment. If the doctor did not know the patient's sex, frequent misdiagnosis was inevitable. Certain urinary changes could even result from a whole range of different diseases. Light-colored, watery urine, for example, could be the result of drinking thin liquids or of obstructed kidneys, which only allowed thin urine to pass. It could also come from a weakened digestion or concoction in the stomach or liver, or, in the case of gangrene, from the fact that bile had risen to the heart.[23]

---

[20]   Botalli, *Commentarioli duo* (1565), 22.

[21]   Hoffmann, *Medicus politicus* (1708), 132; similarly, in France, Finot, *An ex urinis certa valetudinis auguria* (1677).

[22]   Hoffmann, *Medicus politicus* (1708), 132f.

[23]   Beverwijk, *Schat* (1672), 18.

Medical Authority in Jeopardy

When physicians worried that uroscopy harbored a great risk of misdiagnosis and misprognosis—especially in the absence of more precise information about the patient and the many factors that could change the urine—this worry needs to be taken seriously. Yet such concerns can only partly explain the growing and often vitriolic and polemical critique of uroscopy. Very similar criticism had already been put forward and discussed in Antiquity and the Middle Ages without much effect on the great esteem in which uroscopy was held among learned physicians. The cautioning words from some of the leading authors of medieval medicine were well known to Western doctors. The Zurich city physician Clauser, for example, summarized Rhazes's advice as follows: "Do not judge the urine if you do not see the sick man in person and question him and learn from him."[24] All the while it was common as late as the eighteenth century for renowned physicians to treat wealthy patients at a distance, making their diagnoses on the sole basis of letters—some of which were very short—in which the patient described his or her complaints.[25] In no way, then, was a personal encounter, let alone a physical examination, considered indispensable.

As a matter of fact, upon closer examination, numerous medical writings from the early sixteenth century onward leave no doubt that there was another, far more powerful motive, namely physicians' concerns about their authority and status. While uroscopy in the Middle Ages was still extolled as the foundation of medical authority, it now appeared to many physicians as one of the greatest threats to their professional standing.[26]

They had good reason to worry. A first threat to medical authority resulted from the very nature of urine itself. Uroscopy involved close contact with foul, stinking excretions at a time in which, as Norbert Elias has shown in *The Civilizing Process*, human excretions were increasingly perceived as offensive.[27] It is telling that early modern patients or their relatives who mentioned urine or other excretions in their letters, almost routinely added apologetic phrases such as "salva reverentia," "salvo respectu," or "mit Urlob" [with permission]. While examining a clean matula might still be perceived as less damaging to the physician's dignity than diagnosing diseases by poking around in stinking feces with a stick,[28] the contemptuous names given to uroscopists at the time, such as

---

[24]   Clauser, *Betrachtung* ([1531]), no pagination; cf. Costeo's running commentary on the chapter on uroscopy in Avicenna, *Canon* (1595), 149–61.

[25]   On consulting by letter see cf. Stolberg, *Experiencing illness* (2011).

[26]   On the foundations and challenges of early modern learned physicians' authority see Stolberg, *Formen und Strategien* (2003) and Stolberg, *Medizinische Deutungsmacht* (2004).

[27]   Elias, *Civilizing process* (2000).

[28]   Da Monte, *Tractatus de urinis* (sine anno), 2v.

"piss-mongers" or "pis-kijkers" [piss gazers], reveal at least a considerable degree of ambivalence.

Agrippa von Nettesheim's scathing criticism highlights how the physicians' close association with urine and other excretions could indeed jeopardize their status in the academic world. He described them as "usually contagious, stinking of urine and stool, indeed fouler than midwives insofar as they see with their own eyes loathsome and foul things, and must listen to and smell their patients' belches and farts." Like "vultures" they "circle around the sick person's piss pot and outhouse" to turn disgraceful profit. For this reason doctors were not allowed to hold seats in the town council in many places, since they were "usually foul" and, "with [their] constant touching of sick people," befouled themselves, so much so that they even contaminated chairs and benches.[29]

Probably, concerns about their dignity were also a major reason why most physicians were averse to making use of senses other than vision when they examined the urine. "If the physician were not a distinguished and noble man, as he ought to be," wrote Giovanni Argenterio (1513–1572), then he could draw important conclusions from the variations in the taste of urine, but, he continued, "we reject that so as not to turn a noble art into a filthy one."[30] "Who would be so spiritless, so barbaric, and so revolting," asked Scribonius, "that he would examine all the sick people's urine using his sense of taste?"[31] Or to quote Johannes Walaeus's (1604–1649): "Sapor non gustatur," which translates roughly as "the taste is not to be tried."[32]

The problem was that by refusing to taste urine the doctors might maintain their dignity but they risked falling behind in diagnostic acumen. Some of the non-academic uroscopists did not balk at using their gustatory sense,[33] and their Paracelsian competitors were not shy about it either. The Galenic doctors refused to taste even their own urine, huffed van Helmont. If they stooped to taste it, he went on, they would quickly learn that urine did not taste bitter and that its yellow color could thus not arise from admixtures of bile. But no, they would rather put their patients at risk.[34] A proponent of orthodox medicine, Veit Riedlin admitted that at least some additional diagnostic clues could be gained from tasting urine. He told of a clergyman who went so far as to claim that he could tell from the taste of urine whether a person would die, namely, if the urine tasted like a fire that had just been put out. Riedlin emphasized,

29 Nettesheim, *De incertitudine* (1539), vol. 2, 79 and 81.

30 Argenterio, *De urinis* (1591), 18.

31 Scribonius, *De inspectione urinarum* (1585), 44.

32 Walaeus, *Medica* (1660), 76.

33 Saltzmann, *De uromantia* (1651), no pagination; Borrichius, *Itinerarium* (1983), 109, on a local "uromantic" healer, ca 1660.

34 Helmont, *Aufgang* (1683), 393.

however, that he would not put up with the disgusting practice.[35] Thomas Willis (1621–1675), celebrated as the discoverer of the sweet taste of urine in diabetics, was one of the first widely respected early modern doctors who was open and matter-of-fact in pointing out the significance of tasting urine. Presumably the growing appreciation of a strictly empirical, sense-based understanding of nature made this easier.[36] Some of Willis's followers also pointed to the diagnostic significance of sweet-tasting urine. Johan van Dueren, for example, recounted that a patient in his own practice produced urine that was sweet as honey.[37]

These physicians were a minority, however. Even just smelling urine, which Avicenna and even Pinder had advised as a matter of course,[38] seemed a threat to the dignity of early modern doctors, if not a vestige of a barbaric kind of medicine. A Würzburg dissertation by Adriaan van Roomen[39] warned the reader: "To stick one's aquiline nose into the matula (as the Arabs were wont to do)" was "dirty" and dishonored the physician's dignity. Yet the medical tradition that attributed diagnostic significance to different urine odors remained alive. So physicians attempted to maneuver between Scylla and Charybdis: between vulgarity on the one hand and missing out on important diagnostic information on the other. One English introduction to uroscopy, for instance, admonished the reader: "To smell urine is an nasty trick, not fitting the dignity of the physician [...] but sometimes, against our wills, there is a mean odor, especially if the urine is hot or was moved at the fire." For a full page, the reader then learned of the possible significance of a honey-sweet taste in urine, which could result from certain medications for instance, and about the meaning of foul-smelling urine, caused by some foods, humoral changes, or ulcers and other diseases of the urinary organs.[40] Johannes Hornung explained along similar lines that he would rather smell "the excrement of muskrat"—castoreum, that is—than "stinking urine" but then, too, went on to discuss the different odors that could emanate from urine and their diagnostic significance.[41]

The Paracelsians showed even less reserve. Johan Hayne included a small chart in his introduction to uroscopy that was to help uroscopists to identify on the basis of smell three different kinds of putrefied matter, associated with

---

[35]   Riedlin, *Lineae* (1699), 491–5.

[36]   Willis, *Pharmaceutice rationalis* (1674); idem, *Five treatises* (1681), 21f.

[37]   Van Dueren, *Ontdekkinge* (1688), 38f; the patient was a clergyman from Heukelum whom he treated together with Stephan Blankaart.

[38]   Avicenna, *Canon* (1595), 50r, chapter on *De significationibus odoris urine*; Pinder, *Epiphanie medicorum* (1506), 11v.

[39]   Tröstler, *Uroscopia* (1601), 7; it is unclear which of the two was the actual author but probably the text was written by Tröstler's teacher and promoter (*präses*), Adriaan van Roomen.

[40]   Fernel/Cole/Culpeper, *Two treatises* (1662), 45f.

[41]   Hornung, *Uroscopia fraudulenta* (1611), 34f.

the three Paracelsian principles of salt, sulfur, and mercury, respectively. Much as the traditional urinary color charts did, he took recourse here to everyday comparisons, to the stench of onions on glowing embers, for instance.[42]

Patients and families, at times, seem to have drawn conclusions of their own. Kräutermann's *Curieuser und vernünfftiger Urin-Artzt* tells the story of a woman who realized that her husband was dying because his urine smelled as foul as the urine of her previous husband before he died—and indeed he did die soon after.[43]

An even greater threat to the authority and status of academic doctors came, somewhat paradoxically, from the overwhelming trust sick people and their relatives invested in uroscopy. As we have seen, this trust was so deep that patients and their relatives often expected that the uroscopist would identify the illness on the basis of urine alone and withheld information about the patient's age, sex, and complaints. The physicians themselves constantly nourished this trust. They continued to diagnose diseases by uroscopy and prescribed certain drugs based on this diagnosis, and the patient eventually got better, at least for some time, as most patients do in most kinds of diseases no matter how they are treated. As the physicians were well aware, however, there was a high risk of flagrant misdiagnosis under these circumstances. As long as the uroscopist limited himself to expounding morbid processes deep inside the body, the danger of public disgrace was limited. After all, no one could prove or disprove the diagnosis while the patient was still alive. A healer's prediction of the further course of a disease could be evaluated more easily, although, if a prognosis turned out to be wrong, there were still, as we have seen, plausible explanations that could exonerate the uroscopist. Sudden changes in the course of a disease could be explained with the variable nature of diseases and the unpredictable movements of morbid matter in the body. If the disease took a surprisingly favorable turn, this could even cast a flattering light on the therapeutic skills of the uroscopist, who, against all odds, had managed to defeat the disease.

However, , whether or not the physician had identified the age, sex, occupation, and complaints of the patient correctly– as many laypeople expected—could be determined very easily. Critics produced cautionary tales, for example the story of a woman who brought a flask of urine to a doctor, who diagnosed shortness of breath and swollen knees and said that the person in question was unable to walk. The supposed messenger then broke into laughter, telling the shamefaced doctor that the urine was her own and that she suffered nothing of the sort.[44] Hardly less risky, the uroskeptics warned their colleagues,

---

[42]   Hayne, *Drey Tractätlein* (1620), 235.

[43]   Kräutermann, *Curieuser und vernünfftiger Urin-Artzt* (1732), 97f.

[44]   Scribonius, *De inspectione urinarum* (1585), 38.

was the diagnosis of pregnancy: "If then nothing comes of it, since the urine alone cannot be trusted in this respect, he will only be ridiculed."[45]

Even when diseases deep inside the body were at issue, the physician's authority could suffer a severe blow when patients—as Foreest claimed—sent their urine to two or more doctors and then compared their judgments.[46] As doctors knew only too well they could easily come to contradictory conclusions. For good reason the *Curieuse und vernünfftige Urin-Artzt* warned its readers that the physician must generally beware of putting his *judicium* down in writing as he could "thereby disgracefully expose himself" and become the scorn of the community.[47]

Naturally, the numerous lesser-educated, non-physician uroscopists were at no lesser risk of disgracing themselves with a wrong diagnosis. They were not measured by the same standards, however, as the academically educated physicians. Since the physicians missed no opportunity to insist upon their learning and usually charged much higher fees for their services, patients could rightly expect them to prove their superior diagnostic and therapeutic skills in practice.

As critics never tired of warning their colleagues, the danger of an embarrassing misdiagnosis did not only arise from the challenges of interpreting the manifold changes in the urine correctly and from the unwillingness of patients and relatives to give additional information. The physician also always had to be wary that he might be deceived on purpose.[48] Again and again, stories were circulated of doctors who were tricked by patients who foisted the urine of livestock on them in the place of their own, or even wine or other liquids. Since a uroscopic diagnosis cost money, the critics probably exaggerated the extent to which physicians were exposed to such machinations. There were, in fact, only a handful of stories, which authors often only quoted from others or, at most, dressed in a slightly different gown. For historical analysis, these stories are informative not as a source for what actually happened but because they throw light on the complex interplay of trust and mistrust in the premodern doctor-patient relationship and on how doctors perceived it.

In some of the stories, the physician emerges as the winner thanks to his acumen. He beats with their own weapon those who want to deceive him. In one such well-known anecdote, King Heinrich I tries to fool the Abbot Notker, who was known for his medical skills, by replacing his urine with that of a pregnant chamber maid. The wise man predicted that the king would soon give

---

45   Kräutermann, *Curieuser und vernünfftiger Urin-Artzt* (1732), 11.
46   Foreest, *Uromanteia* (1620), 219; Detharding, *Kranken-Wärter* (1679), 69f.
47   Kräutermann, *Curieuser und vernünfftiger Urin-Artzt* (1732), 11.
48   Hornung, *Uroscopia fraudulenta* (1611), 10.

birth.[49] In another story, which comes in various versions, a doctor examines the urine brought to him by a patient, and upon recognizing that the urine had come from a cow, he remarks drily that the patient seems to have eaten too much grass or hay.[50]

In real life, however, the doctor had few chances of exposing such tricks.[51] The urinary treatises did describe the characteristic differences between human and animal urine: Generally the urine of animals was more viscous and cloudier than human urine, smelled "rawer," and featured more sediment.[52] Ultimately, however, it was known that animal urine "was often not unlike human urine."[53] And if it was difficult enough already to make out the differences between healthy human urine and animal urine, how could one tell the urine of a healthy cow from the urine of a sick person? After all, the sick person's urine might look like cow urine due to his or her illness. Hippocrates, for one, and Avicenna, for another, had described the urine of some patients as similar to that of cattle.[54]

It was also difficult to distinguish female and male urine in practice. If the urine of a man was passed off as that of a woman, and the doctor was even explicitly asked to decide about a possible pregnancy, it was very easy to fool him. It was generally accepted that due to the weaker vital heat and reduced power of concoction "the urine of a female person appears usually paler and more watery, with much sediment; while that of males has little or no sediment, and is more colorful."[55] Yet, illnesses or a weakening of the power of concoction with age could easily offset such differences, and the urine of a man dominated by cold, moist "phlegm" or of an "old, worn down man" might resemble very closely female urine in terms of its color.[56]

Thus from the doctor's perspective it was not only unfair but also foolish when people attempted to shame the learned physician in this manner: "The urine of many animals can resemble human urine so closely that even the learned and experienced doctor who is tested by many uncouth and meddlesome people can be tricked and unjustly mocked because of it."[57] "This testing and mocking,"

---

[49]   Cf. Christoffel, *Grundzüge* (1953), 105, note.

[50]   Primrose, *De vulgi erroribus* (1658), 103; Beverwijk, *Schat der ongesontheydt* (1672), 11; Rega, *Tractatus* (1733), 1st treatise, 34.

[51]   Liessell, *Konste* (1668), 28.

[52]   Anonymous, *Key to unknowne knowledge* (1599), ch. 2 and ch. 5; Kräutermann, *Curieuser und vernünfftiger Urin-Artzt* (1732), 102.

[53]   Foreest, *Uromanteia* (1620), 146.

[54]   Hippocrates, *Aphorisms* 4.70 (Littré, vol. 4, 526f); Avicenna, *Canon* (1595), 50r; cf. Foreest, *Uromanteia* (1620), 146f.

[55]   Kräutermann, *Curieuser und vernünfftiger Urin-Artzt* (1732), 6; cf. Henninger, *Theses* (1712).

[56]   Kräutermann, *Curieuser und vernünfftiger Urin-Artzt* (1732), 6f.

[57]   Cordus, *De urinis* (1543), no pagination.

declared Euricius Cordus, "should happen only to the vagrants and vagrant-like who boast that they can see everything in the urine, which no learned or capable doctor does."[58]

The embarrassment was bound to be all the greater when the physician was presented with malmsey, beer, mead, and the like and did not smell or taste it for fear of losing dignity. In this case, he risked becoming the laughing stock of the whole region if he diagnosed a serious illness, only to watch then with his mouth agape as the messenger lifted the matula to his lips and emptied it with demonstrative pleasure.[59]

Attempting Modernization

Weighing

The risk of embarrassing misdiagnosis and the danger that a physician's authority and that of the medical profession as a whole could be greatly harmed did much within sixteenth- and seventeenth-century academic medicine to diminish the great appreciation that uroscopy had enjoyed among medieval physicians. Already, even without taking uroscopy into account, this authority was in peril. In the late Middle Ages, doctors had increasingly succeeded in convincing their contemporaries—especially the lucrative wealthy patients—of the superiority of their art. Uroscopy had played a major part in this by underscoring the physicians' ability to unravel the mysteries of the disease processes deep within the body. But even in the Middle Ages, patients and families, more than anything else, expected a cure. And in this respect doctors, with their bloodlettings, evacuants, and complicated mixtures of herbs, did not—in the eye of the public—perform significantly better than their less learned competitors. So the more they insisted upon their superiority and demanded greater pay, the more a cleft between their highflying claims and the observed outcome of their treatment emerged.

Critics put their finger into the wound. Agrippa von Nettesheim, for instance, attacked the learned physicians who resorted to "ruffled sophisms and deceptive speech" instead of giving sick people "simple and true medicines." At the sickbed, they sought out a cure with "weighty seriousness" and if a sick person happened to recover while under their care, they would sing their own high praises. Yet they blended their medicines all too arbitrarily, he thought. Verily, one saw how "an old farmer's wife would often heal sick people with more certainty using this or that weed than a noble physician with his valuable miracle drugs, which are

---

[58]   Ibid.

[59]   Clauser, *Betrachtung* ([1531]), no pagination; Superville, *Nachricht vom wahren Nutzen* ([around 1732]), 12.

composed according to illusive conjecture." In short, physicians were "expensive murderers," who were "not necessary to those in need of a cure, but rather pernicious."[60] In contemporary art as well, doctors and the discrepancy between the physicians' perceived arrogance and their rather modest successes became the object of scathing satire. Molière's dramas with their presumptuous doctors are a well-known example. Cases of blatant uroscopic misjudgment must have fanned the fires of such criticism.

As physicians increasingly called the diagnostic validity of uroscopy into question, they were robbing themselves of an argument which previously had served to underpin their claim to privileged knowledge of the hidden morbid processes within patients' bodies. Since barber-surgeons, midwives, apothecaries, and countless irregular healers had also taken to uroscopy on a broad scale, however, this argument had lost much of its persuasive power anyway. No longer could learned physicians expect the public to pay great attention to their claim that only a truly learned physician could make a reliable uroscopic diagnosis on the basis of his thorough understanding of human physiology and pathology, supported by a comprehensive knowledge of the medical literature, and thanks to his ability to factor in those diverse individual issues, such as diet and constitution, which critically influence both changes in the urine and the course of disease. In practice, the other healers appeared to come to similarly detailed conclusions and their judgment likewise seemed proven true by numerous patients who recovered from illness whilst following a treatment prescribed on that basis.

One way out of this professional dilemma was to refine uroscopic technique and to modernize it according to the most recent scientific insights. In this way, uroscopy might be made a more reliable procedure and at the same time be turned into an esoteric practice again which could only be mastered by academically trained physicians. This was easier said than done, however. The numerous shades of color or the various *contenta* could hardly be differentiated further. The many nuances commonly described in the literature already put the doctors' sensory and diagnostic abilities to the test.

More likely to help make uroscopy once more primarily the physician's domain, and to place it on the cutting edge of scientific development, were new quantifying techniques. Weighing urine was already recommended by Nicholas of Cusa (1401–1464) in his dialogue between a *mechanicus* and a *philosophus*. According to the *mechanicus*, a doctor could come to a "more truthful judgment" (*verius judicium*) if he took into account not only the deceptive color (*fallax color*) but also the weight (*pondus*) of urine in relation to that of water; the *philosophus* agreed without reservation.[61]

---

60   Nettesheim, *Eitelkeit* (1913), vol. 2, 66–90.
61   Cusanus, *De staticis experimentis* (1543).

Initially, Nicholas of Cusa's suggestion found no detectable resonance in the medical writing of the time, as was similarly the case with his recommendation of enriching pulse diagnosis with pulse counting. By the sixteenth century, however, according to Foreest's account, some uroscopists weighed urine.[62] Although his preferred method was distillation, Leonhard Thurneysser, in the late sixteenth century, occasionally did weigh the urine of his patients.[63] In the early seventeenth century, Johann Baptist van Helmont took up the idea again. "One sure way of examining the urine, however, is through its weight," he wrote. In so doing, he did not appear to be taking recourse to Nicholas of Cusa, but rather to Santorio Santorio's (1561–1636) experiments in Padua, which had caused a sensation. By weighing the entire body, Santorio had aimed to measure the "insensible perspiration" of waste products through the respiratory tract and skin.[64] Van Helmont advised the reader to first determine the weight of an empty glass, then fill it with water and weigh it, then fill it with the same volume of urine and weigh it again. He observed significant differences. The urine of a healthy 35-year-old woman weighed 75 *gran* more than the same volume of pure water. A maiden with a heart tremor, by contrast, excreted urine that looked like water and had the same weight as well. While van Helmont's use of measurement is often looked upon as a milestone on the way to modern urinalysis, van Helmont himself approached it with reserve. The weighing of urine was only a marginal detail in his attempt to put medicine as a whole on a new footing—an attempt, by the way, that met with great skepticism amongst the vast majority of physicians.[65] Helmont had good reasons to remain cautious. After all, it proved very problematic to correlate the various weights of urine to the different pathological conditions.[66] Van Helmont himself revealingly banished his recommendation to the 31st and final section of his chapter on uroscopy and did not want to go into further detail. "Someone else may do more in this respect and do some better thinking," he concluded.[67]

In subsequent times, proponents of iatrochemical approaches above all others continued to recommend the weighing of urine.[68] Some authors actually

---

[62] Foreest, *Uromanteia* (1620), 204.

[63] StB Berlin, Ms. germ. fol. 106, 117r–132r, letter from Thurneysser to Jost Graf zu Barbey, May 1, 1575; ibid., 143r–149r urinalysis (*Harnprobe*) for Graf Wilhelm von Leiteren; in both cases the exact weight of a measure (*mensura*) of the patient's urine is indicated.

[64] Sanctorius, *De statica medicina* (1657).

[65] Helmontianism was more successful in England; cf. Wear, *Knowledge* (2000), 253–98.

[66] Montfalcon, *Urine* (1821), 314.

[67] Helmont, *Aufgang* (1683), 397f.

[68] Henninger, *Theses* (1712), 3; see also the manuscript of Anton R. Martin, *Urostatica, s[ive] de ponderatione urinae*, in: idem, Tractatuli physico-mechan[ici]. Aboai 1772, Milan,

saw a universal diagnostic and prognostic criterion in the varying weight of urine: The more the weight of the urine of a sick person increased, the worse the patient's condition, they thought.[69] This approach was taken particularly far by the anonymous author of a work published in 1718 under the telling title *Mantissa de examinatione naturalium liquidorum et terreorum, praeprimis lotii humani per pondus*, that is roughly "An add-on about the examination of liquid and earthen natural [substances], especially of human urine, by weight." If the person's health was only slightly afflicted and the spirits suffered from the waste materials in the body, then "the urine [is] easily two to three *grans* heavier than healthy urine and up to this weight a person can still make himself useful and likely still walk around. But if the weight is above three to four *gran*, it is dangerous, and as long as this weight increases rather than decreases, the danger persists that the illness is growing perilously and moving toward five *grans* and death. But if the weight slowly decreases, the illness is yielding as well; and there is hope of recovery when this can be observed, a message that cannot be gained with as much certainty from other indications."[70]

In the practice of the majority of physicians, such recommendations appear to have found little reception, however. In the mid-eighteenth century, Johann Friedrich Rübel complained of a "great silence" that still surrounded the question of "how much solid matter is contained in one pound of urine." He himself presented the results of meticulous measurements of his own urine. He found, as did other contemporary authors, that even with healthy urine the proportion of solid matter varied significantly depending particularly on inner heat, physical exercise, fluids consumed, and transpiration. Nevertheless, he saw certain correlations confirmed in the sick body "in practice through various experiences." Lighter urine that contained little matter tended to be present in the case of uterine pain, severe spleen complaints, stomach problems, cramps, stones, and gout; but it could also occur with headaches, dizziness, mania, hot fever, madness, falling sickness, and nervous diseases.[71]

Even if its significance for daily practice was ultimately minimal, the systematic weighing of the urine of healthy and sick people offers a very early example of a tendency that would only later, in the nineteenth and twentieth centuries, emerge on a larger scale: the trend toward measuring and standardizing the healthy and sick body and its functions.[72] By contrast, counting pulse beats with the help of a clock—as opposed to feeling for the various pulse qualities—began to play some role only in the early eighteenth century. Here, English physician John Floyer

---

Biblioteca Universitaria Braidense, Fondo Haller, Ms. AD-XIV-14 n. 4, a work that never seems to have made it into print.

[69]   Kräutermann, *Curieuser und vernünfftiger Urin-Artzt* (1732), 4 and 117–33.

[70]   Anonymous, *Mantissa* (1718), 112.

[71]   Rübel, *Medicinische Abhandlung* (1756), 13f; cf. idem, *Gebrauch* (1762), 84–92.

[72]   See the contributions to Hess (ed.), *Normierung* (1997).

systematically investigated the relationship between pulse frequency and various pathological conditions with the help of a pulse clock. He believed he could prove that a more or less specific correlation existed in the case of many illnesses. According to his experience, a normal pulse beat between 70 and 75 times per minute. A pulse frequency of 96 to 100, by contrast, pointed to an effervescence of the humors which could result in pains, rheumatism, "fluxes," inflammations, asthma, gout, and a whole range of fevers.[73] Routine measurements of the temperature with a clinical thermometer are also a more recent development.[74]

Another comparatively simple quantifying procedure was put forward in 1700 by Friedrich Hoffmann to measure the intensity of the color of the urine. This intensity and its changes over the course of the disease, he claimed, depended critically on vital heat. It could be determined with some precision with a simple experiment (*experimento*). All one had to do was to pour an ounce of urine into a receptacle at various times during the disease and mix in water until the color of the mix matched the color of healthy, natural urine. The amounts of water which had to be added to the urine each time corresponded to the intensity of yellow or red coloring of the urine and indirectly to the inner heat, and thus indicated the degree of inflammation, for example in the case of pleurisy, red murrain, arthritis, or hepatitis.[75]

Chemical Analysis

What met with a much greater response compared to these attempts at quantification were efforts to complement or replace the inspection of urine with the naked eye by chemical analysis. At first, such efforts were advanced primarily by Paracelsians. One of the best known and most successful representatives here was Leonhard Thurneysser, whose technique of distilling urine samples has been described above. Subsequently, it was primarily doctors interested in iatrochemistry who furthered these beginnings and saw their conceptions of physiology and pathology as a whole confirmed in the results of their urinalysis. Thus Otto Tachenius in his *Hippokrates Chymicus* explained that the urine of a dying person contained neither salts nor alkali, taking this as proof of the central role of acid in the body. He held that the vital acid in the stomach turned the chyle to salt, a process that gradually came to a standstill in the body of a dying person.[76]

---

[73] Floyer, *Pulse watch* (1707); see also the manuscript by Anton R. Martin, *Pulsologia, s[ive] de quantitate pulsuum juxta horologium*, in: idem Tractatuli physico-mechan[ici]. Aboai 1772, Milan, Biblioteca Universitaria Braidense, Fondo Haller, Ms. AD-XIV-14 n. 4.

[74] Hess, *Der wohltemperierte Mensch* (2000).

[75] Kongelige Bibliotek Copenhagen, Ms. Thottske S 4 689 (Piper, *Collegium*), 249r–v.

[76] Tachenius, *Hippokrates* (1677), 47–9.

Because of its proximity to Paracelsianism, chemical analysis was initially looked upon with suspicion by many academic physicians. This changed, however, as chemical models and procedures found their way into orthodox medicine. Thus K.B. Behrens criticized Thurneysser's procedure as "very uncertain" in 1668, because the volatile matter would collect in different places depending on the intensity of the heat applied. But he generally praised the distillation of urine as completely sensible: It allowed the solid and fleeting parts, as well as the sulfurous and salty parts, to be separated.[77] In the late seventeenth and early eighteenth centuries such efforts intensified. Lorenzo Bellini (1643–1704) attempted to explain the various colors and qualities of urine via their chemical composition.[78] According to John Munnicks, the natural, yellow color of urine was owed to the salty and sulfurous nutritional constituents that existed as the tiniest dissolved particles in the body and blended with the serum.[79] Johann Sigismund Henninger recommended precipitating urinary contents with the help of chemical substances, then filtering them out so as to make them visible.[80] Herman van Boerhaave carried this work forward.[81] In the mid-eighteenth century, Johann Friedrich Rübel expressed a new optimism in regard to the new physical and chemical procedures. In his view, "the science of urine and urine examination has no small role in medical practice and is not unuseful and should not be decried as false, and even less should be considered contemptible."[82] By the late eighteenth century, chemical urinalysis began to become widely established in academic medicine. Thousands of liters of urine were distilled. Urea was isolated and numerous further contents identified.[83]

However, as Jean-Baptiste Montfalcon lamented as late as the early nineteenth century, all of these efforts hardly yielded results that were relevant to practice. He thought that chemical analysis could be expected to permit a much more precise diagnosis than a judgment based on visible, physical properties. But urine was too diverse, too variable, and each chemist in his analysis came to different conclusions. Chemistry, Montfalcon concluded, had thus ultimately even caused harm in this field by spawning countless ludicrous and indemonstrable theories.[84]

---

77 Behrens, *Wasserbeschawen* (1688), 24–6.

78 Bellini, *De urina* (1718), originally published in idem, *De urinis et pulsibus, de missione sanguinis, de febribus, de morbis capitis et pectoris*. Bologna 1685.

79 Munnicks, *De urinis* (1674).

80 Henninger, *Theses* (1712), 3.

81 On Boerhaave cf. Knoeff, *Boerhaave* (2002).

82 Rübel, *Medicinische Abhandlung* (1756), 58.

83 Cf. e.g. Prochaska, *Dissertatio* (1776).

84 Montfalcon, *Urine* (1821), 329.

Microscopy

Another promising attempt to refine uroscopy, and to make it again the exclusive domain of physicians, was linked to the introduction of microscopes.[85] Although the instruments were continually improved in the course of the early modern period, hopes of attaining useful new diagnostic clues from a microscopic examination of the urine were largely disappointed, however. In retrospect, this disillusionment comes as no surprise. Today the majority of illnesses, apart from those of the kidneys and the efferent urinary tract, are not thought to produce changes in the urine that can be seen under the microscope.

At the time, some authors were more optimistic, however. In the early eighteenth century, one anonymous author ventured furthest in this respect. Under the title *The system of an English doctor on the cause of all sorts of diseases with the surprising appearances of different species of small insects, which can be seen with a good microscope in the blood and in the urine of different patients, even in all those who will become ill,*[86] a Parisian printer and publisher, Alexis-Xavier-René Mesnier, in 1726, published part three of a work that was said to have been extant as a manuscript. He identified the author solely with the initials M.A.C.D. The baroque title said it all: The author was of the opinion that all illnesses were ultimately caused by the smallest insects, which could be seen with the help of a microscope in both the blood and the urine and might also be demonstrable in bodily secretions. He did not content himself with general claims. On some 15 pages he described the shapes of over one hundred small insects, which he claimed to have seen in different diseases, and he included illustrations (see figures 5.1a and 5.1b).

He asked that his readers perform similar examinations themselves. Then they would certainly be amazed that a fact that had been "demonstrated this truthfully" ("si réellement demontré") and was so useful to the advancement of medicine had, to that day, remained unknown to the greatest doctors. He concluded that this showed yet again the power of prejudices over the human mind, just as in the case of the reception of Copernicus's insights or of the discovery of blood circulation.[87]

---

[85]   Cf. Wilson, *Invisible world* (1995)
[86]   M.A.C.D., *Systême* (1726).
[87]   Ibid., 24.

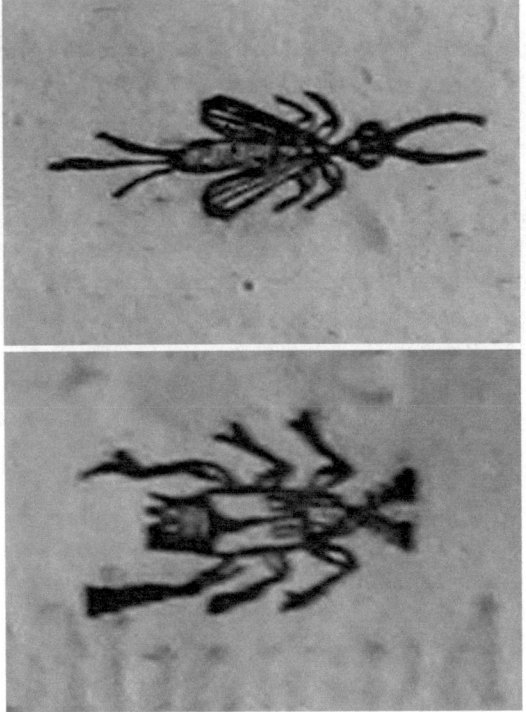

Figures 5.1a and 5.1b   Insects in urine, in: M.A.C.D., *Systême* (1726), p. 8f

Enlightenment and Propaganda

Neither weighing urine nor examining it under a microscope could, at the time, give uroscopy a new and more reliable foundation that would render it once again a privileged realm of the learned physicians. In fact, these attempts at innovation met with little favor even within the medical community, and the population at large appears to have hardly noticed them. Distillation or chemical analysis was a somewhat different case. Leonhard Thurneysser's success goes to show that the examination of urine in the laboratory could also be well received by laypeople and could lend the healer in question the aura of an expert. For a long time, however, most doctors turned their noses up at urine distillation. Probably it was too closely associated with Paracelsianism, which the majority of physician rejected. In addition, practical difficulties of mastering the process of distillation, the need for special equipment, and the repulsive stench may have played a role.

With the major options for developing a modern, more "scientific" version of uroscopy largely exhausted, some medical writers adopted a completely different strategy to protect the physician's authority from the dangers that grew out of the population's unshakable trust in uroscopy. Numerous well- and lesser known medical writers addressed a wide audience and sought to convince them of the limits of uroscopy in general and of the danger of trusting unlearned uroscopists, in particular, whose diagnosis relied exclusively on their examination of the urine. Writing usually in a more or less polemical vein, the authors regularly connected two lines of argumentation. On the one hand they rehearsed the familiar criticisms against uroscopy *per se*, such as the lack of urinary changes in serious and at times fatal diseases and the influence of age, sex, temperament, and lifestyle, which rendered a reliable diagnosis impossible when this information was withheld. On the other hand—and this line of argumentation usually took up far more room—they sought to expose their less learned competitors as charlatans and swindlers. The long titles speak for themselves, for example, *Uromanteia. This is a true and well-founded account of the various judgments and prophecies from urine or water. It explains excellently and proves how false, worthless and deceiving they are and what irreparable harm has often come to those who relied on it.*[88] Or: *De incerto urinarum iudicio; et intolerabili circumforaneorum impostura libellus. This is a short description of today's so-called art of the urine and quackery. It proves thoroughly and in detail that not only [is] today's wrongly called art of the urine used still in many towns by many doctors and physicians now and then to their advantage and to the disadvantage of their neighbor, without shame or shyness; but also [that] the great quackery, which is in fashion with the boasting market criers in the Roman Empire, is nothing else but a lot of irresponsible fraud and damnable imposture.*[89] Or, spread out over 426 pages, *De ontdekkinge der bedriegeryen van de gemeene pizbesienders*, that is "The Exposure of the Deceitfulness of Common Piss Watchers,"[90] or *The pisse-prophet; or, Certain pisse-pot lectures. Wherein are newly discovered the old fallacies, deceit, and jugling of the piss-pot science, used by all those (whether quacks, and empiricks, or other methodical physicians) who pretend knowledg of diseases, by the urine, in giving judgment of the same.*[91]

---

[88]   Foreest, *Uromanteia* (1620); cf. Nutton, *Idle old trots* (1977).

[89]   Himantomus, *De incerto urinarum iudicio* (1657).

[90]   Van Dueren, *Ontdekkinge* (1688).

[91]   Brian, *Pisse-prophet* (1655); see also Ewaldt, *Diatriba* (1718).

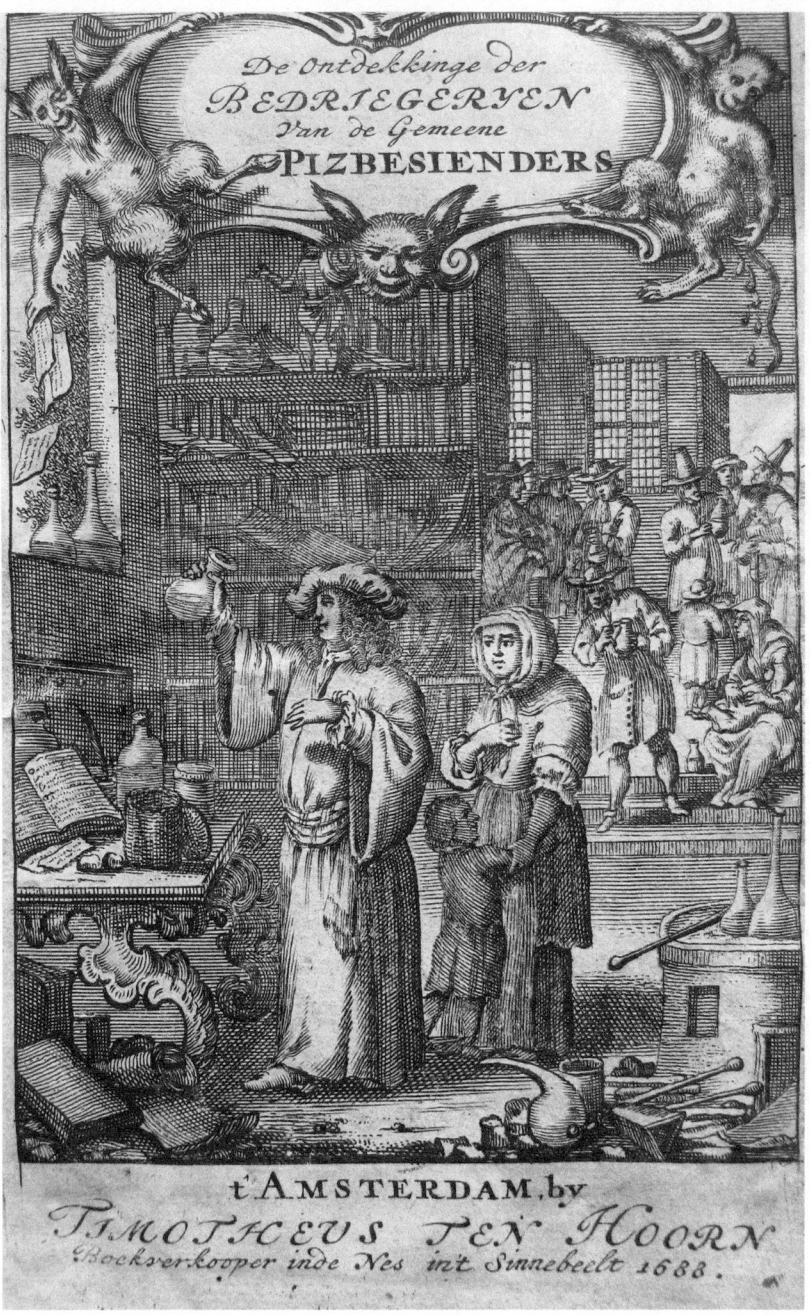

Figure 5.2   Frontispiece of Johan van Dueren, *De ontdekkinge der bedriegeryen van de gemeene pizbesienders* (1688)

Incessantly readers were instructed that the diagnosis of disease on the sole basis of urine was unreliable and that the practice of non-academic uroscopists was based all on speculation and deceit.[92] Some of them were even half blind, like the old "hag" of whom Foreest wrote, who, on account "of her old age and weak sight could hardly tell one person from another."[93] While doctors acknowledged that unlicensed healers sometimes did judge correctly, even naming the right age, sex, and complaints of the patients,[94] they argued that this had nothing to do with their art. These uroscopists, they warned, tricked the patients by secretly gathering information about them and then pretending that they had learned it from the urine. They would, for example, hide behind closed doors while their wife or a maidservant received the sick person or messenger and inquired about the sickness.[95] Or, the physicians thought, they exploited the simple-mindedness of the common people—according to Thoner, urine was usually brought by maids or other naive people[96]—and elicited through clever questions the information which they would later claim to have discerned from the urine.[97] The uroscopist, for instance, might ask the time when the person had passed the water, ascertaining at least the person's sex when the messenger replied and unsuspectingly referred to the patient as "he" or "she."[98]

To what extent non-academic uroscopists actually made use of such tricks must remain open. Certainly using such tricks was not an indispensable prerequisite for the popularity and renown which some of these uroscopists enjoyed among the wider population. Even Thomas Willis conceded that people could easily be convinced of the "mountebanks'" art simply through their own trust in the possibilities of uroscopy.[99] And even without any tricks, especially in the rural areas, many non-academic uroscopists may well have had easier access to additional information about the (presumable) patient. They were better connected to the web of village gossip than were doctors. When a messenger came from a certain village or hamlet, they might already know from another source who had recently fallen ill there and could more easily guess the identity of the patient and his or her complaints.

Doctors also pointed out a strategy employed by non-academic uroscopists to increase the likelihood of a correct diagnosis. According to Foreest, "Such fellows commonly make it their custom, when viewing urine, to give people a long

---

[92] Hart, *Arraignment* (1623), 44.

[93] Foreest, *Uromanteia* (1620), 188; Thoner, *Observationum* (1649), 344, also reports about a highly popular, blind Jewish uroscopist.

[94] Kolreutter, *Von rechten Gebreuchen* (1574), ch. 3.

[95] Thoner, *Observationum* (1649), 344.

[96] Ibid., 342; similarly Rega, *Tractatus* (1733), 1st treatise, 37.

[97] Stahl, *Gründliche Abhandlung* (1739), 4; van Dueren, *Ontdekkinge* (1688), 76–93.

[98] Behrens, *Wasserbeschawen* (1688), 31.

[99] Willis, *Five treatises* (1681), 20.

sermon about it, telling of many things until they finally snatch up something that the sick person can apply to himself."[100] Along similar lines, K.B. Behrens remarked in the late seventeenth century that non-academic uroscopists piled up a lot of "empty words, from which the patient can interpret as much as serves him, and generally these people can count on the good will of their patients to believe that everything was read accurately from the urine when they touch upon the disease with only half a word, even unknowingly."[101]

In the few extant uroscopic *judicia* of non-academic healers we do find, in fact, a whole array of complaints and illnesses listed alongside one another. Without a doubt, this raised the likelihood of the patient recognizing his or her own case in at least some of the conditions the uroscopists had identified. But in this respect learned physicians were hardly different. With or without uroscopy they also frequently listed a whole range of illnesses or symptoms in one and the same patient.

Many of the polemical writings by physicians against non-academic uroscopists were composed in the vernacular, and others were later translated from Latin. This is remarkable in a time in which—at least on the European continent—learned physicians published almost exclusively in Latin. This choice did not only reflect a general desire to reach a wider readership. It also aimed at a particular group. Prefaces and dedications, as well as the body of the texts itself, made no secret that more than anyone, authorities, princes, and magistrates were addressed, the same group that the physicians sometimes also petitioned directly, on a local level.[102] The authorities had a recognized responsibility for a well-ordered health care system. For the benefit of the general public, the physicians called on them to impose draconian punishments on their less learned competitors and put an end to the practice.[103] Cordus argued, for instance, that forgers who defrauded people of their money were burnt at the stake, while fraudulent uroscopists who robbed people not only of their money but also of their lives were allowed to go free or were even held in great respect.[104] To move the authorities to action, Horer similarly argued that someone who falsely pretended to be a baron was severely punished, but not the person who pretended to be a physician.[105]

---

[100] Foreest, *Uromanteia* (1620), 170f.

[101] Behrens, *Wasserbeschawen* (1688), 31.

[102] E.g. StA Nuremberg, B19 184, fol. 18r–19r, letter from the Collegium medicum, March 3, 1709, complaining about a female uroscopist who was said to also prescribe purgatives and medicines which could be used to provoke an abortion.

[103] Foreest, *Uromanteia* (1620), preface by the German translator.

[104] Cordus, *De urinis* (1543), no pagination.

[105] Horer, *Artzney-Teuffel* (1634), 29.

The fight against non-academic uroscopists can thus be recognized as one area of conflict in the fiercely contested health market of the day.[106] In numerous writings, academic physicians attempted to distance themselves and their profession from their less learned competitors. They sought to drive their message home that the most important criterion with which to evaluate medical practitioners—and determine fees—was not the success of the cure, which was ever uncertain, but rather learning, academic training, and theoretical knowledge. A true physician, as Ananius Horer told his readers, had to know Greek and Latin, must have studied rhetoric and dialectic, must be well-versed in natural philosophy and ethics, and have gained extensive botanical and astronomical knowledge.[107] Only someone who knew the laws of the body and its diseases—such was the perpetual argument for the privileged position of academic doctors—could treat illnesses causally, attack them at their roots. Following this argument, the degree of success that non-academic healers could boast of in curing their patients was based on coincidence at best or was, to use contemporary terms, merely "palliative," or "cloaking" in the literal sense: They only made the complaints disappear temporarily, leaving the true cause of the disease untouched so that the disease progressed in secret without any obstacles, and in the long run everything only became worse.[108]

Some authors added a charge which, in the time of witch hunts, came with a particularly explosive power. They accused common uroscopists of using "devilish forbidden substances,"[109] charged them with "dreadful blasphemy" by "arrogating to be physicians" and "doing much wayward and blasphemous, even idolatrous monkey shine with their urine inspection," which endangered not only people's life and limb but also their salvation.[110] Ananius Horer even attributed the widespread trust in uroscopy as such to the devil. The devil had "implanted this opinion not only in the common folk but also in many great people that it is well possible to know and see a patient's illness with all its circumstances simply by examining his urine, no matter whether the patient lives ten or more miles from the doctor, and now they decry anyone who refuses to work like this as a poorly trained and inexperienced doctor—try as one might to contradict."[111]

Capitalizing on prevalent anti-Jewish resentments, some authors described Jewish healers as the embodiment of the deceptive and blasphemous charlatan. Jewish healers as a whole were a preferred target of intense polemics with hardly

---

[106] Elkeles, *Medicus* (1987).
[107] Horer, *Artzney-Teuffel* (1634), 14–20.
[108] Stolberg, *Cura palliativa* (2007).
[109] Oetheus, *Gründtlicher Bericht* (1574), 61v.
[110] Thus the physician Georg Curius in his preface to Cordus, *Kunst* (1536).
[111] Horer, *Artzney-Teuffel* (1634), 61.

concealed religious undertones.[112] They were accused of avarice and a lack of education, and were inculpated with killing their patients.[113] In their criticism, physicians associated Jewish healers in particular with fraudulent uroscopy, and all the other uroscopists, in turn, with the hated Jews. They charged them with overstepping the boundaries of what was allowed by religion and law. There was one main reason, claimed Georg Pictorius in 1557, why "the Jews had [come to enjoy] such authority and trust," a trust so great that "often, learned doctors have to yield to these vagrants." People thought that "they have a secret art in their own secret books that the holy prophet Moses gave them [and] which shall stay with them." In addition, said Pictorius, they actually were "very sure" of examining the water and rarely erred, thanks to all kinds of tricks by which they found out the necessary information about their patients.[114]

Despite the great rhetorical flourish, the physicians' efforts to expose the uroscopic practice of their less-learned competitors as deception or even as sorcery did not meet with much success. Their calls for draconian punishment fell largely on deaf ears. While many laypeople were prepared to acknowledge the superior knowledge of physicians, even highly educated and wealthy contemporaries would consult unlicensed and sometimes illiterate healers, at the latest when the effects of a physician's treatment left something to be desired. Presumably political decision makers saw no reason to deprive themselves and their fellow citizens of this choice. "Why has this admirable and highly necessary art," Ananius Horer asked, "lost so much of its glory and authority today that hardly anyone properly respects and honors it anymore?"[115] He thought he knew the answer. If a healer was considered successful, they cared little about whether or not he had studied. And thus, as Augustin Thoner, for example, found in Ulm,[116] the doctors' efforts did not succeed in garnering the support of authorities in the battle against non-academic uroscopists, against "empirical urine prophets, urine examiners, and seers who persuade the simpletons and the common folk."[117]

Uroscopy and the Anatomical Revolution

The physicians' attempt to persuade the upper classes of the ignorance and wily machinations of the less learned uroscopists failed, just as the attempt failed to modernize uroscopy to make it once more the sole domain of learned physicians.

---

[112] Hortzitz, *"Judenarzt"* (1994).

[113] Pictorius, *Von zernichten Artzten* (1557), preface, IIr.

[114] Ibid., IIIv.

[115] Horer, *Artzney-Teuffel* (1634), 21.

[116] Kutzer, *Herrgott* (2000), 164f.

[117] Horer, *Artzney-Teuffel* (1634), 59.

In this situation, leading medical writers saw hardly any choice but for doctors to forego performing uroscopy as much as possible. Such a view was elaborated at length by no less than Georg Ernst Stahl, professor in Halle and one of the most influential German physicians of his time. He informed his readers that although uroscopy could occasionally be helpful, it was not indispensable, and the doctor should thus keep his authority in mind and distance himself from it. Admittedly one could with the help of uroscopy "judge some illnesses better,"[118] but in most illnesses uroscopy was deceptive and whoever relied on it risked "the disdain and malicious gossip of the ignorant rabble [...], who will decry him as inexperienced when [incorrect judgments] happen." He asked of his colleagues that they limit their use of uroscopy to "reasonable use" in the case of certain diseases such as fever, jaundice, dropsy, and illnesses of the efferent urinary tract, "so the general, indiscriminate prophesying from urine is not given a free pass, gaining repute through the common man's applause."[119] Even in the case of these illnesses, Stahl felt, uroscopy was not essential, not even with the fevers. This raised the question, "whether or not—for the sake of a hardly noticeable benefit which only opens the floodgates to abuse and is not of any real necessity—this malpractice should be tolerated so as not to forego the minor benefit?"[120]

Stahl conceded that an intelligent doctor could request a patient's urine and examine it without abetting "misuse," provided that he made it clear to the patient that uroscopy was only helpful in certain cases, which only the physician could correctly identify.[121] He might also occasionally confirm his tentative diagnosis through uroscopy. But he had to avoid everything that would implicate his practice in uromancy, or urine prophecy. He was not even supposed to ask for or accept "the usual money for the examination of urine."[122] Ultimately, in the interest of "abolishing the far greater misuse" it was preferable to do without "the smaller and also dispensable benefits" which uroscopy could offer in some cases and lay it aside "completely or at least not practice it as often." Only if doctors stopped using uroscopy entirely—and still, thanks to their competence, cured their patients successfully—would commoners understand that uroscopy was not at all needed to diagnose illnesses.[123]

Physicians were further encouraged to turn their back on uroscopy by another development in contemporary medicine, one that held greater promise for their medical authority: the rise of the anatomical and pathological dissection. The rise of anatomy to become the leading medical science of the sixteenth and seventeenth centuries need not be discussed in detail here; it has been

---

118 Stahl, *Gründliche Abhandlung* (1739), 14.

119 Ibid., 14.

120 Ibid., 18.

121 Ibid., 32.

122 Ibid., 32.

123 Ibid., 18f.

described often. First-hand observations gained from numerous dissections of human corpses took the place of the older anatomical treatises written in the Galenic tradition, which, as anatomists had come to realize, were largely based on dissections of pigs and other animals. The new, refined anatomical insights were celebrated and, alongside the knowledge of learned medical literature, were increasingly heralded as the foundation of the superiority of academic medicine. Anatomists such as Andreas Vesalius with his *De humani corporis fabrica libri septem* of 1543,[124] Felix Platter, and Caspar Bauhin became icons of a renewed medicine. Because the best anatomical training was offered at universities in northern Italy, numerous medical students made the move there from north of the Alps. In all of Europe, dissections, staged as impressive public events, attracted not just medical men but also large and sometimes paying audiences who wanted to witness as the anatomist opened up a human body and exhibited and described its internal structures, sometimes in anatomical theaters, sometimes in churches and other public places.[125]

In hindsight, it might appear as something of a mystery that anatomy was held in such high esteem. For the purposes of ordinary, daily practice, the new anatomical knowledge was only of very limited significance. Of course, in surgery, in the treatment of wounds, abscesses, fistulas, and the like, which were accessible from the outside, precise anatomical knowledge was very helpful. But only a small minority of academic physicians, especially north of the Alps, practiced surgery at the time. It was widely considered inferior manual labor and generally left to the hands of barber-surgeons.[126] For the diagnosis and treatment of internal diseases, on the other hand, the principal domain of academic physicians, the new anatomical knowledge was of little help. As long as illnesses were traced first and foremost to corrupted morbid matter, obstructions in the flow of humors, mobile vapors, a weakened vital heat, and related aspects of the humoral body, the best that a more precise anatomical knowledge could do in most cases was determine more exactly where a particular morbid matter had settled. For practical diagnostic and therapeutic purposes, however, it sufficed to know that the morbid matter had, for instance, accumulated near the liver or the kidneys, or in a limb.

Compared to anatomical knowledge, uroscopy promised to give much richer and varied insights into the power of the patient's vital heat, the quality of concoction, the nature of the morbid matter at which a treatment would have to be directed, and any changes in the course of the disease. It was only gradually, and for the most part as a result of the growing esteem for anatomy,

---

[124] Vesal, *Fabrica* (1543).

[125] On the following see Stolberg, *Anatomische Inszenierung* (2011); cf. also Walter, *Ärztliche Selbstdarstellung* (2013).

[126] Among the few famous exceptions are Ambroise Paré and Wilhelm Fabry of Hilden.

that more interest was given to pathological changes in the solid parts of the body that could be observed when the bodies of sick people were dissected after their death.[127]

Thus the high esteem for anatomy can hardly be explained in terms of its concrete, practical usefulness. Rather we have to understand it in a more encompassing way as a cultural phenomenon. The great importance that came to be attributed to dissections reflected the era's new scientific ideals and in turn buttressed them. Throughout the early modern scientific world, the balance shifted from learned commentary on extant writings to empirical research and a striving for new, original insights that were beyond the sphere of traditional book knowledge. Powerful religious motifs came into play as well. Anatomy showed the human body with its complex and ever purposeful construction as the pinnacle of creation, and thus promised to deepen reverence for God and His creation and to strengthen trust in His never-ending love and care.

Seen against the backdrop of an increasing disillusionment with uroscopy, the new anatomy also offered new possibilities for professional self-promotion. The claim to superior anatomical knowledge became a cornerstone of medical authority. It also legitimized physicians' efforts to enter domains like the treatment of wounds which were traditionally considered the privileged realm of other healing professions and to subordinate the barber-surgeons to their supervision even on their very own terrain. It was also above all the doctors' claim to superior anatomical knowledge that allowed them to justify ousting midwives who, until then, had held a near complete monopoly on obstetrics. Despite the fact that most physicians still in the nineteenth century knew little about practical obstetrics and hardly had any relevant experience, a primarily anatomical schooling and examination of midwives by a local physician became obligatory in many places.

Physicians were well aware of the advantages of anatomy when it came to their status and public image. From the sixteenth century on, authors' portraits and other paintings or prints showing an individual physician not only used books to allude to their erudition, but often—and sometimes even exclusively—anatomical preparations, underlining the physician's role as a natural philosopher, as a researcher.[128] Not a single portrait, by contrast, can be found from the time after 1500 in which a physician had himself depicted with a matula.[129]

---

[127] The development was reflected, in particular, in early modern *observationes*; cf. e.g. Tulpius, *Observationum* (1641); on the genre of *observationes* see Stolberg, *Formen* (2007); Pomata, *Sharing cases* (2010).

[128] A famous and influential model was a portrait of Andreas Vesalius which depicted the famous anatomist with a dissected arm, thus presenting him as an anatomical practitioner and researcher (cf. Groß/Steinmetzer, *Coiter*, 2006).

[129] Cf. Jurina, *Vom Quacksalber* (1985), 36.

In terms of the esteem, the professional status, and the authority of learned physicians, the new anatomy had unmistakable advantages over uroscopy. While uroscopy was practiced even by ordinary village healers, performing a real autopsy, examining corpses with one's own hands and eyes, was, with very few exceptions, the exclusive domain of learned physicians. As a rule, only doctors would get permission or be ordered to perform an autopsy. Other healers usually had to content themselves with second-hand knowledge taken from anatomical broadsides or, if they could afford it, from illustrations found in medical textbooks. Only a small elite of non-academic surgeons was taught directly from the corpse, like the surgeons who immortalized themselves in Rembrandt's *The Anatomy Lesson of Dr Tulp*. Yet even in paintings, which the guilds or the portrayed surgeons had commissioned themselves, the learned physician appears as the authority from whose mouth the surgeons learn about the secrets of the human body.[130]

From this perspective, physicians' growing disenchantment with uroscopy may even be understood as an important and unduly neglected driving force of the so-called scientific revolution of the sixteenth and seventeenth centuries. The central place of uroscopy in early modern medical practice reflected the profound belief that true medicine must unveil the secrets inside the body and base treatment on this knowledge of internal processes. The more physicians attacked uroscopy as unreliable the more they needed a new foundation on which to base their claims to a privileged access to the body's interior. They found it in anatomy—which was, in turn, a major element in the early modern shift to more empirical, observational practices. Anatomy might be far less useful for the diagnosis and treatment of illnesses compared to uroscopy, but it gave back to academic medicine that authority, that exclusivity of knowledge, which uroscopy seemed to have once secured for it.

The similar role that uroscopy and anatomy played in the medical profession's quest for authority, status, and an affluent clientele is nicely illustrated by the career of the famous Swiss doctor and anatomist Felix Platter.[131] As he recounted in his memoirs, when he started his practice at the end of 1557 in his home town of Basel, he found himself in a difficult situation due to the great number of physicians in the area. It was clear to him: "I will have to be resourceful if I want to support myself from my practice." He needed to gain a reputation for himself, in other words to stage himself and his abilities in an effective way. According to his own account, he was highly successful as a uroscopist, knowing how to impress people with his uroscopic acumen. They trusted in his ability to find the key to the secret processes within their sick bodies. Soon, however, Platter also found another "art" with which he bolstered his reputation. In Basel there

130 Middelkoop, *Rembrandt* (1998).
131 Platter, *Tagebuch* (1976), 337.

had not been a public dissection since 1543, when Andreas Vesalius publically opened a corpse. While studying in Montpellier, Platter had seen a fair number of dissections and had participated in some. When in April 1559, just a year and a half after receiving his doctorate, a thief was to be executed in Basel, Platter asked permission to dissect the criminal's corpse in public, and permission was granted. After the beheading, the corpse was carried into the Church of St Elizabeth near the city wall. Thus the public execution was followed by the ritual of a public dissection in the sacred space of a church, where doctors and surgeons were invited and came, as Platter wrote, "along with many common people." This public anatomy lasted three days. As he proudly recalled, it brought the 23-year-old Platter great renown. He had not simply put anatomy, the structure of the human body, on center stage, but even more so himself as someone possessing a superior knowledge of the human interior. This act of public self-fashioning did not end with the three-day dissection. Platter subsequently prepared the corpse's skeleton—a laborious and revolting affair. The remains of the rotting flesh, sinews, and bone marrow had to be removed from the bones. In boiling up the bones, a stinking broth was produced on top of which fat and foam floated that had to be skimmed off throughout the process. The cleaned bones finally had to be meticulously put together with wire pulled through hand-drilled holes. Yet Platter apparently felt that such an effort was worth his while. He had a case specifically made for the skeleton and, for many years, it stood in Platter's parlor, by all appearances in the very place where he received those patients who came to see him in his own house. Thus, patients and visitors were always confronted with this proof of Platter's outstanding expertise. Platter was successful. Thanks to both "arts"—uroscopy and anatomy—he was able in the shortest amount of time and in spite of fierce competition to set up an extensive practice and, as he relates, was soon able to count all the noble families among his patients.[132]

Some early modern paintings and prints nicely illustrated the related role of anatomy and uroscopy, presenting them together as different ways of gaining medical knowledge. The third edition of Valentin Kräutermann's *Curieuser und vernünfftiger Urin-Artzt*, for example, includes an etching of a physician performing uroscopy in his own house, with an open book on the table in which the outlines of an anatomical and botanical image can be discerned, and with a full-sized skeleton in the background.[133]

In genre painting—which mirrors primarily the lay perception—we also find indications of this kind of a relationship between uroscopy and anatomy. The famous picture of a "physician" painted by Gerard Dou in 1653 and

---

[132] Ibid., 356 and 369.
[133] Kräutermann, *Curieuser und vernünfftiger Urin-Artzt* (1732), front-leaf.

held today by Vienna's *Kunsthistorisches Museum*[134] shows a uroscopist in his home, in the background a woman, presumably the messenger who brought him the urine (see Plate 30). He concentrates his gaze on the raised matula. In front of him, however, stands an open anatomy book with clear signs that it has been consulted many times: It is Andreas Vesalius's epochal *De humani corporis fabrica libri septem*. While a globe, half hidden by a curtain, represents the healer's erudite knowledge of the natural world, the anatomy book, placed prominently in the foreground, points to his privileged knowledge of the inside of the body, a knowledge which he is staging with his intense gaze at the uroscopy flask, accompanied by an expressive gesture.[135]

Physicians on the Health Market

In this situation, with physicians feeling uneasy about uroscopy while anatomical expertise offered a promising, new foundation for their claims to superior knowledge and privileged status, they might be expected to reject uroscopy outright. This was easier said than done, however. It was extremely difficult to prevail over the expectations and wishes of patients and their relatives. As Augustinus Thoner put it, "the esteem for the doctor is largely dependent on uromancy,"[136] and there was not much he could do about it. Kräutermann's *Curieuser und vernünfftiger Urin-Artzt* from the early eighteenth century got to the heart of it: "And yet, unfortunately, experience tells us that if a doctor completely turned his back on uroscopy, he would certainly not be popular with the country folk, who think highly of it; they would decry him as untrained and would shame him maliciously, as if he didn't know his trade."[137]

Sick people and their relatives routinely expected uroscopy and often, as we have seen, uroscopy alone. They judged the competence and experience of a healer on the basis of his ability to arrive at a precise diagnosis and prognosis

---

[134] Inv. no. GG_592; the bloodletting bowl in the foreground leaves no room for doubt that the title "Arzt" (i. e. physician) is wrong and that the person in question is a barber or barber-surgeon; we find a similar picture in an arched frame, for example, in Dou's portrayal of a wild game butcher in the National Gallery in London (reproduced in Alpers, *Art of describing* (1985), 28).

[135] Bedaux has pointed out a further meaning of this image within the image. Dou chose for his painting the figure of a skeleton with a gravedigger's shovel, which can also be understood as a *memento mori*, as a reference to human mortality (and to the limitations of the healing professions)—although similar elements are found in *De fabrica* quite frequently; Bedaux, *Minnekoorts-, zwangerschaps- en doodsverschijnselen* (1975).

[136] Thoner, *Observationum* (1649), 341.

[137] Kräutermann, *Curieuser und vernünfftiger Urin-Artzt* (1732), 1.

just from the patient's urine and were quick to condemn him when he failed.[138] A physician who wanted to make a name for his practice therefore had to think twice about whether he could afford to do without uroscopy. He risked creating the impression that he did not master the one diagnostic procedure in which the population had the most trust and which many competitors constantly made use of to the satisfaction of their patients. Particularly at the beginning of their career or when they set up practice in a new location, physicians faced a difficult decision. When the Brescian physician Giovanni Francesco Olmo began working in a rural area, the local apothecary gave him the well-meaning advice that he should do as his predecessors and examine the urine that was brought to him. The apothecary advised him to attract the "cloddish" and "uneducated" locals through art and shrewdness. He would soon acquire riches and make a name for himself. By contrast, if he refused to heed the patients' wishes, his art would be of little use to him, because the country folk clung tenaciously to their belief in uroscopy. Olmo remained indignant and steadfast in his refusal. In the end, he boasted, he was able to convince even those who initially thought him ignorant that he was an able doctor. But the first months, he admitted, had indeed been difficult.[139]

There were other physicians, too, who recounted how they had tried to assert themselves and withstand the pressure of the population's expectations. The Zurich town physician, Christoffel Clauser, for example, saw himself subjected to the reproof that he was versed in astrology but did not know medicine very well. It was held against him as a sign of academic arrogance, he complained, that he was not prepared to diagnose and treat illnesses with the sole help of uroscopy.[140]

Such descriptions of individual physicians' heroic resistance against patient expectations give us an impression of their struggle. A doctor who refused to perform the desired urine examination and insisted upon personal visits with sick people instead—generally for significantly higher payment—jeopardized not only his relationship with his patients. He put his reputation and possibly his very livelihood at risk. With this in mind, Jeremias Gebauer, in the early eighteenth century, even publically urged his medical colleagues to study uroscopy in depth. Good uroscopic skills, he claimed, were indispensable to running a successful practice since those who could not predict precisely from the urine what the future held would not be respected as doctors by the common man (*plebejus*) and would not be given any trust.[141] Pointing at

---

[138]   Gabelkover, *Curationum* (1611–1612), preface.

[139]   Olmo, *De certa ratione* (1578), 92r.

[140]   Clauser, *Betrachtung* ([1531]), dedication to his cousin, the pharmacist and member of the town council of Luzern.

[141]   Gebauer, *Uromantiam* (1711), preface.

his own, personal experience, Antonius Eijgel rejected the criticism of Foreest and other uroskeptical authors and stressed that he had gained "great honor" through uroscopy.[142]

The precarious position of academically trained physicians was further aggravated insofar as uneducated uroscopists imitated their learned behavior. "To gain more authority and repute, many of them have all kinds of books and writings lying in front of them," complained Foreest.[143] Contemporary genre painters, in fact, usually presented village healers with a book ostentatiously opened before them, frequently along with several others lying around (see Plate 31). In this manner, they conveyed the impression that they also had access to and applied "book knowledge" and undermined the physicians' claim, namely that these "urine prophets" or "quacks" did not know anything of uroscopy because they lacked the learned knowledge that the doctors had acquired during their long medical studies.

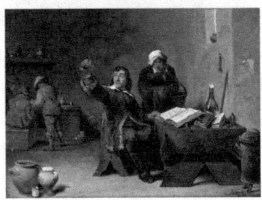

As we have seen, there was the occasional doctor, like Sigmundt Kolreutter in Coburg, Giovanni Francesco Olmo near Brescia, or Clauser in Zurich, who allegedly refused to follow the wishes of their patients and make diagnoses on the sole basis of uroscopy. After certain initial difficulties, they were ostensibly able to convince the population that it was impossible to get a reliable diagnosis from urine alone.[144] Yet it appears they were the rare exception. Haberstroh's suggestion that all the physicians in a certain area should agree not to diagnose illnesses on the sole basis of uroscopy for at least a year went unheard, as did another physician's demand (which Haberstroh mentioned) that all prospective doctors pledge never to base their diagnosis just on uroscopy.[145]

Most physicians ultimately had no choice. As even the critics conceded, most doctors continued to diagnose illnesses from urine and often from urine alone if their clients so desired. The young, prospective physician in particular, often "against his will and most unwillingly had to give in," as Horer put it, if he did not want to alienate the patients and gain a bad reputation with the common man.[146] Along similar lines, Liphimeus wrote that some doctors diagnosed illnesses from urine against their will because they "would otherwise get no patients and have

[142] Eijgel, *Apologema* (1672), 34; Eijgel followed up with a book on the various medicines that could be given, depending on the uroscopic findings (Eijgel, *Nieuwe Genees-konst* (1673)).

[143] Foreest, *Uromanteia* (1620), 203.

[144] Kolreutter, *Von rechten Gebreuchen* (1574), dedicatory epistle; Olmo, *De certa ratione* (1578), 92r–v; Clauser, *Betrachtung* ([1531]).

[145] Jacobus Haberstroh, preface to Himantomus, *De incerto urinarum iudicio* (1657).

[146] Horer, *Artzney-Teuffel* (1634), 62.

no work." He saw part of the fault also with his colleagues, however. "Greed got the better of them," said Liphimeus, when they saw that even noble patients sent their water to the doctors' homes.[147]

In the eighteenth century, many physicians apparently still not only practiced uroscopy and praised its diagnostic potential.[148] Many were also prepared, if necessary, to treat patients on the sole basis of uroscopy without ever having seen them in person. As late as 1736, Daniel de Superville lamented that "this custom has been common for so many years among some doctors [...] that many of them try to find their daily bread in the matula, predicting for little money everything from it for the people, what ails them and how they will fare."[149] According to Stahl, doctors in the eighteenth century felt they had little choice but "to move with the bad times, or to put it better, with the poor habits of the place where they live more than they would like."[150] Disgusted, Johann August Unzer, still in the late eighteenth century, spoke up against the "very debasing rashness" with which "a physician, in order to draw at least even with the charlatan in the art of foretelling, puts up with determining and judging the condition of a patient solely from the natural signs, especially the urine, and from this derives his measures for a cure, without getting involved in a thorough examination." Unzer did not want to accept the physicians' excuse that if they did not do it, somebody else would and take from them "all applause and livelihood." He claimed that there were surely enough wise and generous people who would sustain the livelihood of those steadfast doctors who refused to diagnose diseases just from urine. It seems unlikely, however, that this would have assuaged the concerns of his less successful and prosperous colleagues.[151]

In individual cases, the physicians' willingness to make compromises can be shown concretely. In the practice journal of Johann Friedrich Glaser, a physician in the German town of Suhl, eight cases are documented for the year 1750 in which the doctor made his diagnosis on the basis of uroscopy. In all of these cases, a messenger or another visitor brought the urine into the doctor's practice.[152]

Insofar as many physicians continued to bend to the expectations and demands of their clients, they unintentionally helped assure the survival of this practice. After all, they constantly confirmed people's belief in the paramount diagnostic value of uroscopy, even when used exclusively. As Daniel de Superville

---

[147] Liphimeus, *Warnung* (1626), 71f.
[148] Hederich, *De ambiguitate* (1732), 5 and 17.
[149] Superville, *Gedancken* (1736), 56.
[150] Stahl, *Gründliche Abhandlung* (1739), 7.
[151] Unzer, *Von der Kunst* (1760), 141.
[152] Thümmler, *Rekonstruktion* (2004), 82f; in two cases, we have an extant diagnosis, namely "bilious fever" and "bladder stones" with "tearing" in the back, but we do not know how much information about the patient was relayed orally by the messengers; on Glaser see Schilling/Schlegelmilch/Splinter, *Stadtarzt oder Arzt in der Stadt?* (2011).

concluded in response to the question "How is it possible that the common man gives himself to believe that all diseases can be learned from the urine alone?": "This is the doctors' own fault; they keep people's superstition alive, and although they [...] are convinced that urine alone is a highly uncertain thing in examining illnesses, they prefer to cheat people rather than to let go of the money they can make with piss watching."[153] In 1657 Jacobus Haberstroh had already put it succinctly: "The doctors themselves are the cause of this misuse, because they prostitute themselves without need and against their conscience."[154] Other authors blamed doctors at least in part for the sustained popularity of uroscopy "because many of them, just to make a little money, have no qualms about prattling on about the cause of a disease and its symptoms based only on the water and divine inspiration because they have not seen the patient."[155] The doctor might have discretely "found out much circumstantial information so as to gain knowledge of the illness" and was thus basing his diagnosis on a solid foundation, but he still encouraged his patients' belief in uroscopy.[156]

The pressure was massive though it may not have been the same all over Europe. German physicians like Johannes Lange saw an important reason for the poor reputation of German medicine in foreign countries in the fact that "the majority of common doctors busy themselves almost exclusively with the inspection of putrid water [i.e. urine], claiming to determine the essence of illnesses from it."[157] Similarly the Dutch physician Foreest affirmed that as long as doctors, "especially in our dear fatherland of upper and lower Germany [...] do not disavow the very old and bad habit" of diagnosing illness from urine, it could "never be hoped that this noble and most salubrious of all arts will regain its former dignity and glory."[158] According to Foreest, uroscopy was also practiced by a fair share of "charlatan doctors" in Italy. He even mentioned his teacher Helidaeus Paduanus at the *Ospedale della Vita* in Bologna, to whom farmers brought the urine of sick people "in great amounts at a certain hour." This suggests a kind of uroscopic policlinic, but Foreest added that Helidaeus asked the farmers for details about the sick people and berated them if they would not give him any further information. If necessary, he would send Foreest and other students into the patients' houses to see them in person and learn of "all the signs

---

[153] Superville, *Nachricht vom wahren Nutzen* (around 1732), 9.

[154] Jacobus Haberstroh, preface to Himantomus, *De incerto urinarum iudicio* (1657); he used the German term "prostituieren".

[155] Medical Faculty of the University of Leipzig, preface to Kirstenius, *Trewe Warnung* (1610), 11–14.

[156] Horer, *Artzney-Teuffel* (1634), 62.

[157] Cf. Lange, *Epistolarum* (1589), 49–55; quoted after the German translation in Foreest, *Uromanteia* (1620), 438–59.

[158] Foreest, *Uromanteia* (1620), 273 and 276.

in addition to the disease itself."[159] Among the "righteous and learned" doctors in Italy, claimed Foreest, not a single one would accept the urine of sick people in his own house.[160] It was even deemed "a disgrace" in Italy and France, claimed Johannes Hornung "when the urine of a patient is given to a medical doctor to examine or judge."[161]

How great the difference really was between Germany on the one hand and France and Italy on the other remains an open question in retrospect. Perhaps pointing to the great model of Italy served mainly as a rhetorical device. After all, physicians in Italy such as Giovanni Argenterio likewise complained of colleagues who held that no knowledge of disease was more certain and of more general scope than that which was based on urine.[162] And Leonardo Botalli railed against the many physicians who, in spite of the method's great uncertainty, diagnosed illnesses on the sole basis of uroscopy simply because they were greedy. According to him, many doctors no longer had any shame or piety. To get their hands on a few of their poor patients' coins, they did not shy away from prescribing them—on the sole basis of uroscopy and without demanding any further information—medicines, or would it be more apt to call them poisons, he wondered. Was there anything more brazen? Any abuse more mad? A greed more filthy?[163] Not to offer a diagnostic and therapeutic judgment at all would still be better: As was generally known, Nature herself was a talented physician.[164]

It is revealing that, in the sixteenth and seventeenth centuries, even some of the harshest critics north of the Alps conceded that they had, at least earlier, diagnosed illnesses from urine; and they boasted of their success to top it all off.[165] Pieter van Foreest, for example, the author of the most often quoted work against "uromancy," lamented how in the first years of his practice he had to "accept and examine urine in my parlor against my will following the wicked custom."[166] Some of the critics even admitted that they themselves had used all sorts of those "tricks" to gain additional information, "tricks" which they otherwise attributed to "fraudulent" charlatans and urine prophets. They even went so far as to give the physician advice on how to proceed and get away with it. For example, when a doctor, while examining the urine, laid his hand on that

---

[159] Ibid., 229f.

[160] Ibid., 269.

[161] Hornung, *Uroscopia fraudulenta* (1611), 10; James Primrose (*De vulgi erroribus*, 1658, 93) also claimed, based on Leonhard Fuchs, that uroscopy enjoyed less esteem among Italian and French physicians.

[162] Argenterio, *De urinis* (1591), 3f.

[163] Botalli, *Commentarioli duo* (1565), 22 and 32f (cit.).

[164] Ibid., 35.

[165] Cordus, *De urinis* (1543), no pagination; Hart, *Arraignment* (1623), 42; Brian, *Pisse-prophet* (1655), preface.

[166] Foreest, *Uromanteia* (1620), 145.

part of his own body which he thought might be affected, the messenger or patient would believe that a correct diagnosis had been made and volunteer additional information. According to Roderigo da Castro, the fact that people were only familiar with a few body parts made things even easier: Since they knew only the head, chest, sides, stomach (from the collar bone to the navel), abdomen, back, and joints, the range of possibilities was limited and, on top of that, the physician could assume that in most cases pain was the issue because patients perceived it most readily.[167]

Indeed, some authors also put forward stories of physicians who surprised patients and families with their apparent uroscopic acumen, drawing all the while on their knowledge of the ways of the common people and their life circumstances. Such stories were often retold by other authors. Some were quite simple in nature, such as the anecdote of the physician who recognized that a urine sample had come from a tailor because the flask was closed with various colorful scraps of fabric.[168] Others showcased the doctor's good knowledge of the locality. In one such story, the wife of a sick vintner intends to bring her husband's urine to a physician in Brussels who is renowned as a uroscopist. On the way, she pays a visit to a friend who convinces her to put the doctor to the test. The friend takes the urine to the doctor instead and refuses to give any information about the sick person. The physician, however, recognizes the herbs that have been used to close the flask, and explains to the dumbfounded woman that the urine is not from a townsperson but from a farmer or a vintner. And because he knows exactly where these herbs grow, he can even tell her the gate through which the urine has been carried. The woman is convinced of the physician's abilities and proceeds to tell him everything she knows about the sick man.[169]

Still more sophisticated was the story of the doctor who is shown the urine of a farmer woman. The doctor is provided with no information about the patient or the illness. Yet he is somehow able to find out that he or she has a bruise and guesses correctly that she has fallen down the stairs. When asked about the precise number steps, he initially guesses incorrectly, saying 12 steps based on his knowledge of how low the ceilings in most farmhouses are. The husband asks the doctor to rethink the issue because it was actually more. Bearing in mind the icy roads, the doctor explains to the husband that he, the husband, must have spilled some of the urine on the way. The husband, impressed, confirms this and

---

167 Castro, *Medicus politicus* (1662), 150–52.
168 Beverwijk, *Schat der ongesontheydt* (1672), 11.
169 Foreest, *Uromanteia* (1620), 227; Beverwijk, *Schat der ongesontheydt* (1672), 11.

the physician is able to say that this is the reason why he underestimated the number of steps.[170]

In another case, attributed to Jason Pratensis, a physician recognizes in the urine which two women have brought him that it comes from a man whose pores were open widely due to copious sweating, allowing the cold to move into the body and toward his heart. On this basis he gives an impressive show of his uroscopic talent: He asks the women, to their astonishment, if the person in question is a bridegroom. For, from his knowledge of rural culture, he has good reason to assume that the man in question danced (and sweated) up a storm and then went out into the cold.[171]

The historical accuracy of such anecdotes is more than doubtful. It is surely no coincidence that Foreest, the most important source of these stories, usually remained very vague about their origins and details, while generally giving the names, times, and places in his case histories. He claimed, for instance, that the story of the fall down the stairs had taken place in France and that it had recently been told to him by an apothecary. Some stories even came in variations and were attributed to different medical protagonists. Nevertheless, these stories are very instructive. They served as *exempla* and they show us how learned physicians wanted to present themselves. They showed the learned physicians as smart and quick-witted. They had more than their philosophical abstractions to hold up against the peasants' cunning. They could meet the common folk head on, were a match for them even on their home turf.

This image of the superior intelligence of physicians, which they conveyed to the reader with the help of these stories, seems to have been so important to learned physicians that they were prepared to sacrifice the logical consistency of their polemics against uroscopy. After all, only their readers were informed about the true basis of their diagnostic inferences. The patients and relatives featured in the anecdotes were left believing that the physician had learned everything from the urine, which further strengthened the lay belief in the boundless possibilities of diagnosing illness from urine alone. As late as the early eighteenth century, Georg Ernst Stahl complained about some colleagues, who only pretended to make their diagnoses on the basis of urine and in this way "only feed the entirely ill-founded delusion of the common folk, instead of devoting all their efforts to killing it off."[172]

---

[170] Foreest, *Uromanteia* (1620), 222–5; Beverwijk, *Schat der ongesontheydt* (1672), 10; Thoner, *Observationum* (1649), 343.

[171] Beverwijk, *Schat der ongesontheydt* (1672), 11.

[172] Stahl, *Gründliche Abhandlung* (1739).

Epilogue
Uroscopy and the Disappearance of the Sick Man

A wide range of sources, from patient letters and autobiographies to medical treatises and case histories, show the outstanding place of uroscopy in early modern medicine. Ordinary people held uroscopy in high esteem as the most important diagnostic tool for any kind of disease. For a long time, learned physicians also valued uroscopy as the most certain way of learning about illness and its causes, and at the foremost universities of the time medical students were instructed in the art. In the course of the early modern period, medical writers expressed a growing disenchantment with uroscopy, but their criticism was directed above all against the common practice of diagnosing diseases from the urine in the patient's absence. Many physicians continued to rely on uroscopy and quite frequently, it seems, they bowed to the patients' pressure and prescribed their medicines just based on their uroscopic judgment and without seeing the patient in person. Only very gradually, in the eighteenth century, did uroscopy lose its privileged place in the physicians' diagnostic repertoire.

Ordinary people's deep and pervasive belief in uroscopy and the great difficulties that doctors encountered in trying to make their critique heard, also call on us to revise widely accepted notions about the early modern doctor-patient relationship and the status of the medical profession. Older work in the social history of medicine has described the time around 1800 as a period of radical change in diagnostic practices linked, in turn, to a profound shift in the doctor-patient relationship. Physicians before that time have been said to have very rarely, if at all, performed a physical examination. Their diagnosis, we are told, was based almost exclusively on what the patient told them about the history of the disease, including earlier illness episodes, the major complaints, his or her lifestyle, diet, and so forth. Based on what the patients communicated to them, they would prescribe medicines and give dietetic advice on what to eat and drink, how to structure the day, how much to move, and so forth. Such advice—and this was the physicians' major selling point—was to be tailored as precisely as possible to the patient's individual symptoms, bodily constitution, and life circumstances.

In the wake of two path-breaking articles by English sociologist Nicholas Jewson, this narrative-based medicine that put the individual patient into the center has come to be interpreted as reflecting the predominant type of doctor-patient relationship at the time, namely a relationship based on "patronage." According to Jewson, physicians usually saw only a small number of wealthy and educated patients, on whose benevolence and financial support they depended. To satisfy the needs and expectations of these preeminent patients and to secure their generous gratifications, doctors had to make plenty of time for them, had to listen attentively, and had to take them seriously as individuals with specific bodily constitutions and treat them accordingly. In sum, everything revolved around the patient as a person and his or her subjective descriptions.[1] This situation, the argument continues, changed fundamentally in the late eighteenth and early nineteenth centuries with the rise of clinical medicine.[2] This new medicine was characterized by a focus on objective physical signs and the connection between them and pathological/anatomical changes in the organs, which might later be seen in the dissection room. Physical examination, percussion, and listening with a stethoscope, later the use of the medical thermometer,[3] and around 1900 an increasingly wide spectrum of further technical procedures, such as taking X-rays, measuring blood pressure, and laboratory chemistry, became the cornerstones of medical diagnosis.[4] As Jens Lachmund has argued for stethoscopy, these new diagnostic methods led to "the establishment of a new type of professional expertise that put an end to a relationship of dependency in which the physician around 1800 had still found himself."[5] The new clinical medicine with its focus on organic changes inside the body and the new diagnostic approaches that came with it are thus said to have led to the "demise of the patient narrative,"[6] to the "disappearance of the sick-man from medical cosmology."[7] The patient was turned into a mere case—just like pregnancy, as Barbara Duden and others have claimed, was transformed from the subjective state of being with child into a medical condition identified by means of "objective" diagnosis.

Jewson's claims and their elaboration and reexamination in various national contexts have sharpened our attention to the close links between medical practices and power relations in the doctor-patient relationship. They are to some degree also supported by empirical evidence. Nevertheless, they require

---

[1]   Jewson, *Medical knowledge* (1974); Jewson, *Disappearance* (1976).

[2]   For a still valuable overview see Reiser, *Medicine* (1978); the orientation toward new clinical methods did not by any means come as suddenly, around 1800, as Foucault, *Birth* (1973), claimed in his influential work. It gradually emerged in a process that reaches back at least to the Renaissance and in the course of which the results of anatomical-pathological studies continued to gain significance.

[3]   Reiser, *Medicine* (1978), 110–21.

[4]   Ibid., esp. 1–22.

[5]   Lachmund, *Der abgehorchte Körper* (1997), 11.

[6]   Fissell, *Disappearance* (1991).

[7]   Jewson, *Medical knowledge* (1974); Jewson, *Disappearance* (1976).

substantial modification, not least in the light of the central place that uroscopy held in early modern medical life.

To start with, the old "bedside medicine" or "narrative-based medicine" was not simply displaced or replaced by the new clinical medicine of the nineteenth century. The old "bedside medicine" and the new clinical medicine coexisted for a long time in separate spheres, in terms of both location and social sphere. The increasing significance of nonverbal, physical diagnostic methods such as auscultation and measuring the body's temperature was for quite some time largely restricted to hospital medicine. It was only at the end of the nineteenth century that the new methods found their way into private practice. Yet hospitals as the prime sites of these new diagnostic practices were largely still avoided in the nineteenth century precisely by those affluent patients to whom Jewson referred. Hospitals were increasingly transformed into institutions for the medical care of the sick but they remained, for decades, the refuge of the poor, of workers, of tradespeople, the solitary elderly, and domestic servants.[8] The relationship between the academic hospital physician and his lower-class patients was very different from that in ordinary medical practice. In the hospital, the individual doctor took care of dozens, if not hundreds of sick people, who appeared as recipients of charity rather than clients and who did not have much of a say. The hospital was a place where, as Franz Christoph Karl Krügelstein described it in 1807, "the will of the sick person [is] rather restricted by the physician."[9] The physician was not under pressure to convince the patients or their families of his abilities. Their trust and benevolence—or the lack thereof—had only minimal impact on the doctor's status and income.[10]

Second, the picture of a patronage-type relationship that Jewson has drawn for the time before 1800 must be taken with more than a grain of salt. As early as the sixteenth and seventeenth centuries, doctors, at least in continental Europe, were also routinely treating tradespeople and farmers in their private practices, and published case histories and physicians' practice journals and casebooks

---

[8]   In her ground-breaking work, Mary Fissell (Fissell, *Disappearance* (1991) has traced the disappearance of the patient narrative from English medicine in the early nineteenth century. She has based her findings largely on hospital records, however. Since in hospitals a small number of doctors usually cared for a large number of lower-class and predominantly single patients, it remains doubtful to what degree we can draw more general conclusions from a study of this particular disempowered group.

[9]   Krügelstein, *Handbuch* (1807), 418; contemporary clinical case histories do show, however, that physicians took seriously even their lower class patients' needs and feelings, for instance in the case of a decision whether or not to perform a painful operation (cf. Nolte, *Zeitalter* (2006)).

[10] Lachmund/Stollberg, *The doctor* (1992).

suggest that patients whose social and economic status was lower or, at most, equal to that of the physician were usually a very prominent group.[11]

Third and most fundamentally, a look at the history of uroscopy reveals that ordinary diagnostic practice in the early modern period has been profoundly misrepresented. The widespread and enduring trust that patients and their relatives invested in diagnosis on the sole basis of urine shows that a preference for "objective" diagnostic methods rather than reliance on the patient narrative was by no means an invention of nineteenth-century clinical medicine. Uroscopy was both the most important diagnostic procedure in early modern medical practice and a procedure that could do perfectly well without the patient's narrative. As we have seen, some patients and families, far from insisting on making their own voice heard, even explicitly refused to give any information about the sick person and his or her complaints and history. The skillful physician was to draw his conclusions entirely from what he saw in the urine. There were also other common diagnostic methods that could be performed in the patient's absence, such as astrological diagnosis,[12] and/or did not depend on the patient's narrative. With all its practical difficulties, pulse diagnosis maintained its place in early modern practice, especially in the diagnosis of fevers, and a manual examination was also performed much more frequently than has widely been assumed.[13]

All this casts great doubt on the assumed link between the rise of "clinical medicine" and "objective" diagnostic approaches on the one hand and medical professionalization and the shift in the doctor-patient relationship on the other. Undoubtedly, the position of patients and families in their encounters with academic physicians was comparatively strong in the early modern period. This powerful position did not reflect a relationship of patronage, however. It was due to the varied and largely unregulated health market of the time, in which patients in many places were able to knock on other healers' doors if they were unsatisfied with a physician. The history of uroscopy also makes it clear that we must not take it for granted that patients at all times and in all places wish, above all, to talk extensively about their complaints and therefore will always prefer "narrative-based medicine." In the early modern period, many patients favored a diagnostic approach that called for special technical expertise and was surrounded by a certain mysterious aura rather than the skillful interpretation of what the patient had to tell.

In a sense then, the roles and expectations of physicians and patients were distributed just the other way round. The physicians were the ones who wanted to

---

[11]   This is a major result of the work of a German-Austrian-Swiss research network funded by the Deutsche Forschungsgemeinschaft that brought together eight research projects on the history of medical practices from the seventeenth to the nineteenth centuries (cf. Dinges et alii, *Medical Practice*).

[12]   See e.g. Traister, *Simon Forman* (2001); Kassell, *Medicine and magic* (2005).

[13]   Stolberg, *Examining the body* (2013).

accord a central place to the patient narrative. Of course, physicians occasionally complained about the loquaciousness and know-all manner of some patients or declared their narratives as outright unreliable, because the patients lacked the ability to describe their own perceptions and sensations precisely and impartially. According to G.E. Stahl, one of the greatest difficulties of medical practice was, in fact, "that sick people commonly do not tell the physician what they feel, but have already formed an idea themselves, either using their own bad terms or those of others, giving their illness a name."[14] Antonius Eijgel—a doctor but also a strong proponent of uroscopy—considered uroscopy superior to patient accounts because no patient knew what it was that ailed him, and children or unconscious patients were in no position to express themselves in the first place.[15] Most doctors, however, preferred basing their diagnosis and treatment on the patient's narrative. While they perceived uroscopy increasingly as a threat to their authority, narrative-based medicine allowed them to demonstrate their unique ability to arrive at a diagnostic and therapeutic judgment that took the patient's medical history and current complaints as well as his or her individual constitution, diet, and lifestyle into account. By contrast, a mere look at the matula and nothing else offered little opportunity to put their erudition and superior medical expertise on stage. Yet many physicians found they had no choice. They had to rely primarily on a visual examination of the urine rather than on their interpretation of the patient's narrative. Their patients demanded it.

Only very gradually, and largely limited to the upper classes, the physicians' ideal of an individualized diagnosis and therapy that was tailored to the patient's constitution, history, and lifestyle came to be perceived, in some measure, as indispensable. In the eighteenth century, educated patients occasionally explained how important it was to them that the physician be familiar with their individual physical constitution. Compared to the letters that patients sent to Platter and Thurneysser in the sixteenth century, eighteenth-century patient letters tended to offer much more extensive and detailed accounts, and the urine was no longer routinely sent along. Regarding the wider population, the situation changed only in the course of the nineteenth century. Supported, in some states, by government measures against barber-surgeons and irregular healers, physicians were able to secure an increasing monopoly. At the same time, new conceptions of disease gradually found their way into lay medical culture, taking the place of the traditional humoral medicine which had served as a principal foundation of uroscopy. The triumphant successes of bacteriology, the rise of the pharmaceutical industry, the spread of new alternative healing systems such as homeopathy, and, more than anything, economic and social change, increasing industrialization and urbanization, and the creation of a new

---

14   Stahl, *Gründliche Abhandlung* (1739), 26.
15   Eijgel, *Apologema* (1672), 4.

blue-collar and, later, white-collar class made old conceptions and practices lose significance and pushed them to the margins. This is true for the wide spectrum of magic, sympathetic healing rituals that had been used to confront illnesses, and it is also true for uroscopy. In the end, uroscopy persisted only in the shadows of lay medical culture and irregular medical practice.

The rise of clinical chemistry fostered a renewed interest in the urinary changes associated with different diseases but chemical urinalysis was by no means a substitute for traditional uroscopy. What was largely lost was uroscopy's diagnostic range, the belief that virtually all diseases could be identified from the urine. Except for a few metabolic disorders—in the first place diabetes—chemical urinalysis was useful almost exclusively in diseases of the urinary-genital tract. The visual examination of the patient's urine with the naked eye never disappeared entirely from medical practice.[16] Indeed, the recent renaissance of uroscopy in naturopathic circles suggests that to this day uroscopy continues to have its appeal as a divinatory ritual, as a way of deciphering the mysterious pathological processes within the body in the search for a more profound truth.

---

[16]   This goes, to some degree, even for modern doctors; cf. Krack, *Harnschau* (1982).

Sources

Manuscript Sources

Bamberg, Staatsarchiv (StA): KIII 1481, I–IV.

Basel, Universitätsbibliothek (UB): Ms. Fr. Gr. I 6.

Berlin, Staatsbibliothek zu Berlin—Preußischer Kulturbesitz (StB): Ms. germ. fol. 99, 105, 106, 420a, 420b, 421a, 421b, 422a, 422b, 423a, 423b, 424, 425, 426.

Copenhagen, Kongelige Bibliotek: Ms. Thottske S 4 689.

Erlangen, Universitätsbibliothek (UB), Trewsche Briefsammlung.

Frankfurt, Universitätsbibliothek, Senckenberg Archiv: Ms. 334; Senckenberg correspondence.

Lausanne, Bibliothèque Cantonale et Universitaire (BCU), Lausanne-Dorigny: Fonds Tissot.

Leiden, Universiteitsbibliotheek (UB): Ms. Marchand 3.

London, British Library: Ms. Sloane 94; Ms. Harley 5311.

London, Wellcome Library, Western manuscripts: Ms. 94; Ms. 7117/36.

Ludwigsburg, Staatsarchiv Ludwigsburg: B 412/37.

Memmingen: Stadtarchiv, Bestand A Reichsstadt, Schubl. 408.

Milan, Biblioteca Universitaria Braidense, Fondo Haller: Ms. AD-XIV-14 n. 4; Ms. AE-XI-12 and 13.

Milan, Biblioteca Trivulziana: Ms. 1709.

Munich, Bayerische Staatsbibliothek (BSB): Cgm 6874; Clm 25087.

Munich, Bayerisches Hauptstaatsarchiv (HStA): MInn 61355.

Nuremberg, Stadtarchiv (StA): B19 184.

Paris, Bibliothèque Interuniversitaire de Médecine (BIM): Mss. 5241–5.

Schwäbisch-Hall, Stadtarchiv (StA): Bestand 11, Nr. 84.

Schwerin, Landesarchiv: Altes Archiv 2.12–2/3, 178.

Stuttgart, Hauptstaatsarchiv (HStA): A 213 Bü. 6734; ibid. Bü. 8416; A 282 Bü. 1299.

Stuttgart, Württembergische Landesbibliothek: Cod. med. et phys. 4° 13.

Ulm, Stadtarchiv: Ms. Franc 8a und 8b.

Vienna, Österreichische Nationalbibliothek (ÖNB), Codd. 11198, 11205, 11206, 11210, 11238, 11240.

Zürich, Archiv des Medizinhistorischen Instituts der Universität Zürich: Ms. H 11.

Printed Sources

Academia Leopoldina Naturae Curiosorum Vratisl. (eds): Historia morborum qui annis MDCXCIX. MDCC. MDCCI. MDCCII. Vratislaviae grassati sunt. Lausanne/Geneva 1746.

Ackermann, Michael [i.e. Joseph Xaver Rehmann]: Medicinisches Glaubens-Bekenntniß eines schwäbischen Harnpropheten. Tübingen 1783.

Actuarius, Ioannis Zacharias: De urinis. Transl. by Ambrosius Leo. Venice 1519.

Actuarius, Ioannis Zacharias: De urinis libri VII. Utrecht 1670.

Anonymous: The judycyall of uryns. London [around 1527].

Anonymous: The seinge of urynes, of all the colours that urynes be of, with medecines annexed to euerye urine, and euery uryne his urinall much profitable for euerye manne to knowe. London [around 1550].

Anonymous: Hereafter foloweth the judgment of all urynes: and for to knowe the mannes from the womannes, and beastes both from the mannes and womans with the coloure of everye uryne. London [around 1555].

Anonymous: Le traicté des urines, lequel traicte de leurs couleurs et ce quelles peullent signifier. Paris [before 1567].

Anonymous: The key to unknowne knowledge. London 1599.

Anonymous: Mantissa de examinatione naturalium liquidorum et terreorum, praeprimis lotii humani per pondus. i. e. geringer Zusatz, zu vorigen Blättern von Ausforschung natürlicher Dinge Eigenschafften, zumal des Urins des Menschen, durch subtiles Abwiegen, zur Erkennung eines Gesunden und Ungesunden, des Zu- und Abnehmens der Gesundheit und Kranckheit, und Zeichen des Todes und der Reconvalescenz. In: Anonymous, Relationes curiosae medicae von dem bishero sehr verachteten signo physico dem Urin. Gotha 1718, 101–20.

Anonymous: Onomatologia medico-practica. 4 vols. Nuremberg 1786.

Apollinaris: Tractätlein vom Urin u. Pulß. Ed. by Theodor Majus. Hamburg 1663.

Argenterio, Giovanni: De urinis liber. [Heidelberg] 1591.

Avicenna: Canon medicinae. Venice 1595 (repr. Hildesheim 1964).

Baehrens, Johann Christoph Friedrich: Die Harnlehre des Hippokrates in ihrem wahren Werthe behauptet. Elberfeld 1829.

Becquerel, Alfred: Séméiotique des urines, ou traité des altérations de l'urine dans les maladies. Paris 1841.

Behrens, Konrad Barthold: Ob das Wasserbeschawen in Krankheiten etwas nuze, und wie weit demselben zu trauen. Hildesheim 1688.

Bellini, Lorenzo: De urina, pulsu, sanguinis missione et febribus nec non de capitis pectorisque morbis. 3rd edn. Frankfurt/Leipzig 1718.

Bernd, Adam: Eigene Lebens-Beschreibung. Leipzig 1738 (repr. Munich 1973).

Bertrand, Nicolas: Nova philosophandi ratio de urinis seu paradoxae aliquot de urinis exercitationes. Rhedonis 1630.

Beverwijk, Johann van: Schat der ongesontheyt, ofte genees-konste van de sieckten . In: idem: Wercken der genees-konste. Amsterdam 1672 (part 1 and 2 with separate pagination).

Boerhaave, Herman: Institutiones medicae in usus annuae exercitationis domesticos digestae. Nuremberg 1747.

Boerhaave, Herman: Introductio in praxin clinicam, sive regulae generales in praxi clinica observandae quas praemisit antequam lectiones publicas adgrediebatur in nosocomio Lugdunensi cl. Hermannus Boerhaave a diligente auditore communicatae. Leiden 1740.

Bonacursius, Bartholomaeus: De humano sero. Bologna 1650.

Borrichius, Olaus: Olai Borrichii itinerarium 1660–1665. The journal of the Danish polyhistor Ole Borch. Ed. by H. D. Schepelern. Vol. 1: Introduction. Nov. 1660–Oct. 1661. Copenhagen/London 1983.

Botalli, Leonardus: Commentarioli duo, alter de medici, alter de aegroti munere. Lyon 1565.

Brant, Sebastian: The ship of fools. Transl. by Edwin H. Zeydel. New York 1944.

Brian, Thomas: The pisse-prophet; or, Certain pisse-pot lectures. Wherein are newly discovered the old fallacies, deceit, and jugling of the piss-pot science, used by all those (whether quacks, and empiricks, or other methodical physicians) who pretend knowledg of diseases, by the urine, in giving judgment of the same. London 1655.

Brooke, H.: Hygieine [graece]. Or a conservatory of health. London 1650.

Buck, Michael Richard: Medicinischer Volksglauben und Volksaberglauben aus Schwaben. Eine kulturgeschichtliche Skizze. Ravensburg 1865.

Capivaccius, Hieronymus: De urinis tractatus. Zerbst 1595.

Castro, Roderigo da: Medicus-politicus: sive de officiis medico-politicis tractatus. Hamburg 1662.

Clauser, Christoph: Das die betrachtung des menschenn Harns on anderen bericht unnütz. [Zurich 1531].

Cordus, Euricius: Von der kunst auch missbrauch vnd trug des harnsehens. Magdeburg 1536.

Cordus, Euricius: De urinis, das ist, von rechter besichtigunge des harns, und ihrem mißbrauch. Ed. by J. Dryander. Frankfurt 1543.

Culpeper, Nicholas: Urinalia: or, a treatise of the crisis hapning to the urine: Through default either of the reines, bladder, yard, conduits, or passages. With their causes, signes, and cures. In: Culpeper's semeiotica uranica, or astrologicall judgment of diseases from the decumbiture of the sick much enlarged. London 1655, 151–74.

Cusanus, Nicolaus: De staticis experimentis dialogus (= appended to Vitruvius, De architectura libri decem). Strasbourg 1543.

Da Monte, Giovanni Battista: Lectiones de urinis. Ed. by Franciscus Emericus. Vienna 1552.

Da Monte, Giovanni Battista: De excrementis libri II, alter de fecibus, alter de urinis. Padua 1554.

Da Monte, Giovanni Battista: Tractatus de urinis. Sine loco, sine anno.

Davach de la Rivière, Jean: Le miroir des urines. 3rd edn. Paris 1722.

Detharding, Georg: Der unterwiesene Kranken-Wärter. Kiel 1679.

Dodonaeus, Rembertus: Medicinalium observationum exempla rara, recognita et aucta. 2nd edn. Cologne 1581.

Dueren, Johan van: De ontdekkinge der bedriegeryen van de gemeene piz-besienders. Amsterdam 1688.

Eijgel, Antonius: Apologema pro urinis humanis, of Verantwoordingh voor de Menschelicke Wateren [...] waer in klaerlick bewesen wort, dat de selve verre te boven gaen alle andere Teikenen in de Medicijn [...]. Ten Tweeden: een Beschrijvingh der selver Wateren, soo door eygen Ondervindingen van't Jaer 1636 als door bewijs der autheuren, of Instelleren bevestight. Ten Derden: een Weder-leggingh Tegen de Schriften der Watern van [...] Forestus, en Stretenius. Amsterdam 1672.

Eijgel, Antonius: Nieuwe Genees-konst, of Mantissa medicaminum; dat is, toegift van medicamenten, tegen de siechten, aengewesen zijnde door't Menschelick Water in sijn drie voorgaende Werken. Amsterdam 1673.

Ewaldt, Beniamin: Diatriba semeiotica de uroscopiae usu et abusu, germanice, Vom Gebrauch und Mißbrauch des Wasser-Besehens. Resp. Ernestus Theophilus Friese. Königsberg 1718.

Fernel, Jean: Universa medicina. Geneva 1644.

Fernel, Jean/Cole, Abdiah/Culpeper, Nicholas: Two treatises: The first of pulses, the second of urines. London 1662.

Finot, Raymundus: An ex urinis certa valetudinis auguria? Resp. Jacques des Prez. Paris 1677.

Fletcher, I.: The differences, causes, and judgements of urine according to the best writers thereof, both old and new, summarily collected. London 1641.

Floyer, John: The physician's pulse watch, or an essay to explain the old art of feeling the pulse, and to improve it by the help of a pulse-watch. 2 vols. London 1707.

Foreest, Pieter van: Uromanteia. Das ist, warhafftiger und wolgegründter Bericht, von den vielfaltigen Urtheilen unnd Weissagungen auß den Urinen, oder Wassern. In welchem fürnemblich erkläret unnd bewiesen wirdt, wie falsch, nichtig unnd betrüglich dieselbige seyen, unnd was für unwiderbringlicher Schaden allen den jenigen, so sich darauff verlassen, offt und vielmal daraus erfolg. Frankfurt 1620.

Fries, Lorenz: Spiegel der Artzny. Strasbourg 1518.

Fuchs, Leonhard: Institutionum medicinae, ad Hippocratis, Galeni, aliorumque veterum scripta recte intelligenda mire utiles libri quinque. Lyon 1555.

Gabelkover, Wolfgang: Curationum et observationum medicinalium centuriae IV. Tübingen 1611–1612.

Galen: De crisibus. In: idem: Opera omnia. Ed. by C.G. Kühn. Vol. 9. Leipzig 1825 (repr. Hildesheim 1965), 550–768.

Gebauer, Jeremias: Dissertatio inauguralis medica, proponens uromantiam medicis in certis Silesiae locis summe necessariam. Praes. Joannis Philippus Eyselius. Erfurt 1711.

Gesnerus, Conradus: Compendium ex Actuarii Zachariae libris de differentiis urinarum, iudiciis et praevidentiis. Zurich [around 1541].

Grosshauser, Johann: Praktische Winke zur leichten Erkennung der Krankheiten aus dem Urin. Zusammengestellt auf Grund fremder und eigener Erfahrungen während einer 16jährigen Praxis. Bonn 1901.

Hart, James: The arraignment of urines, wherein are set downe the manifold errors and abuses of ignorant urine-monging [sic] empirickes, cozening quacksalvers, women-physitians and the like stuffe. London 1623.

Harvey, William: Exercitatio anatomica de motu cordis et sanguinis in animalibus. Frankfurt 1628.

Hayne, Johan: Drey unterschiedliche new Tractätlein. Frankfurt 1620.

Hechstetter, Philippus: Rararum observationum medicinalium decades [...]. 2 vols. Augsburg 1624/1627.

Hederich, Carolus Christian: De ambiguitate uroscopiae. Praes. Hermannus Paulus Juchius. Erfurt 1732.

Helmont, Johann Baptist van: Aufgang der Artzney-Kunst. Sulzbach 1683.

Henninger, Joh. Sigismund: Theses miscellaneae circa uroscopiam. Exponit Christianus Fridericus Helwig. Strasbourg 1712.

Himantomus (i.e. Riemschneider), Johann Günther: De incerto urinarum iudicio; et intolerabili circumforaneorum impostura libellus. Quedlinburg 1657.

Hippocrates: Œuvres complètes d'Hippocrate. Ed. by Émile Littré. Paris 1839–1861 (repr. Amsterdam 1978).

Hoffmann, Friedrich: Medicina rationalis systematica. 2nd edn. Halle/ Magdeburg 1729.

Hoffmann, Friedrich: Medicus politicus sive regulae prudentiae secundum quas medicus juvenis studia sua & vitae rationem dirigere debet, si famam sibi felicemque praxin & cito acquirere & conservare cupit. Leiden 1708.

Höfler, Max: Deutsches Krankheitsnamenbuch. Munich 1899.

Horer, Ananius: Artzney-Teuffel, Oder kurtzer Discurs, Darinn diesem Ertzmörder seine Larve abgezogen. Sine loco 1634.

Horlacher, Conradus: Methodus urinoscopiae perfacilis ac perspicua. Ulm 1691.

Hörnigk, Ludwig von: Politia medica Oder Beschreibung dessen was die Medici, so wohl ins gemeins als auch verordnete Hof- Statt- Feldt- Hospital- vnd

Pest- Medici [...] So dann endlichen: Die Patienten oder Krancke selbsten zu thun. Frankfurt 1636.

Hornung, Johannes: De uroscopia fraudulenta discursus. Kurtzer Bericht von dem unvollkommenen und betrüglichen Urtheil des menschlichen Borns oder Harns: wider etliche vermässene Ärtzte, welche allerley Leibsschwachheiten darauß ursprünglichen und gewiß zu erkennen sich fälschlich außthun, dadurch den Patienten nicht allein schädlich und ungewiß gerahten ist, sonder auch der rechte Gebrauch der unaußforschlichen Kunst der Artzney verachtet wirdt. Herborn 1611.

Horst, Gregor: Disputationum medicarum decima quarta, De urinis. Resp. Joachimus Catzschius. Wittenberg 1607.

Horst, Johann Daniel: Manuductio ad medicinam. Marburg 1648.

Hummel, Johannes Heinrich: Historie des Lebens Johannis Henrici Hummelii. Eine Autobiographie aus dem 17. Jahrhundert. Ed. by Chr. Erni. In: Berner Zeitschrift für Geschichte und Heimatkunde 1950, 24–57.

Hygiander: Regeln von dem Urin unbetrüglich zu urtheilen. Nuremberg 1744 (repr. Leipzig 1937).

Isaac Judaeus: Liber de urinis. In: idem: Omnia opera. [Lyon 1515], 157r–203r.

Josselin, Ralph: The diary of Ralph Josselin 1616–1683. Ed. by Alan Macfarlane. London 1976.

Joubert, Laurent: Erreurs populaires au fait de la médecine et régime de santé. Bordeaux 1578.

Ketham, Johannes von [attributed to]: Fasciculus medicinae. Ed. by Karl Sudhoff. Milan 1923 (based on the 1491 edn).

Ketham, Johannes von [attributed to]: Fasciculus medicinae (repr. of a hand-coloured copy in the Biblioteca civica of Bergamo, incunabulo P 3 10, Bergamo 1976). Venice 1493.

Ketham, Johannes von [attributed to]: Fasciculus medicinae. Venice 1495.

Kirstenius, Petrus: Trewe Warnung von rechtem Gebrauch und Mißbrauch der Artzney. Breslau 1610.

Kolreutter, Sigmundt: Von rechten und in der Artzney nützlichen Gebreuchen des Harm [sic] oder Wasser besehens, und dagegen mancherley Mißbreuchen, die darauß ervolget sein. Nuremberg 1574.

Kortum, Karl Arnold: Vom Urin als einem Zeichen in Kranckheiten und von den Kunstgriffen der Harnärzte wenn sie daraus die Krankheiten sagen. Eine Schrift fürs Volk, auch jungen Aerzten nüzlich. Duisburg 1793.

Kräutermann, Valentin (i.e. Christoph von Hellwig): Curieuser und vernünfftiger Urin-Artzt. Arnstadt/Leipzig 1732.

Krügelstein, Franz Christian Karl: Handbuch der allgemeinen Krankenpflege. Zum Gebrauch für Aerzte und Familienväter. Erfurt 1807.

Lange, Johannes: Epistolarum medicinalium volumen tripartitum. Frankfurt 1589.

Liessell, Isaac: Konste om't water te besien, ofte 't rechte oordeel der Wateren. Met reden, en door sesthienjarige experientie gesien. Schoonhoven 1668.

Liphimeus, Sabalathrus: Warnung wider den Harn-Teuffel: Das ist: gründlicher Bericht, von dem Urin deß Menschen, unnd sonderlich wider diejenigen, so vorgeben, daß sie alle unnd jede Kranckheiten auß bloßer Anschawung der Urin erkennen, urtheilen und curiren wollen. Nuremberg 1626.

Loew, Joseph: Ueber den Urin als diagnostisches und prognostisches Zeichen. Landshut [1808].

M.A.C.D.: Systême d'un medecin anglois sur la cause de toutes les especes de maladies: avec les surprenantes configurations des differentes especes de petits insectes, qu'on voit par le moyen d'un bon microscope dans le sang et dans les urines des differens malades, et même de tous ceux qui doivent le devenir. Paris 1726.

Majus, Theodorus: Urin-Büchlein, darinnen einem ieden frommen Menschen, zu seiner Gesundheit, ein fruchtbarer und nöthiger Unterricht mitgetheilet wird, was er sich auf das Wasser oder Urin zu verlassen, und wie dasselbe zu besehen sey, sampt allen Umbständen und Mißbräuchen. Hamburg 1663.

Martini, Heinrich: Anatomia urinae galeno-spagyrica. Ex Doctrina Hippocratis & Galeni nec non recentiorum, imprimis Theophrasti Paracelsi, & Leonhardi Thurnheuseri, aliorumque chymiatrorum principum scriptis adornata. Cui accessit ejusd[em] ars pronuntiandi ex urinis tam rationalis quam mechanica et Caesaris Odoni de urinis libellus posthumus. Frankfurt 1658.

Massaria, Alessandro: Tractatus quatuor utilissimi quorum I. De Peste II. De affectionibus renum & vesicae III. De pulsibus IV. De urinis. Frankfurt 1608.

Melanchthon, Philipp: Commentarius de anima. Wittenberg 1540.

Melanchthon, Philipp: Liber de anima. Wittenberg 1552.

Mérat, [Francois Victor]: Uromancie. In: Adelon et al. (eds): Dictionaire des sciences médicales: Trif–Vap. Paris 1821, 341–8.

Montfalcon, [Jean-Baptiste]: Urine. In: Adelon et al. (eds): Dictionaire des sciences médicales: Trif–Vap. Paris 1821, 307–34.

Munnicks, Johannis: Dissertatio de urinis earundemque inspectione. Utrecht 1674.

Nettesheim, Agrippa von: De incertitudine et vanitate scientiarum. Cologne 1539.

Nettesheim, Agrippa von: Die Eitelkeit und Unsicherheit der Wissenschaft und die Verteidigungsschrift. 2 vols. Ed. by Fritz Mauthner. Munich 1913.

Neubauer, Carl: Anleitung zur qualitativen und quantitativen Analyse des Harns. Wiesbaden 1854.

Neubauer, Carl/Vogel, Julius: Anleitung zur qualitativen und quantitativen Analyse des Harns. Wiesbaden 1858 (7th edn Wiesbaden 1876, 10th edn Wiesbaden 1898).

Odone, Cesare: De urinarum differentiis, causis et iudiciis brevissima et clarissima methodus. Libellus posthumus. Frankfurt 1658.

Oetheus, Jakob: Gründtlicher Bericht, Lehr unnd Instruction von rechtem und nutzlichem Brauch der Artzney, den Gesunden, Krancken und Kranckenpflegern. Dillingen 1574.

Olmo, Giovanni Francesco: De certa ratione iudicandi ex urinis libri quatuor. Venice 1578.

Paracelsus: De urinarum ac pulsuum iudiciis [...] libellus, suis discipulis Basileae [...] anno 1527 praelectus. Cologne 1568.

Paracelsus: De urinis. In: Sudhoff, Karl (ed.): Theophrast von Hohenheim gen. Paracelsus. Sämtliche Werke. Part 1: Medizinische, naturwissenschaftliche und philosophische Schriften. Vol. 4. Munich/Berlin 1931, 623–39.

Paracelsus: Über die Beurteilung der Harne und der Pulse, auch über die Physiognomie, wie viel für einen Arzt notwendig ist. In: idem: Sämtliche Werke. Ed. by Bernhard Aschner. Jena 1928, 777–862.

Paré, Ambroise: Les œuvres. 9th edn. Lyon 1633.

Pfizerus, Johannes Nicolaus: Zwey sonderbare Bücher, von der Weiber Natur, wie auch deren Gebrechen und Kranckheiten. Nuremberg 1673.

Pictorius, Georg: Von zernichten Artzten. Strasbourg 1557.

Pinder, Udalricus: Epiphanie medicorum. [Nuremberg] 1506.

Platter, Felix: Tagebuch (Lebensbeschreibung) 1536–1567. Ed. by Valentin Lötscher. Basel 1976.

Pleier, Cornelius: Examen tractatus Guil. Adolphi Scribonii anno MDXXCV Basileae sub falso prætextu contra uromantes impostores, ipsi uropotas dictos editi. Erfurt 1617.

Primrose, James P.: De vulgi erroribus in medicina libri V. Rotterdam 1658.

Prochaska, Georg: Dissertatio inauguralis medica de urinis. Vienna 1776.

(Pseudo-)Albertus Magnus: Secreta mulierum. London 1485.

Record, Robert: The urinal of physick. London 1651.

Rega, Henricus Jos.: Tractatus duo de urinis. Prior quaestio quodlibetica, an ulla scientiae medicae investigatione aut experimento quispiam possit ex sola urinarum inspectione morborum naturam ad medelam dignoscere? Alter de urinis ut signo. Leuven 1733.

Rhenanus, Johannes: Urocriterium chymiatricum, sive ratio chymiatrica exacte diiudicandi urinas ex tribus principiis activis, et uno passivo. Frankfurt 1614.

Riedlin, Veit: Lineae medicae, singulos per menses quotidie ductae. Augsburg 1699.

Rondelet, Guillaume: De urinis praelectiones. Sine loco, sine anno.

Rübel, Johann Friedrich: Medicinische Abhandlung, wie man in denen Kranckheiten aus dem Urin, Schweiß, und aus dem Stuhlgang ein richtiges Urtheil fällen soll. Augsburg 1756.

Rübel, Johann Friedrich: Von dem rechten Gebrauch und Missbrauch des Urinbesehens. In: idem: Gründliche Abhandlung derer Criminalfälle, welche in das forum juridicum & medicum einschlagen [...]. Nebst einem Anhang: Von dem rechten Gebrauch und Missbrauch des Urinbesehens. Frankfurt/Leipzig 1762, 81–112.

Rusnock, Andrea A.: The correspondence of James Jurin (1684–1750). Physician and secretary to the Royal Society. Amsterdam/Atlanta, GA 1996.

Saltzmann, Rudolph: De uromantia. Subm. Albert Konrad Langenauer. Strasbourg 1651.

Salvianus, Salustius: De urinarum differentiis, causis et iudiciis libri duo. Rome 1587.

Sanctorius, Sanctorius: De statica medicina. The Hague 1657.

Saxonia, Hercules: De urinis. In: idem: Opera practica, books 5 and 6. Padua 1639, 29–59.

Savonarola, Michael: De urinis. In: idem: Practica canonica. Venice 1561.

Schmidt, Johannes: Uromanticus castratus sive tractatus de urinis, earumque inspectione Johannis Munnicks professoris medici Trajectini castigatus. Utrecht 1697.

Schönefeldt, Laurentius: Ein gantz fruchtbar underricht, einem jewelcken minschen tho syner gesuntheit, noedich, unde lustich tho lesen, was hy syck upp de urin effte dat water der minschen tho vorlaten, sampt allen umstendicheden. Lübeck 1534.

Schylander, Cornelius: Medicina astrologica. Antwerp 1577.

Scribonius, Wilhelm Adolph: De inspectione urinarum, contra eos qui ex qualibet urina de quolibet morbo judicare volunt, physiologia cursoria. In: idem: Idea medicinae secundum logicas leges informandae et describendae. Cui accessit de inspectione urinarum. Basel 1585, 11–57.

Scultetus, Johannes: Wund-Artzneyisches Zeug-Hauß. Frankfurt 1666.

Seidel, Bruno: Liber morborum incurabilium causas, mira brevitate, summa lectionis jucunditate exhibens. Leiden 1662.

Stahl, Georg Ernst: De uromantiae et uroscopiae abusu tollendo. Subm. Bernhardus Rappard. Halle/Magdeburg 1711.

Stahl, Georg Ernst: Gründliche Abhandlung von Abschaffung des Missbrauchs, so mit Besehung des Urins, und mit der Wahrsagung aus denselben [sic] in Schwange gehet. Coburg 1739.

Starck, Andreas: Harmspiegel. Das ist: Kurtzer und einfeltiger Bericht, das dem Harm- oder Urin schawen in Pestilentzzeit nicht zu trawen sey. Erfurt 1597.

Starck, Andreas: Krancken Spiegel. Das ist kurtzer Unterricht, wie erstlich ein Krancker, dan ein rechter trewer Artzt sich beyd recht und christlich verhalten mögen, darneben auch, wie in jtziger Pestilentzzeit sich zu bewaren, unnd dem Harm oder Urinschauen nicht zutrawen sey. Mülhausen 1598.

Superville, Daniel de: Gedancken von Quack-Salbern, Medicis und Patienten, woraus sich einjeder belehren kan, wie er sich zu sein selbst Erhaltung vor Quack-Salbern und After-Aertzten hüten, hergegen rechtschaffen- und gewissenhafften Medicis anvertrauen und dieselben ehren solle. Stettin/ Leipzig 1736.

Superville, Daniel de: Nachricht vom wahren Nutzen des menschlichen Urin-Besehens: Worin zugleich der Mißbrauch, so gemeiniglich darbey vorfällt, entdecket, und einjeder sich vor Schaden zu hüten gewarnet wird. Alten Stettin [1732].

Tachenius, Otto: Hippocrates chymicus, which discovers the ancient foundations of the late viperine salt and his clavis therunto. London 1677.

Tentzelius, Andreas: Disputatio medica de urinis. Praes. Philippus Leopoldus. Wittenberg 1609.

Thoner, Augustinus: Observationum medicinalium haud trivialium libri quatuor [...]. Hisce adjuncti sunt consultationum, cum diversarum regionum medicis habitarum, et epistolarum de variis rebus medico-philosophicis disserentium libri duo. Ulm 1649.

Thurneysser, Leonhard: Prokatalepsis [graece] oder Praeoccupatio durch zwölff verscheidenlicher [sic] Tractaten, gemachter Harm Proben. Frankfurt an der Oder 1571.

Thurneysser, Leonhard: Bebaiosis agonismou [graece]. Das ist confirmatio concertationis, oder ein Bestettigung dess Jenigen so streittig, häderig, oder zenckisch ist, wie dann auss Unverstandt die neuwe und vor unerhörte Erfindung der aller nützlichesten [...] Kunst dess Harnnprobirens ein zeitlang gewest ist. Berlin 1576.

Tissot, Samuel Auguste: Abhandlung über die Nerven und deren Krankheiten. Transl. by J. Chr. G. Ackermann, Vol. 1. Leipzig 1781.

Tröstler, Sebastian: Uroscopia seu de urinis theses medicae. Praes. Adriaan van Roomen. Würzburg 1601.

Tulpius, Nicolaus: Observationum medicarum libri tres. Amsterdam 1641.

Turner, Daniel: The modern quack; or, the physical impostor, detected: With a supplement, displaying the present set of pretenders to clap-curing, giving judgment upon urine, etc. London 1718.

Turner, Robert: The compleat bone-setter [...]. Whereunto is added The perfect oculist, and The mirrour of health [...]. Also, The acute judgement of urines. Written originally by Friar Moulton of the Order of St. Augustine. London 1656.

Ulianus, Oswaldus: Difficiliora triginta et unum problemata, circa doctrinam de urinis controversa. Nuremberg 1602.

Unzer, Johann August: Von der Kunst der Aerzte, die Natur der Krankheiten aus den natürlichen Zeichen, besonders aus dem Urine zu beurtheilen. In: Der Arzt (2nd edn) 1 (1760), 129–42.

Valenti, Ernst Joseph Gustav de: Medicina clerica, oder Handbuch der Pastoral-Medizin für Seelsorger, Pädagogen und Aerzte. Part 1. Leipzig 1831.

Vassaeus, Ioannis: De iudiciis urinarum tractatus, ex probatis collectus autoribus, et in tabulae formam confectus, adiectis etiam causis, quae hanc vel illam urinam reddant. Lyon 1553.

Vassaeus, Ioannis: Here beginnith a litel treatise conteyninge the iugeme[n]t of urynes most necessary for al such as be desirouse to knowe the state of their owne bodys or be wylling to helpe their frindes. Transl. by Humfri Lloyd. London 1553.

Vermeer, Hans J.: Ein "Iudicium Urinarum" des Dr. Augustin Streicher aus dem Cod. Wellc. 589. In: Sudhoffs Archiv 54 (1970), 1–19.

Vesal, Andreas: Anatomia Deudsch, Ein kurtzer Auszug der Beschreibung aller Glider menschlichs Leybs aus den Buchern des hochgelerten Hern D. Andree Vesalij von Brüssel. Nuremberg 1551.

Vesal, Andreas: De humani corporis fabrica libri septem. Basel 1543.

Walaeus, Johannes: Medica omnia. London 1660.

Watkyns, Rowland: Flamma sine fumo, or, Poems without fictions hereunto are annexed the causes, symptoms, or signes of serveral diseases with their cures, and also the diversity of urines, with their causes in poeticl [sic] measure. London 1662.

Weinsberg, Hermann von: Das Buch Weinsberg. Kölner Denkwürdigkeiten aus dem 16. Jahrhundert. 5 vols. Leipzig/Bonn 1886–1926 (repr. Düsseldorf 2000).

Willich, Iodocus: Urinarum probationes. Ed. by Hieronymus Reusner. Basel 1582.

Willis, Thomas: Pharmaceutice rationalis. Oxford 1674.

Willis, Thomas: Five treatises, viz. 1. Of urines. 2. Of the accension of blood. 3. Of musculary motion. 4. The anatomy of the brain. 5. The description and use of the nerves. London 1681.

Wirsing, Thomas: Altfränkisches Dorf- und Pfarrhausleben 1559–1601. Ein Kulturbild aus der Zeit vor dem 30jährigen Krieg. Dargestellt nach den Tagebüchern des Pfarrherrn Thomas Wirsing von Sinbronn. Ed. by August Gabler. Nuremberg 1952.

Wittich, Johannes: Consilia, observationes atque epistolae medicae. Leipzig 1604.

Wood, Owen: An epitomie of most experienced, excellent and profitable secrets appertaining to physick and chirurgery alphabetically, for all those diseases that are most predominant and dangerous (curable by art) in the body of man, as by the table appears. Also, the judgement of urines. For the benefit of such discreet ladies, gentlewomen, and others which labour to do good in that art, mysterie, and profession. 4th edn. London 1653.

Zacchia, Paolo: Quaestiones medico-legales. 3rd edn. Amsterdam 1651.

Zedler, Johann Heinrich: Grosses vollständiges Universal-Lexikon aller Wissenschafften und Künste. Vol. 51. Leipzig/Halle 1747.

Ziegler, Adolf: Die Uroscopie am Krankenbette. Zum Gebrauch für Aerzte bearbeitet. Erlangen 1865.

Zimmermann, Johann Georg: Von der Ruhr unter dem Volke im Jahr 1765, und denen mit derselben eingedrungenen Vorurtheilen, nebst einigen allgemeinen Aussichten in die Heilung dieser Vorurtheile. Zurich 1767.

Zwinger, Theodor: Dissertatiuncula medica de uromantias usu et abusu. Subm. Joh. Rodolphus Staegerus. Basel 1705.

Secondary Literature

Aalkjaer, V.: Uroscopia. A historical and art historical essay. In: Acta chirurgica scandinavica 433, Suppl. (1973), 3–11.

Alexander, Jeffrey C.: Cultural pragmatics: Social performance between ritual and strategy. In: Alexander, Jeffrey C./Giesen, Bernhard/Mast, Jason L. (eds): Social performance. Cambridge 2006, 29–90.

Alexander, Jeffrey C./Giesen, Bernhard/Mast, Jason L. (eds): Social performance. Symbolic action, cultural pragmatics, and ritual. Cambridge 2006.

Alexander, Jeffrey C./Mast, Jason L.: Introduction: symbolic action in theory and practice: the cultural pragmatics of symbolic action. In: Alexander, Jeffrey C./Giesen, Bernhard/Mast, Jason L. (eds): Social performance. Cambridge 2006, 1–28.

Alpers, Svetlana: The art of describing. Dutch art in the seventeenth century. Chicago 1985.

Anonymous: The evolution of urine analysis. An historical sketch of the clinical examination of urine. Lecture memoranda. British Medical Association Birmingham. London 1911.

Baigrie, Brian S. (ed.): Picturing knowledge. Historical and philosophical problems concerning the use of art in science. Toronto 1996.

Bautier, Pierre: Les petits maîtres anversois du XVIIIe siècle. Gérard Thomas et Balthazar van den Bossche. In: La revue de l'art 46 (1924), 131–8.

Bedaux, Jan Baptist: Minnekoorts-, zwangerschaps- en doodsverschijnselen op zeventiende-eeuwse schilderijen. In: Antiek 10 (1975), 17–42.

Belliger, Andréa/Krieger, David J. (eds): Ritualtheorien. Ein einführendes Handbuch. Opladen/Wiesbaden 1998.

Belting, Hans: Bild-Anthropologie. Entwürfe für eine Bildwissenschaft. Munich 2001.

Berg, Alexander: Der Krankheitskomplex der Kolik- u. Gebärmutterleiden in Volksmedizin und Medizingeschichte unter besonderer Berücksichtigung der Volksmedizin in Ostpreußen. Ein Beitrag zur Erforschung volkstümlicher Krankheitsvorstellungen. Berlin 1935.

Berger, Johanna: Die Entwicklung der Harndiagnostik aus der Harnschau zur Harnuntersuchung. Münster 1966.

Berger, Peter L./Luckmann, Thomas: The social construction of reality. A treatise in the sociology of knowledge. London 1966.

Bernabeo, Raffaele: Paracelso, urologo ed uroscopo. In: Pagine di storia della medicina 10:2 (1966), 17–21.

Beyer, Andreas/Lohoff, Markus (eds): Bild und Erkenntnis. Formen und Funktionen des Bildes in Wissenschaft und Technik. Munich 2005.

Bleker, Johanna [née Berger]: Von der Uroscopie zur Urochemie. In: Hippokrates 37 (1966), 653–7.

Bleker, Johanna: Die Harndiagnostik des Leonhard Thurneysser am Thurn. In: Deutsches Ärzteblatt 67 (1970), 320–29.

Bleker, Johanna: "Die Kunst des Harnsehens—ein vornehm und nötig Gliedmaß der schönen Artzeney." In: Hippokrates 41 (1970), 385–95.

Bleker, Johanna: Chemiatrische Vorstellungen und Analogiedenken in der Harndiagnostik Leonhart Thurneissers (1571 und 1576). In: Sudhoffs Archiv 60 (1976), 66–75.

Boehm, Gottfried: Was ist ein Bild? Munich 1995.

Bourdieu, Pierre: Outline of a theory of practice. Cambridge 1977.

Breidbach, Olaf: Bilder des Wissens. Zur Kulturgeschichte der wissenschaftlichen Wahrnehmung. Munich 2005.

Brinkman, A.A.A.M.: Brueghel's "Alchemist" and its influence, in particular on Jan Steen. In: Janus (1974), 233–69.

Brockliss, Laurence W. B./Jones, Colin: The medical world of early modern France. Oxford 1997.

Brusati, Celeste: Natural artifice and material values in Dutch still life. In: Franits, Wayne (ed.): Looking at seventeenth-century Dutch art. Realism reconsidered. Cambridge 1997, 144–57.

Bury, M. R.: Social constructionism and the development of medical sociology. In: Sociology of health & illness 8 (1986), 137–69.

Buvelot, Quentin (ed.): Frans van Mieris 1635–1681. Zwolle 2005.

Bynum, William F./Nutton, Vivian (eds): Theories of fever from antiquity to the Enlightenment. London 1981.

Bynum, William F./Porter, Roy/Wear, Andrew (eds): Companion encyclopedia of the history of medicine. London/New York 1993.

Cheymol, Jean: Le diagnostic de grossesses au temps des mireurs d'urines. In: Histoire des sciences médicales 7:1 (1973), 7–28.

Christoffel, Hans: Grundzüge der Uroskopie. In: Gesnerus 10 (1953), 89–122.

Clark, Stuart: Thinking with demons. The idea of witchcraft in early modern Europe. Oxford 1997.

Clericuzio, Antonio: Elements, principles and corpuscles. A study of atomism and chemistry in the seventeenth century. Dordrecht 2000.

Condrau, Flurin: The patient's view meets the clinical gaze. In: Social history of medicine 20 (2007), 525–40.

Conrad, Lawrence I. et al.: The Western medical tradition 800 BC to AD 1800. Cambridge 1995.

Cook, Harold J.: The decline of the old medical regime in Stuart London. Ithaca/New York 1986.

Crohns, Hjalmar: Zur Geschichte der Liebe als Krankheit. In: Archiv für Kultur-Geschichte 3 (1905), 66–86.

Csordas, Thomas J. (ed.): Embodiment and experience. The existential ground of culture and self. Cambridge 1994.

Darmon, Pierre: Le tribunal de l'impuissance. Paris 1979.

Debus, Allen G.: The chemical philosophy. Dover 2002.

Dimitriadis, Konstantin: Byzantinische Uroskopie. Diss. med. (typescript). Bonn 1971.

Dinges, Martin: Social history of medicine in Germany and France in the late twentieth century. From the history of medicine toward a history of health. In: Huisman, Frank/Warner, John Harley (eds): Locating medical history. Baltimore/London 2004, 209–36.

Dinges, Martin et alii (eds): Medical practice, 1600–1900. Physicians and their patients. Leiden/Boston 2015 [forthcoming]

Dixon, Laurinda S.: Perilous chastity. Women and illness in pre-Enlightenment art and medicine. Ithaca/London 1995.

Dixon, Laurinda S.: Together in misery. Medical meaning and sexual politics in two paintings by Jan Steen. In: Carroll, Jane L./Stewart, Alison G. (eds): Saints, sinners, and sisters. Gender and Northern art in medieval and early modern Europe. Aldershot/Burlington, VA 2003, 247–68.

Duden, Barbara: The woman beneath the skin. A doctor's patients in eighteenth-century Germany. Cambridge 1991.

Duden, Barbara: Die "Geheimnisse" der Schwangeren und das Öffentlichkeitsinteresse der Medizin. Zur sozialen Bedeutung der Kindsregung. In: Hausen, Karin/Wunder, Heide (eds): Frauengeschichte Geschlechtergeschichte. Frankfurt 1992, 117–28.

Duden, Barbara: Der Frauenleib als öffentlicher Ort. Vom Mißbrauch des Begriffs Leben. Munich 1994.

Duden, Barbara: Zwischen "wahrem Wissen" und Prophetie: Konzeptionen des Ungeborenen. In: Duden, Barbara/Schlumbohm, Jürgen/Veit, Patrice (eds): Geschichte des Ungeborenen: zur Erfahrungs- und Wissenschaftsgeschichte der Schwangerschaft, 17.–20. Jahrhundert. Göttingen 2002, 11–48.

Elias, Norbert: The civilizing process. Sociogenetic and psychogenetic investigations. Revised edn. Oxford 2000.

Elkeles, Barbara: Aussagen zu ärztlichen Leitwerten, Pflichten und Verhaltensweisen in berufsvorbereitender Literatur der Frühen Neuzeit. Hannover 1979.

Elkeles, Barbara: Medicus und Medikaster: Zum Konflikt zwischen akademischer und "empirischer" Medizin im 17. und frühen 18. Jahrhundert. In: Medizinhistorisches Journal 22 (1987), 197–211.

Ernst, Katharina: Patientengeschichte. Die kulturhistorische Wende in der Medizinhistoriographie. In: Bröer, Ralph (ed.): Eine Wissenschaft emanzipiert sich. Die Medizinhistoriographie von der Aufklärung bis zur Postmoderne. Heidelberg 1999, 97–108.

Fichtner, Gerhard: Neues zu Leben und Werk von Leonhart Fuchs aus seinen Briefen an Joachim Camerarius I. und II. in der Trew-Sammlung. In: Gesnerus 25 (1968), 65–82.

Fissell, Mary E.: The disappearance of the patient's narrative and the invention of hospital medicine. In: French, Roger/Wear, Andrew (eds): British medicine in an age of reform. London/New York 1991, 91–101.

Fissell, Mary E.: Making meaning from the margins. The new cultural history of medicine. In: Huisman, Frank/Warner, John Harley (eds): Locating medical history. Baltimore/London 2004, 364–89.

Ford, Brian J.: Images of science. A history of scientific illustration. London 1992.

Foucault, Michel: The birth of the clinic. An archeology of medical perception. London 1973.

Franits, Wayne (ed.): Looking at seventeenth-century Dutch art. Realism reconsidered. Cambridge 1997.

Franits, Wayne: Dutch seventeenth-century genre painting. Its stylistic and thematic evolution. New Haven/London 2004.

Frisch, Anton von: Historischer Rückblick über die Entwicklung der urologischen Diagnostik. In: Wiener klinische Wochenschrift 40 (1907), 1191–8.

Geyl, A.: Un traité de médecine du quartorzième siècle. In: Janus 14 (1909), 354–89.

Gils, J.B.F. van: De dokter in de oude Nederlandsche tooneelliteratuur. Haarlem 1917.

Gils, J.B.F. van: Een detail op de doktersschilderijen van Jan Steen. In: Oud Holland 38 (1920), 200f.

Gombrich, Ernst Hans: The uses of images. Studies in the social function of art and visual communication. London 1999.

Good, Byron J.: Medicine, rationality and experience. An anthropological perspective. Cambridge 1994.

Grell, Ole Peter (ed.): Paracelsus: The man and his reputation, his ideas and their transformation. Leiden 1998.

Groß, Dominik/Steinmetzer, Jan: Volcher Coiter (1534–1576) und die Konstituierung ärztlicher Autorität in der Vormoderne. Aachen 2006.

Gudlaugsson, Sturla J.: Ikonographische Studien über die holländische Malerei und das Theater des 17. Jahrhunderts. Würzburg 1938.

Gudlaugsson, Sturla J.: Gerard ter Borch. The Hague 1959.

Gudlaugsson, Sturla J.: The comedians in the work of Jan Steen and contemporaries. Soest 1975.

Guerrino, Antonio A./Kohn Loncarica, Alfredo G.: La uroscopia en la edad media. In: Episteme 7 (1973), 289–97.

Hacke, Daniela: Von der Wirkungsmächtigkeit des Heiligen: Magische Liebeszauberpraktiken und die religiöse Mentalität venezianischer Laien in der frühen Neuzeit. In: Historische Anthropologie 3 (2001), 311–32.

Heintz, Bettina/Huber, Jörg (eds): Mit dem Auge denken. Strategien der Sichtbarmachung in wissenschaftlichen und virtuellen Welten. Zurich 2001.

Hellens, Franz: Gérard Terborch. Brussels 1911.

Helm, Jürgen: Die Galenrezeption in Philipp Melanchthons "De anima" (1540/1552). In: Medizinhistorisches Journal 31 (1996), 298–321.

Herzlich, Claudine/Pierret, Janine: Kranke gestern, Kranke heute. Die Gesellschaft und das Leiden. Munich 1991.

Herzog, Markwart: Scharfrichterliche Medizin. Zu den Beziehungen zwischen Henker und Arzt, Schafott und Medizin. In: Medizinhistorisches Journal 29 (1994), 309–22.

Hess, Volker (ed.): Normierung der Gesundheit. Messende Verfahren der Medizin als kulturelle Praktik um 1900. Husum 1997.

Hess, Volker: Der wohltemperierte Mensch. Wissenschaft und Alltag des Fiebermessens (1850–1900). Frankfurt 2000.

Heßler, Martina (ed.): Konstruierte Sichtbarkeiten. Wissenschafts- und Technikbilder seit der frühen Neuzeit. Munich 2006.

Homblé, A.G.: Uromantie ofte piskijkerij in volkskundige kontekst. In: Brabantse Folklore 201 (1974), 42–66.

Horine, Emmet Field: An epitome of ancient pulse lore. In: Bulletin of the history of medicine 10 (1941), 209–49.

Hortzitz, Nicoline: Der "Judenarzt." Historische und sprachliche Untersuchungen zur Diskriminierung eines Berufsstands in der frühen Neuzeit. Heidelberg 1994.

Huisman, Frank/Warner, John Harley (eds): Locating medical history. The stories and their meanings. Baltimore/London 2004.

Jankrift, Kay Peter: Krankheit und Heilkunde im Mittelalter. Darmstadt 2003.

Jansen, Guido M. C. (ed.): Jan Steen. Maler und Erzähler. Stuttgart/Zurich 1996.

Jenkins, Glen P.: Diagnosis by diagram. The matulae disc from Johannes de Ketham's "Fasciculus medicinae," 1495. In: Journal of laboratory and clinical medicine 114 (1989), 439–40.

Jewson, Nicholas D.: Medical knowledge and the patronage system in 18th century England. In: Sociology 8 (1974), 369–85.

Jewson, Nicholas D.: The disappearance of the sick man from medical cosmology, 1770–1870. In: Sociology 10 (1976), 225–44.

Jordanova, Ludmilla: Medicine and the visual culture. In: Social studies of medicine 3 (1990), 89–99.

Jordanova, Ludmilla: The social construction of medical knowledge. In: Social history of medicine 8 (1995), 361–81.

Jütte, Robert: Ärzte, Heiler und Patienten. Medizinischer Alltag in der frühen Neuzeit. Munich/Zurich 1991.

Jurina, Kitti: Vom Quacksalber zum Doctor medicinae. Die Heilkunde in der deutschen Graphik des 16. Jahrhunderts. Cologne 1985.

Kaplan, Edward: Robert Recorde and the authorities of uroscopy. In: Bulletin of the history of medicine 37 (1963), 65–71.

Kaplan, Steven L. (ed.): Understanding popular culture. Europe from the Middle Ages to the nineteenth century. Berlin 1984.

Kaptchuk, Ted J.: Intentional ignorance: a history of blind assessment and placebo controls in medicine. In: Bulletin of the history of medicine 72 (1998), 389–433.

Kassell, Lauren: Medicine and magic in Elizabethan London: Simon Forman. Astrologer, alchemist, and physician. Oxford 2005.

Keil, Gundolf: Die urognostische Praxis in vor- und frühsalernitanischer Zeit. Medical Habilitationsschrift (typescript). Freiburg 1970.

Keil, Gundolf: Harnschriften. In: Gerabek, Werner et al. (eds): Enzyklopädie Medizingeschichte. Berlin 2005, 533–5.

Kemp, Martin: Bilderwissen. Die Anschaulichkeit naturwissenschaftlicher Phänomene. Cologne 2003.

King, Lester S.: The medical world of the eighteenth century. Chicago 1958.

King, Lester S.: The road to medical Enlightenment 1650–1695. London/New York 1970.

Kinzelbach, Annemarie: Gesundbleiben, Krankwerden, Armsein in der frühneuzeitlichen Gesellschaft. Gesunde und Kranke in den Reichsstädten Überlingen und Ulm, 1500–1700. Stuttgart 1995.

Kleinman, Arthur: Patients and healers in the context of culture. An exploration of the borderland between anthropology, medicine, and psychiatry. London 1980.

Knoeff, Rina: Herman Boerhaave (1668–1738). Calvinist chemist and physician. Amsterdam 2002.

Konert, Jürgen/Dietrich, Holger G. (eds): Illustrierte Geschichte der Urologie. Berlin/Heidelberg 2004.

Krack, Niels: Die Harnschau. Heidelberg 1982.

Krafft, Fritz: Christus als Apotheker. Ursprung, Aussage und Geschichte eines christlichen Sinnbildes. Marburg 2001.

Kuriyama, Shigehisa: The expressiveness of the body and the divergence of Greek and Chinese medicine. New York 1999.

Kutzer, Michael: Herrgott, Heiler und Harnschau: Das Vermächtnis des Ulmer Stadtarztes Augustin Thoner (1567–1655). In: Medizinhistorisches Journal 35 (2000), 149–73.

Labouvie, Eva: Andere Umstände. Eine Kulturgeschichte der Geburt. Cologne 1998.

Labouvie, Eva: Verbotene Künste. Volksmagie und ländlicher Aberglaube in den Dorfgemeinden des Saarraumes (16.–19. Jahrhundert). St. Ingbert 1992.

Lachmund, Jens: Der abgehorchte Körper. Zur historischen Soziologie der medizinischen Untersuchung. Opladen 1997.

Lachmund, Jens/Stollberg, Gunnar (eds): The social construction of illness. Illness and medical knowledge in past and present. Stuttgart 1992.

Lachmund, Jens/Stollberg, Gunnar: The doctor, his audience, and the meaning of illness: The drama of medical practice in the late 18th and early 19th centuries. In: iidem, Social construction, 53–66.

Lachmund, Jens/Stollberg, Gunnar: Patientenwelten. Krankheit und Medizin vom späten 18. bis zum frühen 20. Jahrhundert im Spiegel von Autobiographien. Opladen 1995.

Latour, Bruno: Science in action. How to follow scientists and engineers through society. Cambridge, MA 1987.

Lebrun, François: Se soigner autrefois. Médecins, saints et sorciers aux 17e et 18e siècles. Paris 1983.

Lenhardt, Friedrich: Blutschau. Untersuchungen zur Entwicklung der Hämatoskopie. Pattensen 1986.

Lennep, Jacques van: Alchimiste. Origine et développement d'un thème de la peinture du dix-septième siècle. In: Revue belge d'archéologie et d'histoire d'art 35 (1966), 149–68.

Lennep, Jacques van: Alchimie. Paris 1985.

Lindemann, Mary: Health and healing in eighteenth-century Germany. Baltimore/London 1996.

Lindemann, Mary: Medicine and society in early modern Europe. 2nd edn. Cambridge 2010.

Lock, Margaret: Cultivating the body. Anthropology and epistemologies of bodily practice and knowledge. In: Annual review of anthropology 22 (1993), 133–55.

Lumme, Christoph: Höllenfleisch und Heiligtum. Der menschliche Körper im Spiegel autobiographischer Texte des 16. Jahrhunderts. Frankfurt 1996.

Lupton, Deborah: Medicine as culture. Illness, disease and the body in Western societies. London 1994.

Maar, Christa/Burda, Hubert (eds): Iconic turn. Die neue Macht der Bilder. Cologne 2005.

Maclean, Ian: Logic, signs and nature in the Renaissance. The case of learned medicine. Cambridge 2002.

Mazzolini, Renato (ed.): Non-verbal communication in science prior to 1900. Florence 1992.

Meige, Henri: Les peintres de la médecine. Samuel van Hoogstraten. In: La nouvelle iconographie de la Salpêtrière 8 (1895), 192–204.

Meige, Henri: Le mal d'amour. In: La nouvelle iconographie de la Salpêtrière 12 (1899), 57f, 340–52 and 420–32.

Meige, Henri: Les médecins de Jan Steen. Part 1, 2. In: Janus 5 (1900), 187–90 and 217–26.

Meige, Henri: Les urologues. In: Archives générales de médecine, N. F. 3 (1900), 760–64.

Middelkoop, Norbert E. et al. (eds): Rembrandt under the scalpel. The anatomy lesson of Dr Nicolaes Tulp dissected. Amsterdam 1998.

Moehsen, J. C. W.: Leben Leonhard Thurneyssers zum Thurn. Ein Beitrag zur Geschichte der Alchemie wie auch der Wissenschaften und Künste in der Mark Brandenburg gegen Ende des 16. Jahrhunderts. Berlin/Leipzig 1783.

Moulinier-Brogi, Laurence: L'uroscopie au moyen âge. "Lire dans un verre la nature de l'homme." Paris 2012.

Moulinier-Brogi, Laurence: L'uroscopie en vulgaire dans l'occident médiéval: un tour d'horizon. In: Goyens, Michèle/De Leemans, Pieter/Smets, An (eds): Science translated. Latin and vernacular translations of scientific treatises in medieval Europe. Leuven 2008, 221–41.

Moulinier-Brogi, Laurence: Un flacon en point de mire. La science des urines, un enjeu culturel dans la société médiévale (XIIIe–XVe siècles). In: Annales. Histoire, science sociales (2010), N° 1, 11–37.

Murray Jones, Peter: Medieval medicine in illuminated manuscripts. Revised edn. London 1998.

Naumann, Otto: Frans van Mieris the Elder (1635–1681). Doornspijk 1981.

Neumann, Julius: Geschichte der Uroskopie. In: Zeitschrift der Heilkunde 15 (1894), 53–74.

Nicholson, Malcolm: The art of diagnosis. Medicine and the five senses. In: Bynum, William F./Porter, Roy (eds): Companion encyclopedia of the history of medicine. London/New York 1993, 801–25.

Nolte, Karen: Zeitalter des ärztlichen Paternalismus? Überlegungen zu Aufklärung und Einwilligung von Patienten im 19. Jahrhundert. In: Medizin, Gesellschaft und Geschichte 25 (2006), S. 59–89.

Nowosadtko, Jutta: Wer Leben nimmt, kann auch Leben geben. Scharfrichter und Wasenmeister als Heilkundige in der Frühen Neuzeit. In: Medizin, Gesellschaft und Geschichte 12 (1993), 43–74.

Nowosadtko, Jutta: Scharfrichter und Abdecker. Der Alltag zweier "unehrlicher Berufe" in der Frühen Neuzeit. Paderborn 1994.

Nutton, Vivian: Idle old trots, coblers and costardmongers. Pieter van Foreest on quackery. In: Bosman-Jelgersma, Henriette A. (ed.): Petrus Forestus medicus. Amsterdam [1977], 243–55.

Osborne, Jonathan: A sketch of the physiology and pathology of urine; with an historical introduction. London 1820.

Pagel, Walter: Das medizinische Weltbild des Paracelsus: seine Zusammenhänge mit Neuplatonismus und Gnosis. Wiesbaden 1962.

Park, Katharine: Secrets of women. Gender, generation, and the origins of human dissection. New York 2006.

Paster, Gail Kern: The body embarrassed. Drama and the disciplines of shame in early modern England. Ithaca 1993.

Paul, Norbert/Schlich, Thomas (eds): Medizingeschichte: Aufgaben, Probleme, Perspektiven. Frankfurt/New York 1998.

Pergens-Maeseyck, Ed[uard]: Eine Urinschautafel aus Cod. Brux. Nr. 5876 nebst Kommentar. In: Archiv für Geschichte der Medizin 1 (1908), 393–402.

Petterson, Einar: Amans amanti medicus. Die Ikonologie des Motivs "Der ärztliche Besuch." In: Bock, Henning/Gaehtgens, Thomas W. (eds): Holländische Genremalerei im 17. Jahrhundert. Berlin 1984, 195–224.

Petterson, Einar: Amans Amanti Medicus. Das Genremotiv "Der ärztliche Besuch" in seinem kulturgeschichtlichen Kontext. Berlin 2000.

Pomata, Gianna: La promessa di guarigione. Malati e curatori in antico regime. Bologna XVI–XVIII secolo. Bari 1994.

Pomata, Gianna: Sharing cases: The "Observationes" in early modern medicine. In: Early science and medicine 15 (2010), 193–236.

Pomata, Gianna: Observation rising. Birth of an epistemic genre, 1500–1600. In: Daston, Lorraine/Lunbeck, Elizabeth (eds): Histories of scientific observation. Chicago/London 2011, 45–80.

Porter, Dorothy/Porter, Roy: Patient's progress. Doctors and doctoring in eighteenth-century England. Stanford 1989.

Porter, Roy: The patient's view. Doing medical history from . In: Theory and society 14 (1985), 175–98.

Porter, Roy (ed.): Patients and practitioners. Lay-perceptions of medicine in preindustrial society. London 1985.

Porter, Roy/Porter, Dorothy: In sickness and in health. The British experience, 1650–1850. New York 1989.

Principe, Lawrence M./DeWitt, Lloyd: Transmutations: Alchemy in art. Selected works from the Eddleman and Fisher Collections at the Chemical Heritage Foundation. Philadelphia 2002.

Probst, Christian: Der Weg des ärztlichen Erkennens am Krankenbett. Herman Boerhaave und die ältere Wiener medizinische Schule. Wiesbaden 1972.

Probst, Christian: Fahrende Heiler und Heilmittelhändler. Medizin von Marktplatz und Landstraße. Rosenheim 1992.

Pyle, Andrew: Atomism and its critics. From Democritus to Newton. Bristol 1997.

Reichardt, Sven: Praxeologische Geschichtswissenschaft. Eine Diskussionsanregung. In: Sozial.Geschichte 22 (2007), 43–65.

Reiser, Stanley Joel: Medicine and the reign of technology. Cambridge 1978.

Riha, Ortrun: Die mittelalterliche Blutschau. In: Gadebusch Bondio, Mariacarla (ed.): Blood in history and blood histories. Florence 2005, 49–67.

Rosenberg, Charles E./Golden, Janet (eds): Framing disease. Studies in cultural history. New Brunswick 1992.

Rubin, Lewis P.: A young woman taken to the doctor by her family. Mezzotint by Johann Andreas Pfeffel after an original painting by Jan Josef Horemans. In: Journal of the history of medicine and allied sciences 36 (1981), 489.

Ründal, Erik O.: "daß seine Mannschaft gantz unvollkommen sey": Impotenz in der Frühen Neuzeit—Diskurse und Praktiken in Deutschland. In: Österreichische Zeitschrift für Geschichtswissenschaften 22 (2011), 50–74.

Ruisinger, Marion Maria: Patientenwege. Die Konsiliarkorrespondenz Lorenz Heisters (1683–1758) in der Trew-Sammlung Erlangen. Stuttgart 2008.

Sander, Sabine: Handwerkschirurgen. Sozialgeschichte einer verdrängten Berufsgruppe. Göttingen 1989.

Sarasin, Philipp/Tanner, Jakob (eds): Physiologie und industrielle Gesellschaft. Studien zur Verwissenschaftlichung des Körpers im 19. und 20. Jahrhundert. Frankfurt 1998.

Schadewaldt, Hans: Die Geschichte des Urins in der Medizin. In: Thomas, Carmen (ed.): Saft. Munich/Zurich 1999, 158–93.

Schatzki, Theodore R./Knorr Cetina, Karin/Savigny, Eike von (eds): The practice turn in contemporary theory. London/New York 2001.

Schilling, Ruth/Schlegelmilch, Sabine/Splinter, Susan: Stadtarzt oder Arzt in der Stadt? Drei Ärzte der Frühen Neuzeit und ihr Verständnis des städtischen Amtes. In: Medizinhistorisches Journal 46 (2011), 99–133.

Schlegelmilch, Sabine: "What a magnificent work a good physician is." The medical practice of Johannes Magirus (1615–1697). In: Martin Dinges et alii: Medical practice, 1600–1900. Physicians and their patients. Leiden/Boston 2015 [forthcoming].

Schlich, Thomas: Wissenschaft: Die Herstellung wissenschaftlicher Fakten als Thema der Geschichtsforschung. In: Paul, Norbert/Schlich, Thomas (eds): Medizingeschichte. Frankfurt/New York 1998, 107–29.

Schmelzer, Kurt: Ein Vergleich der Harnschau des Paracelsus mit der Uroskopie vor Paracelsus und der heutigen, auf Grund der Schrift Paracelsus': "De urinarum ac pulsuum indiciis libellus." Munich [1943].

Schummer, Joachim/Spector, Tami I.: The visual image of chemistry. Perspectives from the history of art and science. In: Hyle—International journal for philosophy of chemistry 13 (2007), 3–41.

Siegel, Rudolph E.: Galen's system of physiology and medicine. Basel/New York 1968.

Snoep-Reitsma, Ella: De waterzuchtige vrouw van Gerard Dou en de betekenis van de lampetkan. In: Album amicorum J.G. van Gelder. The Hague 1973, 285–92.

Spitzer, Gabriele: "…und die Spree führt Gold." Leonhard Thurneysser zum Thurn. Astrologe—Alchimist—Arzt und Drucker im Berlin des 16. Jahrhunderts. Berlin 1996.

Stolberg, Michael: "Mein askulapisches Orakel!": Patientenbriefe als Quelle einer Kulturgeschichte der Krankheitserfahrung im 18. Jahrhundert. In: Österreichische Zeitschrift für Geschichtswissenschaft 7 (1996), 385–404.

Stolberg, Michael: A woman's hell? Medical perceptions of menopause in preindustrial Europe. In: Bulletin of the history of medicine 73 (1999), 408–28.

Stolberg, Michael: The monthly malady: A history of premenstrual suffering. In: Medical history 44 (2000), 301–22.

Stolberg, Michael: An unmanly vice: Self-pollution, anxiety, and the body in the eighteenth century. In: Social history of medicine 13 (2000), 1–21.

Stolberg, Michael: Der gesunde Leib. Zur Geschichtlichkeit frühneuzeitlicher Körpererfahrung. In: Münch, Paul (ed.): "Erfahrung" als Kategorie der Frühneuzeitgeschichte (= Historische Zeitschrift, Beiheft 31). Munich 2001, 37–57.

Stolberg, Michael: Formen und Strategien der Autorisierung in der frühneuzeitlichen Medizin. In: Oesterreicher, Wulf/Regn, Gerhard/Schulze, Winfried (eds): Autorität der Form—Autorisierungen—institutionelle Autorität. Münster 2003, 124–52.

Stolberg, Michael: Erfahrungen und Deutungen der weiblichen Monatsblutung in der Frühen Neuzeit. In: Mahlmann-Bauer, Barbara (ed.): Scientiae et artes. Die Vermittlung alten und neuen Wissens in Literatur, Kunst und Musik. Wolfenbüttel 2004, 913–31.

Stolberg, Michael: Medizinische Deutungsmacht und die Grenzen ärztlicher Autorität in der Frühen Neuzeit. In: Dülmen, Richard van/Rauschenbach, Sina (eds): Macht des Wissens. Entstehung der modernen Wissensgesellschaft 1500–1820. Cologne/Weimar 2004, 113–30.

Stolberg, Michael: "Zorn, Wein und Weiber verderben unsere Leiber." Krankheit und Affekt in der frühneuzeitlichen Medizin. In: Steiger, Johann Anselm (ed.): Passion, Affekt und Leidenschaft in der Frühen Neuzeit. Wiesbaden 2005, 1033–59.

Stolberg, Michael: The decline of uroscopy in early modern learned medicine, 1500–1650. In: Early science and medicine 12 (2007), 313–36.

Stolberg, Michael: "Cura palliativa." Begriff und Diskussion der palliativen Krankheitsbehandlung in der vormodernen Medizin (ca. 1500–1850). In: Medizinhistorisches Journal 42 (2007), 7–29.

Stolberg, Michael: Lukas Cranachs "Melancholia"-Darstellungen und die zeitgenössische Medizin. In: Oehmig, Stefan (ed.): Medizin und Sozialwesen in Mitteldeutschland in der Reformationszeit. Leipzig 2007, 249–71.

Stolberg, Michael: Formen und Funktionen ärztlicher Fallbeobachtungen in der Frühen Neuzeit (1500–1800). In: Süßmann, Johannes/Scholz, Susanne/Engel, Gisela (eds): Fallstudien: Theorie—Geschichte—Methode (= Frankfurter Kulturwissenschaftliche Beiträge, Vol. 1). Berlin 2007, 81–95.

Stolberg, Michael: Eine anatomische Inszenierung: Felix Platter (1536–1614) und das Skelett der Frau. In: Schramm, Helmar/Schwarte, Ludger/Lazardig, Jan (eds): Spuren der Avantgarde: Theatrum anatomicum. Frühe Neuzeit und Moderne im Kulturvergleich. Berlin/New York 2011, 147–67.

Stolberg, Michael: Experiencing illness and the sick body in early modern Europe. Basingstoke/New York 2011 (orig. German publ. Cologne 2003).

Stolberg, Michael: Examining the body (c. 1500–1750) In: Toulalan, Sarah/Fisher, Kate (eds): The Routledge history of sex and the body, 1500 to the present. Oxford 2013, 91–105.

Stolberg, Michael: Bedside teaching and the acquisition of practical skills in mid-sixteenth-century Padua. In: Journal of the history of medicine and allied sciences 68 (2013), 633–64.

Stone-Ferrier, Linda: From shrew to poetess. Two non-traditional female roles evoked by a curious painting by Gabriel Metsu. In: Carroll, Jane L./Stewart, Alison G. (eds): Saints, sinners, and sisters. Gender and Northern art in medieval and early modern Europe. Aldershot/Burlington, VA 2003, 223–45.

Stukenbrock, Karin: Abtreibung im ländlichen Raum Schleswig-Holsteins im 18. Jahrhundert. Eine sozialgeschichtliche Untersuchung auf der Basis von Gerichtsakten. Neumünster 1993.

Sudhoff, Karl: Die Harnglasscheibe im 15. Jahrhundert. In: idem: Tradition und Naturbeobachtung in den Illustrationen medizinischer Handschriften. Leipzig 1907, 13–18.

Sudhoff, Karl: Ein ärztlicher Brief aus dem Anfange des 16. Jahrhunderts. In: Archiv für Geschichte der Medizin 8 (1915), 450f.

Sudhoff, Karl: Harnglas und Harnglaskorb. Etwas aus dem ABC der medizinischen Realienkunde des Mittelalters. In: Archiv für Geschichte der Medizin 17 (1925), 292–8.

Talbot, Charles: A mediaeval physician's vade mecum. In: Journal of the history of medicine 16 (1961), 213–33.

Tambiah, Stanley J.: A performative approach to ritual. London 1981.

Thomas, Carmen (ed.): Ein ganz besonderer Saft—Urin. Munich/Zurich 1999.

Thümmler, Andrea: Rekonstruktion des Alltags eines thüringischen Arztes im 18. Jahrhundert anhand seines Praxistagebuches 1750–1763. Med. diss. (typescript). Berlin 2004.

Traister, Barbara Howard: The notorious astrological physician of London: Works and days of Simon Forman. Chicago/London 2001.

Vieillard, Camille: L'urologie et les médecins urologues dans la médecine ancienne. Paris 1903.

Voswinckel, Peter: Der schwarze Urin. Vom Schrecknis zum Laborparameter. Berlin 1993.

Walter, Tilmann: New light on antiparacelsianism (c. 1570–1610). The medical republic of letters and the idea of progress in science. In: Sixteenth century journal 43 (2012), 701–25.

Walter, Tilmann: Ärztliche Selbstdarstellung im Zeitalter der Fugger und Welser. Epistolarische Strategien und Repräsentationspraktiken bei Felix Platter (1536–1614). In: Westermann, Angelika/Welser, Stefanie (eds): Personen und Milieu. Individualbewusstsein? Persönliches Profil und soziales Umfeld. Husum 2013, 285–314.

Wear, Andrew: Knowledge & practice in English medicine, 1550–1680. Cambridge 2000.

Wear, Andrew/French, Roger K./Lonie, Ian M. (eds): The medical Renaissance of the sixteenth century. Cambridge 1985.

Wehren, Eugen: Das medizinische Werk des Wundarztes Michel Schüppach (1707–1781) an Hand seiner Rezept- und Ordinationsbücher. In: Berner Zeitschrift für Geschichte und Heimatkunde 47 (1985), 85–166.

Wershub, Leonard Paul: Urology. From antiquity to the 20th century. St Louis, MO 1970.

Westermann, Mariet: The amusements of Jan Steen. Comic painting in the seventeenth century. Zwolle 1997.

Wiedemann, Theodor: Geschichte der Reformation und Gegenreformation im Lande unter der Enns. Vol. 3: Die reformatorische Bewegung im Bisthume Passau. Prague 1882.

Wiesemann, Marjorie E.: Caspar Netscher and late seventeenth-century Dutch painting. Doornspijk 2002.

Wilson, Catherine: The invisible world. Early modern philosophy and the invention of the microscope. Princeton, NJ 1995.

Winn, Peter A.: Rechtsrituale. In: Belliger, Andréa/Krieger, David J. (eds): Ritualtheorien. Opladen/Wiesbaden 1998, 449–69.

Wolff, Eberhard: Perspektiven der Patientengeschichtsschreibung. In: Paul, Norbert/Schlich, Thomas (eds): Medizingeschichte. Frankfurt/New York 1998, 311–30.

Wright, P./Treacher, A. (eds): The problem of medical knowledge. Examining the social construction of medicine. Edinburgh 1982.

Zaun, Stefanie/Geisler, Hans: Die Harnfarbenbezeichnungen im "Fasciculus medicine" und ihre italienischen und spanischen Übersetzungen. In: Bennewitz, Ingrid/ Schindler, Andrea (eds): Farbe im Mittelalter. Materialität—Medialität—Semantik. Vol. 2. Berlin 2011, 969–85.

Zglinicki, Friedrich von: Die Uroskopie in der bildenden Kunst: eine kunst- und medizinhistorische Untersuchung über die Harnschau. Darmstadt 1982.

Zimmermann, Albrecht: Der Arzt in der niederländischen Malerei des 17. Jahrhunderts. In: Medizin in Historie und Kunst. Sammlung Niederländischer Meister der Bezirksärztekammer Nordwürttemberg. Stuttgart 1970, 22–39.

Index

acrimony, 21, 92, 95

Actuarius, Johannes, 123

Agrippa von Nettesheim, Heinrich
    Cornelius, 129, 134

age, 15, 18, 52, 126–7, 131, 133, 142, 144

alchemy, 7, 67, 101, 115–7, 120

anatomy, 3, 7, 67–8, 118, 147–53, 162

animal urine, 5, 46, 133

Apollinaris, 34, 41, 82

apoplexy, 41, 72–3, 97, 125

apothecaries, 9–10, 29, 75, 79–80, 87, 135,
    154, 160

Argenterio, Giovanni, 42, 129, 158

arthritis, 125; *see also* joint pains

ascites, 113; *see also* dropsy

asthma, 26, 54, 138

astrology, 56, 101, 154, 164

atoms, 42–3

auscultation, *see* stethoscope

authority of, 5, 24, 128–134, 142, 148–155

Avicenna, 32, 38, 63, 65, 82, 130, 133

barber-surgeons, 5, 29, 57, 78–80, 89, 91,
    114, 135, 149–50, 153n., 165

Baehrens, Johann Christoph Friedrich, 28

Bauhin, Caspar, 149

Behrens, Konrad Barthold, 15, 75, 84,
    100n., 139, 145

Bellini, Lorenzo, 33, 139

Bernd, Adam, 21–2

Beverwijk, Johann van, 107, 112

bile, 27, 41, 48, 50–1, 55, 69, 88–9, 96–7,
    127, 129

bladder, diseases of 20, 42, 52–3, 95,
    124–5; *see also* bladder stone

bladder stone, 2, 43, 63, 156n.

blood, 13, 26–7, 48–52, 59–66, 69, 73, 78,
    82–3, 85–6, 88, 90–1, 95–8, 109n.,
    124, 126, 140

blood circulation, 65, 97, 100, 124, 126,
    140

blood-letting, 49, 56, 64, 74, 87, 91, 134,
    153n.

Boerhaave, Herman, 27, 57, 139

Bossche, Balthasar van den, 115–6

Botalli, Leonardo, 126–7

Brakenburg, Richard, 116

cachexia, 63; *see also* consumption

Castro, Roderigo da, 53–4; 159

chlorosis, 54, 63, 108, 119,

Christus medicus, 110, **111**

chyle, 26, 48, 50, 59, 96, 138

Clauser, Christoph, 128, 154–5 ,

clergy, 11, 21, 30, 60, 92, 113, 129–30

Collenberg, Hermann, 10

color charts, 36–8, 151

color wheels, 33–4, 36, 38, 50

concoction, 21, 27, 33, 41, 43, 48–52,
    59–63, 66–7, 92–3, 96, 124–5,
    127, 133, 149

consultation by letter, 11–22, 41, 60,
    68–70, 73–4, 91, 102, 128, 165

consumption, 23, 41–2, 51, 53–4, 56, 59,
    76, 78, 94, 125

convulsions, 26, 72–3, 76, 102; *see also*
    epilepsy

Cordus, Euricius, 13, 44, 77, 102, 133–4,
    145,

court proceedings, 6, 23–4, 29–30, 102–4

Culpeper, Nicholas, 55–6

Da Monte, Giovanni Battista, 33, 44, 47, 64, 66

Davach de Rivière, Jean, 36, 38

Detharding, Georg, 17

diarrhea, 51, 55, 103; *see also* dysentery

dietetics, 9–10, 17, 59, 94, 135, 161, 165; *see also* food

digestion, 16, 23, 48, 50, 55, 59, 62, 92, 94, 96; *see also* concoction

dissections, 3n., 7, 67–8, 148–152, 162; *see also* anatomy

divination, *see* uromancy

Dixon, Laurinda, 108n., 109, 113n., 119–20

doctor-patient relationship, 124, 161–2, 164

Dou, Gerard, 109, 113–4, 152–3,

dropsy, 5–6, 26, 87, 109, 113–4, 125, 158

Dueren, Johan van, 77n., 130

dying, 9–10, 20, 113–4, 131, 138

dysentery, 55, 125

Eijgel, Antonius, 15, 155, 165

Elias, Norbert, 128

emetics, 60, 74, 92, 94, 103, 124

epilepsy, 26, 79

fees, 75–78, 88, 103

fetus, 85, 130; *see also* pregnancy

fevers, 23, 31, 41, 43, 54–56, 72, 75–6, 83, 96–7, 103, 137–8, 148, 156n., 164

fever thermometer, 8, 138, 162

fluxes, 51, 69, 92–3, 126, 138

food, 16, 41, 43, 46, 48, 50–51, 55, 59–63, 66, 85, 92, 96, 103, 124–5, 127, 130

Foreest, Pieter van, 13, 34, 77, 80, 100, 102, 112, 132, 136, 144, 155, 157–8, 160

Fracastoro, Girolamo, 43

France, 20n., 22, 25, 47, 137, 158, 160

Frank, Johannes, 26

French disease, 125

Fries, Lorenz, 13n., 14–5, 49, 80, 102, 126

Galen, 3n., 31–2, 41, 48, 56, 63, 65–68, 109, 116, 124–5, 149

gender, 15, 18, 44, 52, 55, 83, 94, 117, 127, 131, 142, 144

genre painting, 6–7, 65, 105–22, 152–3, 155

gout, 125, 137–8; *see also* podagra

Grosshauser, Johann, 28

Haberstroh, Johannes, 155, 157

hangmen, 96–7, 103–4

Harvey, William, 65, 124

Hayne, Johan, 44, 57, 67, 130

heart, 9, 11, 13, 17, 20, 54, 65–6, 69, 73, 90, 108, 127, 136, 160

Heemskerk, Egbert van, 113

Helidaeus Paduanus, 157

Helmont, Johann Baptist van, 129, 136

Henninger, Joh. Sigismund, 84n., 139

Heurne, Johan van, 12

Hippocrates, 28, 31, 39, 63, 107, 133

Hoffmann, Friedrich, 15, 26, 53–4, 127, 138

Hoogstraten, Samuel van, 119

Horer, Ananius, 14, 99, 125, 145–7, 155

Horlacher, Konrad, 39

Hornung, Johannes, 49, 130, 158

hysteria, 26, 94, 108–9

iatrochemistry, 66, 125, 136, 138–9, 141; *see also* alchemy

injuries, 29, 52, 72n., 125, 149–50

irregular healers, 4–7, 18, 23–25, 29–30, 57, 75–79, 86, 88, 91, 95–7, 99–104, 114–5, 129, 135, 144–7, 151, 153, 155, 165

Italy, 33, 57, 126, 149, 157–8

Jason Pratensis, 160

jaundice, 5, 9, 48, 62, 73, 148

Jews, 77, 100, 144, 146–7

Jewson, Nicholas, 161–3

joint pains, 42, 92, 159

Joubert, Laurent, 84, 86

judicium, 92–3, 97, 101, 127, 132, 144

Juncker, Justus, 116
Jurin, James, 21

kidneys, 12, 20, 27–8, 41–3, 48–50,
    52–3, 63, 66–7, 69, 74, 77, 95–6,
    124–127, 140, 149
knackers, 24, 30
Kräutermann, Valentin, *see* Valenti

Lange, Johannes, 77, 157,
Lasster, Johann, 58–61
laxatives, 10, 47, 60, 74, 87, 103, 114, 145n.
lifestyle, 13, 17, 52, 80, 87, 116, 142, 161,
    165
liver, 10, 13, 41–3, 48–50, 52–3, 55,
    59–61,66–7, 69, 71, 77, 83, 96–7,
    124–7, 149
Loew, Joseph, 28
lovesickness, 54, 65, 107–113, 117–120,

magic, 98, 102, ; *see also* sympathetic
    healing
magistrates, 23, 30, 89–90, 129, 145, 147
Massaria, Alessandro, 64, 125
masturbation, 22
matula, 1, 16, 22, 25, 34, 36–7, 39, 41–2,
    45, 47, 67–8, 99, 101, 105, 110,
    113, 115–6, 120–1, 128, 130, 134,
    150, 153, 156, 165
medical market-place, 4–5, 146, 153, 164,
medieval medicine, 2, 33, 48, 57–8, 82,
    101, 124–5, 128, 134
melancholy, 25, 53, 55–6, 127
menstruation, 21, 62, 85–6, 93, 118–9,
messengers, 6, 12, 14–7, 23, 26, 45–6, 53,
    58, 79–80, 88–9, 106, 114, 131,
    134, 144, 153, 156, 159
    baskets, 46, 105, 107, 113–4, 116
Munnicks, John, 139
Metsu, Gabriel, 115
microscopy, 140–1
midwives, 30, 87–8, 129, 135, 150
Mieris, Frans van, 6, 113, 115
mirrors, 6, 19, 47, 99–100, 152

misdiagnosis, 43, 46, 75, 86, 94, 127–8,
    131–4

nervous diseases, 22, 94–5, 109n., 125, 137
Netherlands, 15, 79, 96, 105, 116–9, 157
Netscher, Caspar, 105, 112
Nicholas of Cusa, 135

obstructions, 16, 87–88, 94–6, 127, 149
Olmo, Giovanni Francesco, 154–5
Ostade, Adriaen van, 6, 112, 115

pain, 12, 20, 41, 50–1, 55, 58–9, 75, 92–3,
    95–7, 102, 121, 137, 159
paracelsism, 11, 56, 66–70, 113n., 125,
    129–131, 138–9, 141; *see also*
    alchemy *and* iatrochemistry
patients' families, 4, 8, 11, 31, 53, 64, 78,
    91, 131, 134, 159, 163–4
Pictorius, Georg, 147
plague, 5, 10, 22, 51, 75
Platter, Felix, 11–2, 14–15, 17, 20, 149,
    151–2, 165
pneumonia, 125
podagra, 42, 125; *see also* gout
pregnancy, 10, 16, 29n., 30, 54, 79–80,
    82–91, 93, 95, 108–9, 118–121,
    127, 131–3, 162
prognosis,1– 2, 5, 9, 31, 55–6, 59, 64,
    71–73, 75, 91, 94, 101, 128, 131,
    137, 153–4, 156
pulse diagnosis, 13, 32, 56, 63–66, 106–7,
    110, 112–3, 118–9, 136–8, 164
purgatives, *see* laxatives

regimen, *see* dietetics
religion, 9, 75, 99, 114, 147, 150
Rhazes, 128
rheumatism, 138
Riedlin, Veit, 129
ritual, 7, 97–104, 114–5, 152, 166
Rondelet, Guillaume, 125
Rübel, Johann Friedrich 5, 14, 137, 139

St Jerome, 115

Santorio, Santorio, 135
Savonarola, Michele, 42n., 50, 125
Schönefeldt, Lorenz, 44–5
Schüppach, Michel, 18
scientific revolution, 151
Scribonius, Wilhelm Adolph, 15, 17, 129
Senckenberg, Johann Christian, 20–1
Sennert, Daniel, 43
shame, 44, 79, 97, 128, 131, 133, 153
skin, 32, 48–9, 55, 136; *see also* ulcers *and* sweat
Soranos, 107
spirits, 45, 47, 55, 61, 65–6, 68–9, 109, 137
spleen, 48, 55, 77, 96, 137
Stahl, Georg Ernst, 15–7, 45n., 100n., 148, 156, 160, 165
Starck, Andreas, 14
Steen, Jan, 6, 105, 108, 110, 112–3, 115–6, 118, 120
stethoscope, 8, 84, 162–3
stomach, 13, 16, 20n., 22, 33, 41, 48, 50, 53, 55, 59–63, 66–7, 69, 89, 92–3, 95–7, 103–4, 124–5, 127, 137–8, 159
stones, 2, 43, 62–3, 74, 137, 156n.
stroke, *see* apoplexy
Superville, Daniel de, 79–80, 156
surgeons,; *see* barber-surgeons
sweat, 10, 49, 51–2, 87, 160
sympathetic healing, 24, 98, 166
syphilis, *see* French disease

Tachenius, Otto, 138
temperament, 13, 17, 52, 126–7, 142
Teniers, Daniel, 115
Thomas, Gerard, 115
Thoner, Augustinus, 77, 84, 86, 144, 147, 153
Thurneysser, Leonhard, 11–14, 20, 67–70, 73–4, 92n., 136, 138–9, 141, 165
Tissot, Samuel Auguste, 21–2
town councils, *see* magistrates
tumors, 21, 51, 125

ulcers, 2, 29, 42, 52, 130
Unzer, Johann August, 16, 156
unlicensed healers *see* irregular healers
urine
    bubbles, 41, 46, 52–54, 62, 77, 82, 152
    chemical analysis, 27–9, 97, 166; *see also* iatrochemistry *and* alchemy
    contents, 20, 32, 39–42, 44–8, 51–3, 60, 63, 135, 139; *see also* urine – sediment
    color, 12, 20, 20–9, 31-39, 41–2, 46n., 47–51, 53–7, 62–3, 67, 82–4, 93–4, 101, 104, 106, 120, 127, 129, 133, 135, 138–9
    distillation, 69, 93, 99–100, 136, 138–9, 141
    foam, *see* bubbles
    sediment, 21, 26, 31, 39, 43, 46–7, 49, 52, 54, 67–8, 133
    smell, 21, 32, 66–7, 99–100, 130–1, 133–4
    sound, 21, 32–3
    weight, 99–100, 135–138, 141
urine glass, *see* matula
uromancy, 25, 28, 99–101, 123, 125n., 139n., 148, 153, 158
uterus, 10, 54, 82, 93–4, 109, 118

Valenti, E. J. Gustav de, 22, 83, 152,
vapors, 9, 22, 51, 53, 62–2, 73, 92–4, 109n., 149
Vesal, Andreas, 42, 149, 150n., 152–3

Walaeus, Johannes, 129
Watkyns, Rowland, 82
Willis, Thomas, 130, 144,
Wirsing, Thomas, 9–10, 17, 73, 79
wounds, *see* injuries
Wood, Owen, 54, 83–4, 118

Zacchia, Paolo, 83n., 84
Zimmermann, Johann Georg, 16